FASCIAL DYSFUNCTION

Manual Therapy Approaches

FASCIAL DYSFUNCTION
Manual Therapy Approaches

Edited by

Leon Chaitow ND DO

State Registered Osteopathic Practitioner (UK), Honorary Fellow and formerly Senior Lecturer, University of Westminster, London, UK; Editor-in-Chief *Journal of Bodywork and Movement Therapies*; Director, Ida P Rolf Research Foundation (USA); Member Standing Committees, Fascia Research Congress & Fascia Research Society (USA)

With contributions by

Julian M. Baker
Stefano Casadei
Leon Chaitow
Julie Ann Day
John Dixon
César Fernández-de-las-Peñas
Willem Fourie
Sandy Fritz
Warren I. Hammer
Elizabeth A. Holey

Jonathan Martine
Divo Gitta Müller
Thomas W. Myers
Alessandro Pedrelli
Andrzej Pilat
Robert Schleip
Antonio Stecco
Carla Stecco
Paolo Tozzi
Michelle Watson

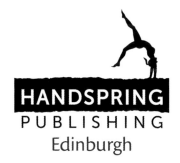

HANDSPRING
PUBLISHING
Edinburgh

HANDSPRING PUBLISHING LIMITED
The Old Manse, Fountainhall,
Pencaitland, East Lothian
EH34 5EY, United Kingdom
Tel: +44 1875 341 859
Website: www.handspringpublishing.com

First published 2014 in the United Kingdom by Handspring Publishing

ISBN 978-1-909141-10-0

British Library Cataloguing in Publication Data
A catalogue record for this book is available from the British Library

Important notice

It is the responsibility of the practitioner, employing a range of sources of information, their personal experience, and their understanding of the particular needs of the patient, to determine the best approach to treatment.

Neither the publishers nor the authors will be liable for any loss or damage of any nature occasioned to or suffered by any person or property in regard to product liability, negligence or otherwise, or through acting or refraining from acting as a result of adherence to the material contained in this book.

Commissioning Editor Mary Law, Handspring Publishing Limited
Text design by Pete Wilder, Designers Collective
Cover design by Bruce Hogarth, KinesisCreative
Artwork by Bruce Hogarth, KinesisCreative
Copy editing by Lynn Watt
Typeset by DiTech Process Solutions
Printed and bound in Great Britain by Martins the Printers Ltd

The
Publisher's
policy is to use
paper manufactured
from sustainable forests

CONTENTS

CONTRIBUTORS

Julian M. Baker
Bowen Technique Practitioner
Owner and Principal Instructor
The European College of Bowen Studies
Frome, UK

Stefano Casadei BSc, PT
Physiotherapist and Fascial Manipulation Teacher
Cesena, Italy

Leon Chaitow ND, DO
State Registered Osteopath (UK)
Honorary Fellow, University of Westminster, UK;
Editor-in-Chief, Journal of Bodywork and Movement Therapies;
Director, Ida P. Rolf Research Foundation (USA);
Member Standing Committees:
Fascia Research Congress and Fascia Research Society, USA

Julie A. Day PT
Certified teacher of Fascial Manipulation® (Stecco Method);
Secretary of Fascial Manipulation Association
Vicenza, Italy

John Dixon PhD, BSc (Hons)
Reader in Rehabilitation Science, School of Health and Social Care
Teesside University, Middlesbrough, UK

César Fernández-de-las-Peñas
PT, DO, PhD, DMSc
Head of Department, Department of Physical Therapy,
Occupational Therapy, Physical Medicine and Rehabilitation,
Universidad Rey Juan Carlos Alcorcón, Madrid, Spain;
Centre for Sensory-Motor Interaction (SMI), Department of Health
Science and Technology, Aalborg University, Aalborg, Denmark

Willem Fourie PT, MSc
Practitioner
Roodeport, South Africa

Sandy Fritz BS, MS, NCBTMB
Founder, Owner, Director, and Head Instructor
Health Enrichment Center
School of Therapeutic Massage and Bodywork
Lapeer, MI, USA

Warren I. Hammer DC, MS, DABCO
Postgraduate faculty, New York Chiropractic College
Seneca Falls, NY;
Northwestern Health Sciences University, Bloomington, MN, USA

Elizabeth A. Holey
MA, Grad Dip Phys, MCSP, Dip TP, FHEA
Pro Vice-Chancellor, Teesside University, Middlesbrough, UK
Previously Deputy Dean of Health and Social Care and Physiotherapy
Subject Leader, Teesside University, Middlesbrough, UK

Jonathan Martine BA, CAR, CMT
Certified Advanced Rolfer™
Boulder, CO, USA

Divo Gitta Müller HP
Continuum movement teacher
Somatics Academy GbR
Munich, Germany

Thomas W. Myers LMT, NCTMB
Director: Kinesis LLC,
Walpole, Maine, USA

Alessandro Pedrelli
Doctor of physical therapy, BA
Certificate teacher of Fascial Manipulation® (Stecco Method);
Vice-president of Fascial Manipulation Association
Vicenza, Italy

Andrzej Pilat PhD, PT
Director, 'Tupimek' College of Myofascial Therapy;
Lecturer, School of Physical Therapy, Universidad Autónoma
Madrid, Spain

Robert Schleip PhD, MA
Director, Fascia Research Project
Institute of Applied Physiology
Ulm University, Ulm;
Research Director, European Rolfing Association eV
Munich, Germany

Antonio Stecco MD
Specialist in Physical Medicine and Rehabilitation
University of Padova, Italy

Carla Stecco MD
Assistant Professor, Molecular Medicine Department
University of Padova, Italy

Paolo Tozzi MSc Ost, DO, PT
School of Osteopathy CROMON
Rome, Italy

Michelle Watson MSc, CertEdHE, MCSP
Former Senior Lecturer, Department of Physiotherapy, Coventry
University, Coventry;
Managing Director and Clinical Lead, Therapy Fusion Ltd
Stratford upon Avon, UK

PREFACE

For generations anatomists have carefully been trimming away and discarding connective tissues in order to reveal attractive images of muscles, joints and organs that appear in textbooks – images that are often unrecognizable to anyone who has observed the same structures during dissection.

Quite literally, fascia ended up on the cutting-room floor in the interests of presenting a coffee-table artwork, unrelated to physical reality.

Noted Dutch anatomist Jaap van der Wal has even suggested (2009a) that major anatomy texts should be located on the fiction shelves of book stores! He reports: *'I was trained to consider fasciae as connective layers that had to be removed, because they 'covered' something... one had to separate, to dis-sect and the revealed structures ('organs') had to be 'cleaned,' 'cleared' of connective tissue. Connective tissue was something like a covering or sleeve over and in between the dissected structures, often it had to be removed during the dissection procedure.'*

Fascia/connective tissue was seemingly a nuisance to the anatomist, with very little effort by scientists to study or understand its multiple functions.

Research into fascia was therefore largely neglected for decades, with some notable exceptions – including Grinnell (2007): fibroblast mechanics; Hinz & Gabbiani (2010): fibrosis and wound healing; Huijing (1999): force transmission; Ingber (2010): mechanotransduction and tensegrity; Langevin (2006): signaling mechanisms; Purslow (2002): connective tissue structure; Reed & Rubin (2010): fluid dynamics; Solomonow (2009): ligaments; Stecco et al. (2009): continuity of fascial anatomy; Tesarz et al. (2011): neurology of fascia;

van der Wal (2009a, 2009b): architecture of fascia; Willard (2007): fascial continuity.

While these examples may seem to indicate a rich degree of research activity, the reality was that for many years, in the main body of science, fascia had been the forgotten tissue – an apparently unimportant, unexciting and superfluous structure that needed to be removed (during dissection) in order for the more glamorous organs, muscles, nerves etc. to be observed and examined.

And then – in 2007 – the first multidisciplinary international congress on Fascia Research (FRC1) was organized and held at Harvard Medical School Conference Centre, Boston.

The event was conceived by clinicians, therapists, practitioners – mainly but not exclusively from the Rolfing/Structural Integration, osteopathic and massage professions. The concept was simple: to invite the best research scientists in the world to come to an event where they could present their findings to an audience of mainly, but not entirely, practitioners who were anxious to understand what mechanisms were producing the clinical results they were seeing daily with their patients – and that remained largely unexplained.

To the genuine surprise of the organizers, most scientists agreed to present – and the event was a phenomenal success.

Scientists were surprised to find an enthusiastic audience of non-scientists and clinicians who were thrilled to be able to pose questions to scientists, many of whom had little idea of the relevance of their studies to manual therapists.

After Boston came Amsterdam (at the Free University, 2009) and then Vancouver (2012). A 4th FRC will take place in 2015 in Washington DC.

The effects of these conferences on worldwide fascia study has been astonishing.

For example, in 2012 the scientist/clinician (and one of the driving forces in the initiation of the Fascia Research Conferences), Tom Findley MD PhD, noted that *'the number of peer-reviewed scientific papers on fascia indexed in Ovid Medline or Scopus has grown from 200 per year in the 1970s and 1980s to almost 1000 in 2010'* – and this trend has continued.

Each of the fascia research events has built on previous ones, with an increasing dialogue emerging between practitioners and scientists, as they inform and question and learn, from each other.

However, a negative effect has also emerged – the misinterpretation of evidence, a sort of pop-version of fascia research, in which complex processes and mechanisms have been over-simplified to the point of the absurd, frequently by under-informed therapists and practitioners, and this is the main reason for compiling this book.

The book aims to explain the clinical relevance of the avalanche of complex scientific information that has emerged from the research conferences in particular, and recent fascia research (which has exploded into action) in general.

The multiple roles of fascia in the body, and what can go wrong, are outlined in the first section of this book, as are chapters describing assessment and palpation methods, and a summary of mechanisms that might explain the effects of various forms of manual treatment.

Section II contains a series of chapters that individually detail a number of the major fascia-related methods of treatment, with evidence for their usefulness, and proposed mechanisms of action.

This book should be seen as work in progress – a translation of current research-based knowledge, designed to counterbalance the plethora of misinformation related to fascial function, dysfunction and treatment.

As new evidence emerges, a currently constant process, so will there be a need for ongoing translation – so that science continues to inform practice.

Leon Chaitow
Corfu, Greece 2014

References

Findley T 2012 Editorial: Fascia science and clinical applications: a clinician/researcher's perspectives. J Bodyw Mov Ther 16:64–66

Grinnell F 2007 Fibroblast mechanics in three dimensional collagen matrices. First International Fascia Research Congress, Boston

Hinz B, Gabbiani G 2010 Fibrosis: recent advances in myofibroblast biology and new therapeutic perspectives. F1000 Biology Reports 2:78

Huijing PA 1999 Muscle as a collagen fiber reinforced composite: a review of force transmission in muscle and whole limb. J Biomech 32(4):329–345

Ingber DE 2010 From cellular mechanotransduction to biologically inspired engineering: 2009 Pritzker award lecture, BMES annual meeting October 10, 2009. Annals of Biomedical Engineering 38(3):1148–1161

Langevin HM 2006 Connective tissue: a body–wide signaling network? Med Hypotheses 66(6):1074–1077

Purslow PP 2002 The structure and functional significance of variations in the connective tissue within muscle. Comp Biochem Physiol A Mol Integr Physiol 133 (4):947–966

Reed, R Rubin K 2010 Transcapillary exchange: role and importance of the interstitial fluid pressure and the extracellular matrix. Cardiovascular Research 87(2):211–217

Solomonow M 2009 Ligaments: a source of musculoskeletal disorders. J Bodyw Mov Ther 13(2):136–154

Stecco A et al 2009 Anatomical study of myofascial continuity in the anterior region of the upper limb. J Bodyw Mov Ther 13(1):53–62

Tesarz J et al 2011 Sensory innervation of the thoracolumbar fascia in rats and humans. Neuroscience 194:302–308

van der Wal J 2009a The architecture of connective tissue as a functional substrate for proprioception in the locomotor system. Second International Fascia Research Congress, Amsterdam, October 27–30

van der Wal J 2009b The architecture of the connective tissue in the musculoskeletal system – an often overlooked contributor to proprioception in the locomotor apparatus. Int J Ther Massage Bodywork 4(2):9–23

Willard F 2007 Fascial continuity: four fascial layers of the body. First International Fascia Research Congress, Boston

COLOR PLATE SECTION

All of the illustrations in this colour plate section are also printed in black and white at the point in the main text where they are referred to (see Figure numbers).

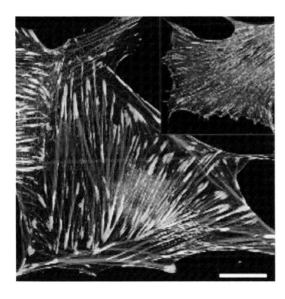

Plate 1 (Fig. 1.2) Myofibroblast on hard base (left) and soft base (right).

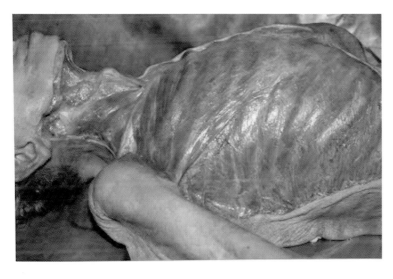

Plate 2 (Fig. 1.6) Epimysial fascia of the pectoralis major and serratus anterior muscles – note the continuity of superficial fascia between these and the cervical fascia. *Photo courtesy of Carla Stecco.*

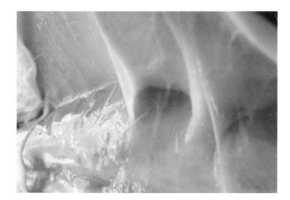

Plate 3 (Fig. 3.3) Fascial adhesion in dissection. Felt-like fascial adhesions are palpable in the living body and visible in the cadaver. *Photo courtesy of Robert Schleip.*

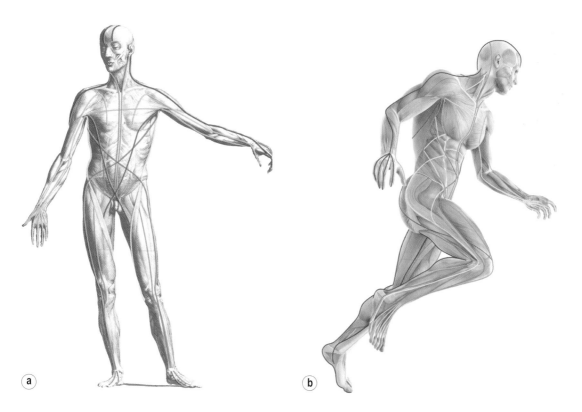

Plate 4 (Figs 3.7a & b) Anatomy Trains' myofascial meridians map continuous lines of myofascial tension that generally run longitudinally along the body's musculature.

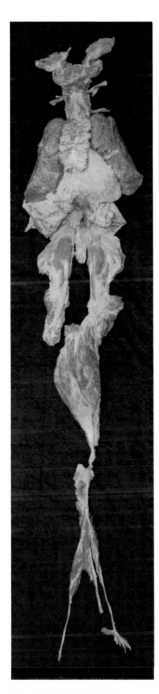

Plate 5 (Fig. 3.11b) The Deep Front Line dissected as one myofascial meridian (at least for the left leg) including the hyoid and jaw bone as 'sesamoids' within the line.

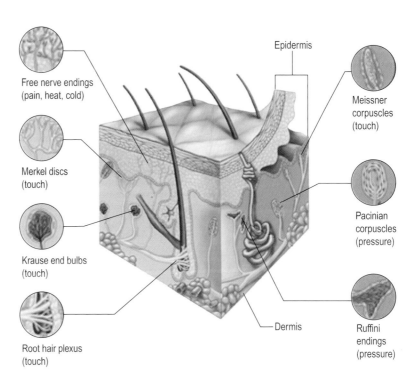

Free nerve endings
(pain, heat, cold)

Merkel discs
(touch)

Krause end bulbs
(touch)

Root hair plexus
(touch)

Epidermis

Meissner
corpuscles
(touch)

Pacinian
corpuscles
(pressure)

Dermis

Ruffini
endings
(pressure)

Plate 6 (Fig. 6.3) Diagram of receptors within skin and superficial fascia. *From Constantin 2006 Inquiry into biology. McGraw-Hill Ryerson, p.429, Fig. 12.27. Reproduced with permission of McGraw-Hill Ryerson Ltd.*

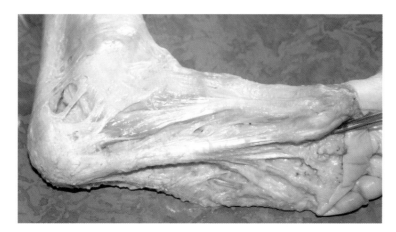

Plate 7 (Fig. 9.4) Dissection of the plantar aponeurosis. While a longitudinal continuity along the main axis of the foot is evident, the plantar aponeurosis also continues with the medial and lateral fasciae of the foot (fascia of the abductor hallucis and abductor digiti minimi muscles, respectively).

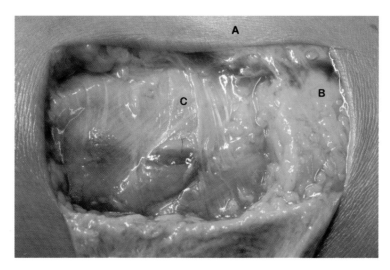

Plate 8 (Fig. 14.4) Fascia as a matrix (note the high level of hydration). This shows the left cubital fossa region on a fresh cadaver dissection. A: skin; B: superficial fascia level; C: deep fascia level.

SECTION I

FASCIAL FOUNDATIONS

The clinical relevance of the flood of recent fascial research demands and deserves clarification. This section provides a summary of the key areas of current fascial research and the evidence this offers relative to manual therapy. The opening chapters therefore evaluate the multiple roles of fascia and the ways in which dysfunction emerges, followed logically by insights into assessment method and the evidence as to which types of manual therapy have been shown to positively influence fascial behavior. The ways in which recent research has offered insights into fascial function, dysfunction, evaluation and treatment are therefore presented from an evidence-informed background, allowing the reader to extract what is most relevant to his/her work. The subsequent section provides examples of numerous fascia-related approaches where there is evidence of therapeutic value.

Chapter 1

THE CLINICAL RELEVANCE OF THE FUNCTIONS OF FASCIA: TRANSLATING THE SCIENCE

Leon Chaitow

This chapter explores fascia's remarkable functions from the perspective of the manual therapist, highlighting the clinically relevant connections between fascial function, dysfunction, and fascia's anatomical and physiological features.

As outlined in this chapter, fascia has multiple functions, and maintaining and restoring these when they are disturbed – for a variety of reasons ranging from aging to trauma – should be a primary focus of practitioners/therapists.

Definitions - what fascia is and what it does

At present there is no generally accepted way of categorizing fascia. Schleip (2012a) has noted there are currently at least three common ways of codifying fascia:

- The Federative International Committee on Anatomical Terminology (1998) describes fascia as *'sheaths, sheets or other dissectible connective tissue aggregations'* including *'investments of viscera and dissectible structures related to them'* (Terminologia Anatomica 1998)
- *Gray's Anatomy for Students* (Standring et al. 2008) describes fascia as *'masses of connective tissue large enough to be visible to the unaided eye'* noting that *'fibres in fascia tend to be interwoven'* and that it includes *'loose areolar connective tissue'* such as the subcutaneous *'superficial fascia'*
- The most recent international Fascia Research Congress (Schleip et al. 2012b) characterizes fascia as: *'fibrous collagenous tissues which are part of a body wide tensional force transmission system.'*

In order to enhance fascial function when it has been lost or is under strain, we need to:

- Understand the roles of fascia – what it is and what it does (Ch. 1)
- Be aware of how fascia can become dysfunctional – and what symptoms are then likely to result (see Ch. 2)
- Have the ability to evaluate, observe, palpate and assess fascial function and dysfunction, which is the theme of Chapters 3 and 4 (by Tom Myers and this author)
- Be aware of methods that can prevent dysfunction, as well as being able to effectively restore and/or enhance its functionality. Detailed evaluations of 15 separate models of fascial care and treatment are offered in Chapter 5, and in Section 2 (comprising Chs 6-20). These chapters examine what is known about the most widely used fascia-focused therapeutic methods – their methodologies, mechanisms (as far as these are currently understood) as well as the evidence of therapeutic effects (as far as this is available).

An evidence-informed picture should emerge that can be used in clinical reasoning when deciding on therapeutic choices, as well as providing the basis for explaining possible fascial-involvement to patients/clients. Effective clinical choices in management of existing fascia-related problems should therefore result.

This book's terminology

Taking account of the various definitions listed above, and where appropriate, this book describes individual fascial tissues and structures by considering:

- The functional role of particular tissues, for example *separating* fascia
- The anatomical structures related to the tissues under discussion, for example *cervical* fascia
- Additional descriptors may be given, for example *loose* or *dense* connective tissue
- The relative hierarchical position may be described, for example *superficial* or *deep* fascia.

Note: In this book, due to the current lack of universal agreement regarding terminology, the following descriptors may be found in different chapters or quotes, all referring to the same connective tissue layer: superficial, subcutaneous, loose, non-dense, areolar, pannicular.

The importance of clinically relevant (and accurate) translation of research

The increased interest in fascia, resulting from recent research congresses and symposia and the explosion of research-based publications on the subject, has led to the development and promotion of a variety of 'new' methods of treatment. Many of these attempt to validate themselves via reference to research studies, with a significant number being trademarked (™), or in attempting to protect their uniqueness, by adding a registration symbol (®).

Some of these copyrighted, registered modalities are included as individual chapters in Section 2. The authors of those chapters have explained the methods and the foundations on which the modality has been constructed – that is, the way in which scientific research has been translated into a clinical approach.

This trend towards copyrighting methods emphasizes the need for practitioners, clinicians, and therapists to have the ability to exercise critical

evaluation of the evidence presented to them, and be able to then make informed decisions. One of the main aims of this book is to provide the tools that will lead to sound judgments being exercised.

Clinical practice informed by research evidence

Apart from a summary of fascia's anatomical and physiological features, this chapter outlines key aspects of recent fascial research, while also offering translation of new information where this is potentially clinically relevant.

In order to successfully achieve prevention, assessment and successful treatment of fascial dysfunction, we depend on accurate interpretation of basic science findings. The more clearly that we understand fascial anatomy and physiology, and the more we are aware of the implications of research findings, the better able we will be to recognize the roles fascia may play in a variety of painful and dysfunctional conditions.

- What do studies on cells and tissues in a lab actually mean, when it comes to management of fascia-related pain and dysfunction?
- What can we learn from mathematical modeling evaluations of fascial function (see Ch. 5)?
- How do such studies inform treatment methods (see Chs 2 and 4)?
- How does anatomical research, for example emerging from dissection findings, translate into clinical reasoning (see Chs 3 and 4)?
- How might information deriving from imaging studies offer the manual clinician information that is clinically useful (see Chs 3 and 4)?

(Bio)Tensegrity defined

- 'Tensegrity' is an invented word that combines elements of 'tensional integrity.' It describes a structural shape that is determined by the closed, continuous, tensional behaviors of the components of the system – rigid struts and flexible connecting elements, which respond compliantly to tension and compression (Fig. 1.1).
- Levin and Martin (2012) observe that biotensegrity: *'reverses the centuries-old concept*

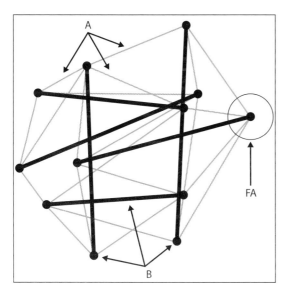

FIGURE 1.1 Biotensegrity model. A pre-stressed tensegrity model representing biotensegrity architecture at all size scales throughout the body – at molecular, tissue, organ and organ system levels – all with compression and tension elements. A = tension features: microfilaments cells, muscle, tendon, ligament, fascia. B = compression: DNA helix, microtubules, extracellular matrix, ribs, bones, fascia. FA = focal adhesion: points of integration between tensional and compressive elements at a cellular level. *Adapted from Swanson 2013.*

that the skeleton is the frame upon which the soft tissue is draped, and replaces it with an integrated fascial fabric with "floating" com- *pression elements (bones in vertebrates), enmeshed within the interstices of the tensioned elements.'*

- Ingber (1993) has demonstrated that cells function as independent pre-stressed tensegrity structures, and that molecules, tissues and organs can all be viewed as tensegrity complexes.
- Within these hierarchical biological tensegrity systems (biotensegrity), individual pre-stressed cells are poised and ready to receive mechanical signals and to convert them into biochemical changes, termed mechanotransduction (see below).

The concept of fascially-linked, continuous chains, slings, trains and loops of myofascial structures is discussed later in this chapter. See Box 1.1 for a summary of some of the main functional features of fascia.

Key Point

The (Bio)tensegrity model should remind us that compressive or tensional load has mechanical (and chemical) *mechanotransduction* effects – and that architectural shape matters – and that as it changes so do its functions (see Fig. 1.1). (Mechanotransduction is described later in this chapter. It refers to the ways cells convert mechanical stimuli into chemical activity.)

Box 1.1

Examples of functional characterizations of fascia (Kumka & Bonar 2012)

- **Linking fascia:** This comprises dense connective tissue which can be classified as active or passive, and which 'includes fasciae of muscles, fasciae of regions (head and neck, trunk, limbs), aponeuroses, tendinous arches and neurovascular sheaths.' (Terminologia Anatomica 1998).
  - o **Active linking fascia:** contains numerous pain and mechanoreceptors; is active during movement and in stabilizing of joints, and critical for force-transmission (see later in the chapter). It

  may have the ability to contract to offer pretension to muscles. Example: thoracolumbar fascia; IT tract.
  - o **Passive linking fascia:** maintains continuity between structures; has proprioceptive functions; it is passively involved in force transmission via loading from muscles. Examples: ligamentum nuchae, plantar aponeurosis.
- **Fascicular fascia:** This comprises a mixture of both loose and dense connective tissues that provide the architectural shape of muscles:

o It surrounds muscles (epimysium), as well as separating muscle fibers (perimysium), while covering each muscle fiber (endomysium).

o Fascicular fascia merges to form dense myotendinous structures. This intramuscular fascicular fascial network acts to both spread and focus forces inside muscles, as well as between synergistic muscles – and via linking fascia – to antagonist muscles. In addition, it provides a range of protective tunnels and pathways for nerves, blood vessels and lymphatic structures.

- **Compression fascia :** This dense connective tissue structure envelops and compartmentalizes the limbs involving sheet-like layers.

o For example, the crural fascia of the lower limb exists as stocking-like coverings that variously offer compression and tension, while strongly affecting muscular efficiency and venous return. The dense layers are separated by loose connective tissue that facilitates sliding, gliding motions between them, allowing differential actions of individual strata.

- **Separating fascia :** Largely comprising loose connective tissue, this sometimes gossamer-thin material creates envelopes, bags, compartments, tunnels, sheaths and linings that separate organs and body regions, reducing friction while offering shock-absorbing and sliding potentials, in response to movement, tension and distension.

o Examples include pericardium, peritoneum and synovial sheaths.

Kumka and Bonar (2012) emphasize the ubiquitous nature of fascia when they offer an example of all four of these suggested categories – in the thigh:

- *'Illiotibialband (Linking)*
- *Perimysium of the quadriceps femoris muscle (Fascicular)*
- *Fascia lata (Compression)*
- *Subcutaneous tissue (Separating).'*

Key Point

The clinical relevance of the notes in Box 1.1 relate to concepts of continuity – of chains, strings and slings, involving fascial connections. Specific clinical implications for manual therapies are discussed in this chapter under subheadings such as *Force transmission* and *Mechanotransduction*.

Fascia: *resilience* as a descriptor

Schleip et al. (2012a) describe fasciae as: ...'*The soft-tissue component of the connective tissue system that permeates the human body. One could also describe them as fibrous collagenous tissues that are part of a body wide tensional force transmission system. The complete fascial net then includes not only dense planar tissue sheets (like septa, muscle envelopes, joint capsules, organ capsules and retinacula), which might also be called 'proper fascia', but it also encompasses local densifications of this network in the form of ligaments and tendons. Additionally it includes softer collagenous connective tissues like the superficial fascia or the innermost intramuscular layer of the en-domysium...the term fascia now includes the dura mater, the periosteum, perineurium, the fibrous capsular layer of vertebral discs, organ capsules as well as bronchial connective tissue and the mesentery of the abdomen.'*

Fascia is part of all the soft tissues of the body:

- Fascia binds, packs, protects, envelopes and separates tissues.
- Fascia invests and connects structures, providing the scaffolding that permits and enhances transmission of forces.
- Fascia has sensory functions, from the microscopic level (for example, individual cell-to-cell communication) to the involvement of large fascial sheets, such as the thoracolumbar fascia (TLF).
- Fascia provides the facility for tissues to slide and glide on each other.

- Fascia also offers a means of energy storage – acting in a spring-like manner via pre-stressed fascial structures, such as the large tendons and aponeuroses of the leg, during the gait-cycle, for example. Think of kangaroos or cats!
- The multiple functions of the connective tissue matrix, with its combined qualities of strength and elasticity – of biotensegrity – can be described by the single word *resilience*. This can be defined as having the ability to adapt to distorting forces and, where appropriate, the ability to return to the original form and position, which is very much the quality of the fascial web. *Resilience* also describes the ability to rapidly recover from illness or injury (see Box 1.2).

Fascia's functional characteristics

The definitions and concepts relative to fascia (above) offer useful ideas as to how we might make clinical sense of the fascial components of the body (Langevin et al. 2011a, Swanson 2013). What emerges is that:

- Fascia is connected to all other tissues of the body, microscopically and macroscopically – so that its three-dimensional collagen matrices are architecturally continuous – from head to toe, from individual cells to major organs.
- Fascia has important colloidal viscoelastic, elastic and plastic properties (see Box 1.2).
- Fascia is richly innervated – participating in proprioception and sensing of pain (see Box 1.3).
- Fascia is functional, not passive. It is dynamic and active – participating in movement and stability.

> **Key Point**
>
> Kumka (personal communication, 2013) offers a clinician's perspective: *'morphological characteristics of fascia – its location, relationships, innervations etc. – are the 'highways' through which fascia should be approached by clinicians.'*

Box 1.2

Fascial properties – thixotropy, plasticity, elasticity, viscoelasticity and the processes of drag, hysteresis and creep

Fascia has a remarkably diverse set of properties – and these have implications for manual therapists. Two key principles should be kept in mind when considering fascial characteristics:

Hooke's Law: Stress imposed on tissues (that is, the degree of force being applied) is directly proportional to the strain produced (e.g. change in length) within the elastic limits of the tissues. See elasticity and plasticity discussion below.

Wolffe's Law: Tissues (e.g. bone, fascia) remodel in response to forces or demands placed upon them. Chen and Ingber (2007) describe how mechanical forces are transmitted into the cytoskeleton and the nuclear matrix of cells, where biochemical and transcriptional changes occur through the process of mechanotransduction.

- Fascia is a **colloid**, defined as comprising particles of solid material, suspended in fluid. The amount of resistance colloids offer to applied load increases proportionally to the velocity of force application. For a simple example of colloidal behaviour, consider a thick mixture of flour and water. If the resulting colloid is slowly stirred with a stick or spoon, movement will be smooth, but any attempt to move it rapidly will be met with a semi-rigid resistance (known as '**drag**'). This quality of colloids is known as **thixotropy** – most evident in the extracellular matrix (described later in this chapter).
- **Collagen** is the most widely distributed protein in the body and this is responsible for the colloidal properties of fascia.
- The thixotropic property of colloids means that the more rapidly force is applied (load), the more rigidly will the tissue respond – hence the likelihood of fracture when rapid force meets the resistance of bone. If force is gradually applied, 'energy' is absorbed by, and stored in, the tissues, with

potential therapeutic implications (Binkley & Peat 1986).

- **Energy-storage** is also a feature of preparation for movement – as explained below (Schleip et al. 2012a).

Gentle, sustained, manual load is a requirement if drag and resistance are to be reduced when attempting to induce changes in those fascial soft-tissue structures most amenable to change i.e. the more superficial, loose fascial layers, rather than the dense, deeper, fasciae.

- Soft tissues display variable degrees of **elasticity** (springiness, resilience or 'give') in order to withstand deformation when load is applied. The elastic property of fascia is possible because these tissues have the ability to store some of the mechanical energy that is applied to them. They are then able to utilize this when returning to their original shape and size when load is removed.

- This process of energy storage, and energy loss, is known as **hysteresis** (Comeaux 2002). The properties of hysteresis (and creep, described below) offer possible explanations for myofascial release (or induction, see Ch. 14) methodology, as well as aspects of neuromuscular therapy (Ch. 15). These qualities should be taken into account during technique application.

- If load is excessive or frequently repeated, it may overcome the elastic potential of tissues, leading to plastic deformation. Permanent change, or a semi-permanent **plastic** distortion, of the connective tissue matrix may result, with a return to normal only achievable with the introduction of sufficient energy to allow a reversal of the deformation process, ideally by means of slowly applied manual therapies (Doubal & Klemera 2002).

- Olson and Solomonow (2009) offer a potent example of the effects of exhausted elasticity resulting from repetitive load: *'viscoelastic tissue properties becomes compromised by prolonged repetitive cyclic trunk flexion-extension which in turn influences muscular activation. Reduction of tension in the lumbar viscoelastic tissues of humans occurs during cyclic flexion-*

extension and is compensated by increased activity of the musculature in order to maintain stability. The ligamento-muscular reflex is inhibited during passive activities but becomes hyperactive following active cyclic flexion, indicating that moment requirements are the controlling variable. It is conceived that prolonged routine exposure to cyclic flexion minimizes the function of the viscoelastic tissues and places increasing demands on the neuromuscular system which over time may lead to a disorder and possible exposure to injury.'

- Greenman (1996) has described how fascia manages loads and stresses, in both plastic and elastic ways, with its responses depending – variously – on the type, speed, duration and amount of the load. When load is gradually applied to fascia, elastic reactions follow in which slack is reduced as tissues respond. Persistent load leads to what is colloquially referred to as '**creep**', in which the shape of tissue slowly lengthens or distorts, due to the viscoelastic property of connective tissue. An example of creep is the process of gradual compression affecting intervertebral discs when standing upright.

- Stiffness of any tissue relates to its viscoelastic properties and, therefore, to the thixotropic colloidal nature of collagen/fascia.

- Cantu and Grodin (2001) use the term '**deformation characteristics**' to describe what they see as the 'unique' feature of connective tissue. This term incorporates the combined **viscous (permanent, plastic)** deformation characteristic, as well as the spring-like **(temporary, elastic)** deformation potentials, as summarized above.

Key Point

Awareness of these multiple fascial qualities offers clinicians insights into the multiple ways in which mechanical load can influence what they are touching. Another aspect of that contact is of course how the nervous system is influenced, and also by fluid dynamics – both of which are discussed later in this chapter.

Box 1.3
Major fascial reporting stations

- **Golgi receptors:** These are plentiful in dense connective tissue. In myotendinous junctions and ligaments of peripheral joints they are known as **Golgi tendon organs**, where they respond to muscular contraction. Other Golgi receptors respond to active (but probably not passive) stretching movements – with immediate tonus decrease in related motor fibers. The extent to which manually applied load can elicit Golgi responses remains unclear (Schleip 2003).

- **Pacini and Paciniform mechanoreceptors:** These intrafascial receptors are found in dense connective tissue. Pacini bodies in muscle fascia, myotendinous junctions, deep capsular layers and spinal ligaments are reported to respond to changes in pressure and vibration – but not sustained compression – with effects leading to enhanced proprioceptive feedback and motor control.

- **Ruffini mechanoreceptors:** These are located in dense connective tissue, ligaments of the peripheral joints, dura mater, and outer capsular layers. Some respond to rapid pressure changes, but the majority are affected by sustained pressure, or slow rhythmic – deep – strokes, as well as to lateral (tangential) stretch forces. The effects include reduced sympathetic activity.

- **Interstitial (e.g. Types 3 and 4) mechanoreceptors:** These offer sensory information, and are far more plentiful in – for example – muscle spindles and fascia – than are Pacini and Ruffini reporting stations. The highest density is located in the periosteum. Ten percent are myelinated (Type 3), the remaining being unmyelinated (Type 4). Some are responsive to rapid pressure, others to fascial (and skin) stretching. Others are low threshold – responding to touch that is 'as light as a painter's brush' (Mitchell & Schmidt 1977). They are also known as *interstitial myofascial* tissue receptors (interoceptors). Schleip (2011) suggests that these interoceptors have autonomic influences – on blood pressure, for example.

- The clinical employment of suitable manual strategies in order to influence different neural receptors is explored further in Chapter 5.

Key Point

Awareness of the ways in which different degrees, durations and directions of load may influence the neural structures within fascia offers clinically relevant therapeutic options; for example, light, brief, tangential load (affecting Pacini mechanoreceptors), as compared with moderate, sustained stretch (affecting Golgi tendon organs). A sharp 'cutting/pricking' sensation is a commonly reported sensation when dysfunctional fascia is being stretched or compressed.

Innervation of fascia

- Leaving aside the processes of mechanotransduction (as mentioned above and described more fully below), how the body regulates itself and adapts to its environment depends, to a large extent, on neural reporting that offers the brain information regarding internal and external requirements. Interpretation of such information, received from pain receptors and mechanoreceptors of varying types, determines the way the body responds to the demands of life.

- Proprioceptors are mechanoreceptors that constantly monitor joint position, tendon load, ligament tension, and the status of muscle-tone and contraction. Golgi tendon organs (see Box 1.3) are examples of specialized proprioceptors that are involved in preservation of joint integrity. Proprioception from fascia is largely provided by the mechanoreceptors located within fascial structures, as well as from what has been termed the 'ectoskeleton' (Benjamin 2009). This describes a virtual 'soft tissue skeleton' in which mechanoreceptors in muscles connect to the fascial layers to which muscle fascicles insert, as part of the process of force transmission (discussed later in this chapter).

- Stecco et al. (2007) have demonstrated the presence of a variety of neural structures in deep fascia – including Ruffini and Pacini corpuscles. This strongly suggests that fascia participates in perception of posture, as well as motion, tension and position (see Box 1.3).

- Additionally, the TLF is densely innervated with marked differences in the distribution of the nerve endings, over various fascial layers: the subcutaneous tissue (superficial fascia) contains a dense presence of sensory mechanoreceptors, such as Pacini receptors and Ruffini endings (see Box 1.3). Substance P-positive free nerve endings – assumed to be nociceptive – are exclusively found in these layers: *'The finding that most sensory fibers are located in the outer layer of the fascia, and the subcutaneous tissue, may explain why some manual therapies that are directed at the fascia and the subcutaneous tissue (e.g. fascial release) are often painful'* (Tesarz et al. 2011).

Note: The TLF is described further and is given particular attention in Chapter 9, The Fascial Manipulation® method applied to low back pain.

Key clinically relevant fascial features

As noted, fascia provides structural and functional continuity between the body's hard and soft tissues, as an ubiquitous elastic–plastic, sensory component that invests, supports, separates, connects, divides, wraps and gives cohesion to the rest of the body – while sometimes allowing gliding, sliding motions – as well as playing an important role in transmitting mechanical forces between structures (Huijing 2007).

The individual elements contained in that summary ('elastic', 'plastic', 'sensory', 'separating', 'gliding' etc.) need to be unravelled and individually discussed – as they are in the opening chapters of the book and in many of the discussions of clinical methods in Section 2.

All of these functions and attributes of fascia are interesting; however, some have greater clinical relevance than others. Potentially clinically relevant fascial features that deserve attention include the ways in which fascial cells respond to different forms and degrees of mechanical load (mechanotransduction), as well as the multiple connecting, wrapping and linking aspect of fascia and how these impact therapeutic assessment and treatment.

Mechanotransduction

Mechanotransduction describes the multiple ways in which cells respond to different degrees of load: torsion, tension, shear, ease, compression, stretch, bending and friction – resulting in rapid modification of cellular behaviour and physiological adaptations – including gene expression and inflammatory responses. Mechanotransduction in connective tissues involves both physical and chemical communication processes that take place between specialized cells, such as myofibroblasts, and their immediate environment, including the soup-like extracellular matrix (ECM) network in which they function. Mechanotransduction processes that involve collagenase and TGF-β1 (transforming growth factor beta-1) are of particular importance and are explained below.

> **Key Point**
>
> The extent to which mechanotransduction effects (due to different forms and degrees of load on cells) can be influenced by manual therapy remains speculative. However, there is evidence that alteration of local tissue tension can influence post-traumatic healing, via mechanotransduction, by means, for example, of changes in collagenase and/or TGF-β1 production. These fascial features are discussed below and more fully in Chapter 5.

Extracellular matrix (ECM)

The ECM is the physical microenvironment in which cells operate. The ECM also provides the opportunity for cells to anchor themselves (using *adhesion complexes* – described below).

The space around and between cells comprises an intricately organized elastic mesh of locally secreted protein, collagen fibers and polysaccharide molecules, as well as ion-rich water and glycosaminoglycans (GAGs) – such as hyaluronic acid – that make up the ECM. Fascia's key cells, the fibroblasts, synthesize the ECM and collagen in response to load.

- The surface of the cells that produce the ECM's constituent materials – fibroblasts – are directly connected to it by GAGs and collagen fibers
- Extracellular collagen fibers in the matrix turn over rapidly, up to 50% in just 24 hours, demonstrating an active ever-changing nature (Hocking et al. 2009)
- Two principle factors drive the development of myofibroblasts: mechanical stress and transforming growth factor beta-1 (TGF-β1):
  o Myofibroblasts feel stress using specialized matrix adhesions (see below)

Cell matrix adhesion complexes (CMACs)

Cells anchor themselves to the scaffolding of the ECM using soluble adhesive substances. These tie proteoglycans and collagen fibers to receptors on the cell surface. Using this structural architectural framework (see notes on tensegrity, earlier in the chapter), cells sense and convert mechanical signals into chemical responses allowing them to instantly react to external load. Therefore – in addition to their adhesive functions – cell adhesion molecules help to modulate signal transduction:

- *'CMACs are exceptionally flexible and dynamic complexes, and their components undergo rapid and regulated turn-over to maintain delicately balanced streams of mechanical and chemical information. Besides the critical role of CMACs in cell migration, signalling through these complexes provides influence over virtually every major cellular function, including for example cell survival, cell differentiation and cell proliferation.'* (Lock et al. 2008)
- Quite literally cells inform adjacent cells of their physical and chemical responses to altered load. In this process physical load is also transferred to adhesion complexes – the virtual 'limbs' of cells that 'anchor' to the ECM.

- This is particularly relevant during wound healing. When myofibroblasts are activated to perform as structural/architectural stabilizers of the repairing wound, it has been found that they perform these roles most efficiently when the tissues they are operating in are firm/tense, rather than being flaccid/relaxed – with these features (firm/soft) being recognized by their surface receptors, the adhesion features.
- Wipff and Hinz (2009) note that when placed on rigid plastic, myofibroblasts respond by enlarging and developing thick stress-fiber bundles – but when placed on a soft surface their focal adhesions do not develop, remaining relatively small (see Fig. 1.2 and Plate 1).

The therapeutic relevance of fluid dynamics and the ECM are described below.

Key Point

The clinical relevance of an understanding of the nature and functions of the ECM includes awareness that, for example, various forms of load modify its behavior with profound effects on structure and function. Manual therapy's influence on such processes is discussed in Chapter 5, while chapters in Section 2 outline individual therapy models.

Specialized cells, structures and functions of fascia (Benjamin 2009)

Fascia holds the body together, involving a body-wide tensional network of sometimes dense and fibrous, and sometimes elastic and flimsy (gossamer thin), collagenous, soft tissues.

Note: This list is not comprehensive, but highlights the major elements involved in fascial structure and function:

- **Collagen:** Derived from the classical Greek word for glue, kola, collagen is made up of different combinations and concentrations of proteins, bundled together in a variety of fibers. The architecture of collagen is sometimes described in terms of the directions of these fibers, as well as the thickness and density of the resulting structure. Collagen provides support, shape, and stability, while the ratio with which it is merged with elastin (see below) determines its degree of flexibility (Langevin & Huijing 2009). Tissue features, such as fiber directions, are largely dependent on the tensional and compressive demands to which they are being adapted. Most collagen (around 90%) in the body is Type 1 – for example, found in skin; however, there are many other collagen types (Ross & Pawlina 2011). Purslow and Delage (2012) report that cross-linkages stabilize collagen molecules in muscular fascia, but that these cross-links can become excessive due to aging – as well as being influenced by diet, and the toxic effects of, for example, tobacco smoke. Nutritional and lifestyle influences on fascial function – and the emergence of dysfunction through aging or trauma – are discussed in Chapter 2. Major influences on collagen production involve substances discussed later in this section – see information under the subheadings *Collagenase* and *Transforming growth factor beta-1 (TGF-β1)*.

- **Fibroblasts:** These are the commonest cell-type in connective tissue. They secrete collagen proteins that maintain the structural framework of the extracellular matrix – that remarkably diverse mesh that surround cells, which provides scaffolding as well as being a communication network. Fibroblasts alter their function in response to activity and load that modifies their shape (see discussion on mechanotransduction). Kumka and Bonar (2012) have noted that:

  '*Fibroblasts are highly adaptable to their environment, and show a capacity to remodel in response to the direction of various mechanical stimuli, producing biochemical responses. If function changes, as with increased mechanical stress, or prolonged immobilization, deoxyribonucleic acid (DNA) transcription of procollagen in the fibroblasts will change types (e.g., collagen type I into collagen type III), or undifferentiated cell types may adapt towards a more functionally appropriate lineage.*'

- **Collagenase:** When fibroblasts are subjected to either continuous or cyclical load (stretch, shear forces or compression - mechanical –

or, for example, involving edema) they secrete collagenases, enzymes that break the peptide bonds in collagen, preventing excessive connective tissue formation, for example during wound healing (Tortora et al. 2007).

- Cyclical stretching (or compression) of fibroblasts – involving approximately 10% of available elasticity – doubles collagenase production.
- In contrast, continuous stretching is only 50% as effective (Langevin 2010, Carano & Siciliani 1996). Additionally, Bouffard et al. (2009) report that brief, light, stretching of tissues that house fibroblasts promotes collagenase production, decreasing the formation of new collagen structures, therefore reducing the likelihood of fibrosis. There are numerous other mechanotransduction processes; however, the example given here offers a sense of the potentials for mechanical (via exercise and/or manual therapy and/or acupuncture) influences on cell behavior.

Key Point

Of potential clinical importance is the observation that lightly loaded cells lose their sensitivity to mechanical deformation after 10–15 minutes, requiring a rest period or a different stimulus to recommence collagenase secretion.

The observation that intermittent load has a greater influence on collagenase production than sustained load, is also clinically relevant.

In general, varying degrees and forms of load – including exercise, light, heavy, sustained, cyclical mechanical stimulus – modifies cellular behaviour and gene expression, influencing tissue remodelling – involving enzymes and various growth factors such as TGF-β1.

Unsurprisingly, exercise enhances collagen formation, while inactivity dramatically diminishes this, in muscles but not in tendons.

- **Myofibroblast:** These derive from fibroblasts that have been stimulated to change their form and function, as a result of mechanical load and consequent deformation. Myofibroblasts have some of the characteristics of smooth-muscle cells, containing actin and myosin, so that they have the ability to contract. Myofibroblasts help in repair, reconstruction and remodeling of injured tissue by secreting new ECM (see above) and by exercising high contractile force. If these processes become unregulated, tissue contracture (as in Dupuytren's disease) and development of fibrosis may result. Fibrosis is discussed further in Chapter 2. The two key features that are involved in transformation of fibroblasts to myofibroblasts are mechanical load, and the chemical TGF-β1. Particular levels of stress are required to induce myofibroblast development, such as occur in trauma. Myofibroblasts sense changes in load/tension using specialized matrix adhesions – the structures that allow them to stick to surfaces (see Fig. 1.2 and Plate 1).

Key Point

Different forms of load application will have mechanotransduction effects on myofibroblasts, with significant influence on remodeling and rehabilitation.

- **Smooth muscle cells:** Unsurprisingly, these are located in smooth muscle tissue,

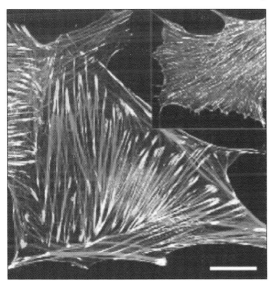

FIGURE 1.2 Myofibroblast on hard base (left) and soft base (right). See also Plate 1 (Wipff & Hinz 2009).

as found in the walls of viscera and blood vessels. Perhaps more surprisingly, they are also embedded in connective tissues. These non-striated, spindle-shaped cells are capable of slow rhythmic involuntary contractions. Schleip et al. (2006) suggest that their presence in fascia may relate to fascial tone, influencing musculoskeletal dynamics.

Key Point

In Chapter 2 there is a short discussion of the effects of altered pH on fascia – sometimes resulting from patterns of overbreathing (such as hyperventilation). This causes smooth muscles to constrict, with potential relevance for fascial tone.

- **Integrins:** Aerial-like protein projections, vital for cell-to-cell and cell-to-ECM communication. Myers (2012) has explained this superbly: *'The ECM is connected to cell membranes and through them to the cytoskeleton via hundreds or thousands of binding integrins on the cell surface. Forces from outside the cell are transmitted via these adhesive connections to the inner workings of the cell. Thus, we can now understand that each cell, as well as "tasting" its chemical milieu, is "feeling" and responding to its mechanical environment ... forces also move in the other direction – from the cell to the ECM – in the case of muscular or (myo)fibroblast contraction that gets conveyed through the membrane to the surrounding ECM.'*
- **Fibronectin:** This is a glue-like substance that, for example, binds to integrins, the cell-spanning receptor proteins.
- **Elastin:** This allows tissues in the body to resume their shape after stretching or contracting; for example, where superficial fascia needs to allow significant sliding motion, as on the dorsum of the hand, levels of elastin are increased to allow for restoration of position and shape, following movement.
- **Fibrillin:** This constituent of the ECM is essential for the formation of elastic fibers that provide strength and flexibility to connective

tissue. When it is genetically mutated, Marfan syndrome results.

- **Fat (adipose tissue):** Superficial fascia (see below for more on this topic) in different areas of the body contains distinctive layers of fat that provides insulation and cushioning. In the heel this cushioning is in the form of fibro-adipose tissue.

- **Transforming growth factor beta-1 (TGF-β1):** This is a secreted protein that performs many cellular functions, including the control of cell growth, cell proliferation and cell differentiation. New collagen is formed in response to mechanical loading (as in exercise or manual therapy) that stimulates, among other substances, TGF-β1. According to Langevin (2006), brief stretching decreases the effects of TGF-β1 in production of additional collagen – which may be relevant to manual therapy techniques aimed at reducing the risk of scarring/fibrosis. Inactivity has been shown to dramatically reduce collagen proliferation function in muscle tissues – but not in tendons (Kjaer et al. 2009).

Fascial lubricants

- **Proteoglycans (PG), glycosaminoglycans (GAG):** These water-loving, mucus-like substances, largely made up of protein and sugar molecules in varying combinations, form the ground substance – a loosely packed feature of the ECM. These substances have important roles in assisting diffusion of nutrients and waste products, as well as offering a home for chondroitin and other sulfates, and various collagen fibers with stabilizing, compressive or tensile functions.

- **Hyaluronic acid (HA):** This component of PG and GAG has lubricating functions and assists in maintaining the viscosity of the ECM. A layer of lubricating hyaluronic acid lies between the deep fascia and muscle (Langevin 2009).

- **Load effects on HA:** Using sophisticated mathematical modelling methods, Roman et al. (2013) compared the lubrication ef-

fects of HA when three different forms of manual load were applied: constant sliding, perpendicular vibration, tangential oscillation. The degree of effectiveness was judged by increased fluid-pressure of HA, since *'the pressure generated in the fluid between the muscle and the fascia... [during treatment]... causes the fluid gap to increase.'* The findings were that *'perpendicular vibration and tangential oscillation may increase the action of the treatment in the extracellular matrix, providing additional benefits in manual therapies that currently use only constant sliding motions.'*

- Langevin et al. (2011b) have shown that reduction of fascia's gliding potential in the thoracolumbar area (described technically as 'reduced thoracolumbar shear strain') correlates with increased thickness of the TLF, and in males, seems to predispose to low back pain. This gender-specific link between a free sliding motion of fascia in the TLF, the thickness of the connective tissue layers, and low back pain, remains unexplained.

Guimberteau's alternative sliding model

A different model is suggested (Guimberteau & Bakhach 2006, Guimberteau 2012) in which it is observed that:

'The traditional notion of different fascias or the sliding, gliding, collagenous system...focuses on the separateness of these structures. Electron scanning microscopy suggests that this system does not consist of different, superimposed layers. In reality, there is a single, tissular architecture with different specializations. To emphasize its functional implications, we call this tissue the multimicrovacuolar collagenous (dynamic) absorbing system (MVCAS).'

Guimberteau and colleagues' detailed observations suggest that:

- This intercellular environment contains a highly hydrated proteoglycan gel, with high lipid content. Its sides comprise intertwined vacuoles composed of collagen and elastins.

- The MVCAS is seen as the building block of: *'an inter-organic network, functioning at different levels and performing three major mechanical roles: (i) responding to any kind of mechanical stimulus in a highly adaptable and energy-saving manner; (ii) preserving the structures, providing information during action and springing back to its original shape; (iii) ensuring the interdependence and autonomy of the various functional units.'*

They also note that:

- *'...the microvacuolar system's function is to maintain the peripheral structures close to, but not mechanically affected by the body action in progress. Conversely, it also offers resistance, first minimally then increasing as the load increases.'*

- A practical example is offered in which finger flexion is observed, during which: *'the movement of the flexor tendon is barely discernible in the palm. It is the same under the skin areolar tissue, which is the connective link between muscle, tendon, fat, aponeurosis and subdermal areas. The MVCAS system situated between the tendon and its neighboring tissue seems to favor optimal sliding. Tendon excursion can be large and rapid without resistance and without provoking any movement in neighboring tissue, thus accounting for the absence of any dynamic repercussions of such movement on the skin surface.'*

- The ability of the MVCAS to respond resiliently is altered when negative influences such as edema, trauma, inflammation, obesity and/or aging occur, creating changes in microvacuolar shape.

> ## Key Point
>
> The clinical relevance of knowledge of the ECM and of GAGs (such as hyaluronic acid) highlights the importance of sliding/gliding functions – whether between fascial layers or involving a different mechanism. In essence, the ability for frictionless muscular activity is the ideal. There is some evidence that different forms of therapeutic load may help to create enhanced sliding potential. See Chapter 5 for more on the specific forms of load.

Fluid dynamics and fascia

- When Klingler and colleagues (2004) examined the effects of stretching on the water-binding capabilities of ground substance of pig connective tissue, they found that the water content reduced – as though squeezing a sponge. This effectively eased the stiffness of the tissues. After around 30 minutes the water content increased again, so that several hours after the stretch there was an increase in the elastic stiffness of the tissue. They concluded that fascia seems to adapt hydrodynamically in response to mechanical stimuli, such as compression and stretch, largely due to a sponge-like mechanical squeezing and refilling effect in the bioarchitecture of water-loving GAGs and proteoglycans. This suggests that at least some of the effects of manual therapy and exercise – relative to ease of movement, stiffness etc. – relates to changes in the water content of connective tissues. This has potential relevance for reducing edema, as well as for increasing the water supply to under-hydrated proteins, allowing for increased extensibility of the tissues.

- Reed et al. (2010) studied the ways in which fluid moves between peripheral lymph and blood vessels and the interstitial tissues. During inflammation, for example, they found that the physical properties of the loose connective tissues (involving GAGs and hyaluronic acid, as described above) can change within minutes, resulting in as much as a hundred-fold increase in fluid flow. They propose that: *'connective tissue cells apply tensile forces on ECM fibres that in turn restrain the under-hydrated ground substance from taking up fluid and swelling.'* Connective tissue is seen to be an active feature of fluid balance and physiology.

- Meert (2012) notes that the fluid in the ECM: *'creates a transport space for nutrients, waste materials and messenger substances and actually facilitates homeostasis between the extracellular and the intracellular region. In addition, the lymphatic system filters this supply out of the ocean of interstitial fluids and drains it into the venous system.'*

- *'Fibroblasts respond to connective tissue tension by homeostatic adjustment of interstitial fluid pressure and transcapillary fluid flow. Transmission of forces from fibroblasts to the extracellular matrix...causes changes in interstitial hydrostatic pressure...influencing the response to injury and inflammation'* (Langevin et al. 2005).
- Fryer and Fossum (2009) suggest that the isometric contractions used in muscle energy techniques (MET; see Ch. 13) *'increase drainage from interstitial spaces reducing concentrations of pro-inflammatory cytokines.'*
- Fascial fluid dynamics, and intramuscular fascial changes, help explain effects of modalities involving isometric contractions (such as MET and proprioceptive neuromuscular facilitation).

> ### Key Point
> The clinical relevance of fluid dynamics and fascia points to fluid/water having a major influence on flexibility and stiffness, as well as on the distribution of substances, such as nutrients, pro- and anti-inflammatory products, and the drainage of debris during processes such as inflammation and tissue repair – with influences on homeostatic function.

The bigger picture: structural characteristics of fascia

Describing the different fascial structures independently, as below, may detract from the reality that the fascial network is continuous; every part of it is joined to every other part, structurally and functionally.

This has been succinctly expressed as follows by Schleip et al. (2012, Introduction):

'The fascial body is one large networking organ, with many bags and hundreds of rope-like local densifications, and thousands of pockets within pockets, all interconnected by sturdy septa as well as by looser connective tissue layers.'

The text below describes some of the different forms, types and locations of fascia and its geography (see also Box 1.1 for 'functions of fascia') followed by a summary of how this translates into one of the most clinically useful aspects of current research evidence – load transfer.

Fascial layers and bags (Willard 2012a)

Tensional forces resulting from muscular contractions and load-demands are spread to adjacent – and distant – tissues via fascial sheets, as well as by means of densified threads, strings, straps, wrappings, and rope-like connections (tendons, ligaments, retinacula etc.).

Fascia also comprises a complex variety of bags, septa, pockets and envelopes that contain, separate and divide tissues and structures – while in many instances allowing a sliding, gliding, facility that provides the basis for frictionless movement between soft tissue layers. This can be lost or reduced by adhesions and increased density.

The geography of fascia can be broken into broad functional categories:
1. Superficial or areolar or pannicular (loose) fascia
2. Deep axial (or investing) fascia
3. Meningeal fascia (surrounds nervous system)
4. Visceral fascia (surrounds and supports organs).

1. Superficial (loose or areolar or pannicular) fascia

A superficial layer of loose connective tissue and fat surrounds the torso and extremities, but not the external orifices. This allows sliding between itself and denser, deeper fascia that wraps and invests muscle.

Blood vessels and nerves pass to and from deeper structures, through the superficial fatty layer.

This loosely-packed subcutaneous – superficial – fascia is the connective tissue that is most accessible (and amenable) to manual therapy interventions (see Box 1.4 on stretching and superficial fascia).

Box 1.4
Loose connective tissue and stretching

- Langevin et al. (2005) reported that sustained, light (under 20% of available elasticity) stretch produced a significant time-dependent increase in fibroblast cell body perimeter and cross-sectional area: *'this study [has] important implications for our understanding of normal movement and posture, as well as therapies using mechanical stimulation of connective tissue, including physical therapy, massage, and acupuncture.'*

- Fourie (2009) notes that animal and human studies indicate that the ideal degree of stretch, required to lengthen *loose connective tissue*, should not exceed 20% of the available elasticity, with 5% to 6% usually being adequate.

- *'When connective tissue stretches (e.g. via physical extension or mechanical stimulation with an acupuncture needle) fibroblast cells that help produce and maintain the connective-tissue matrix, enlarge and flatten. We suggest that focal adhesion complexes on the surface of the fibroblasts detect stretching, and initiate signaling mediated by the protein Rho. The cell then releases ATP into the extracellular space encouraging a change in cell shape, possibly involving breakdown products with analgesic effects. In addition, the Rho pathway instigates remodeling of the cell's focal adhesions, which mediate where and how the cell attaches to the extracellular matrix, leading to relaxation of connective tissue'* (Langevin 2013).

- See subheading, Cell matrix adhesion complexes (CMACs), for explanation of 'focal adhesions'.

- When subjected to mechanical strain (such as light sustained stretch), fibroblasts within muscle fascia secrete interleukin-6, which has been shown to significantly influence differentiation that is essential for muscle repair, and to powerfully influence inflammatory processes (i.e., it has the potential to trigger either pro- or anti-inflammatory effects depending on other factors) (Hicks 2012).

- Fibroblasts synthesize the ECM and collagen in response to load such as stretch.

Major features of superficial fascia

- Contains lymphatic channels
- Has a shock-absorbing function – for example, in the heel
- Acts as a heat insulator and thermal regulator
- Stores energy in the form of triglycerides
- Provides channels for veins and, in some areas, well-protected, large nerve fibers, as well as containing numerous mechanoreceptors (Schleip et al. 2012b)
- Sometimes houses vestigial muscle structures – for example the platysma in the neck
- Contains elastic fibers that allow skin (dermis, epidermis) stretching, and which also create tensile and elastic properties that facilitate a degree of lengthening followed by a return to the original state
- Connects deeper fascia with the body surface; housing fatty lobules (small subdivisions)
- Contains ground substance – the ECM – that fills the spaces between cells, and which has multiple properties that determine the orientation of collagen fibrils, as well as various fluids that allow movement such as the sliding, gliding functions of these tissues (see notes on ECM earlier in this chapter, and notes on GAGs)
- Reed et al. (2010) have summarized major features of the ground substance of superficial fascia, as follows:

'The ECM of the loose connective tissue, constituting the interstitial matrix, has three principal components:
a. collagens constituting the stiff scaffolding for organs and organisms
b. elastic fibers and microfibrils
c. the ground substance composed from proteoglycans and hyaluronan, as well as glycoproteins.

This interstitial matrix provides the route of transport for nutrients and waste materials between the abluminal side of the endothelial barrier to the parenchymal cells of any tissue.

- Superficial fascia also contains various important cell types including:
  o adipocytes for fat storage
  o fibroblasts (see notes earlier in the chapter)
  o various protective blood cells, such as neutrophils and macrophages
  o mast and plasma cells
  o sweat glands.

> ### Key Point
>
> Clinically significant aspects of loose, superficial, connective tissues lie in its relative accessibility to compression, stretching and/or needling – as examples. Load aiming to enhance length has been suggested to require light elongation pressure (well under 20%) – sustained for minutes not seconds.

2. Deep (axial or investing) fascia

Axial fascia extends deep into the body, surrounding the major muscles, tendons, ligaments, and aponeuroses (flat, broad tendon-like sheets that join muscles and the body parts that muscles act on) of the trunk, extending into the limbs, providing protection and lubrication. Force transfer during muscle contraction is an important feature of deep fascia.

3. Meningeal fascia (surrounds nervous system)

This is encased within the axial fascia, surrounding and protecting the structures of the nervous system.

4. Visceral and mediastinal fascia

Willard (2012b) has summarized the visceral fascia, thus: *'Visceral fascia can be traced from the cranial base into the pelvic cavity. It forms the packing surrounding the body cavities where it is compressed against the somatic body wall. It also forms the packing around visceral organs, many of which it reaches by passing along the suspensory ligaments such as the mesenteries. This fascia also functions as a conduit for the neurovascular and lymphatic bundles as they radiate outward from the thoracic, abdominal, and pelvic mediastinum to reach the specific organs.'*

Visceral fascia surrounds and supports organs and provides the 'packing tissue' for the midline structures of the body (Drake et al. 2010) – it is continuous from the nasopharyngeal and cervical region, all the way through the thorax (mediastinum), passing via the diaphragm, through the abdomen, to the pelvic floor. In the midline, in addition to the abdominal plexus and the autonomic nerves, it houses major vessels, such as the aorta, and the caval venous systems, as well as the thoracic duct. The visceral fascia effectively envelopes all the major organs, invests the pleural and peritoneal linings, and forms the neurovascular sheaths. The mediastinal fascia, largely comprising loose connective tissue, therefore forms the central compartmental cavity of the thorax, housing major organs as well as neural and vascular structures.

Manual therapy methods exist that have potential therapeutic influences for the mediastinum (Barral & Mercier 2004).

> ### Key Point
>
> The forms and locations of the various fascial features are clinically relevant because of the potentials offered to the manual therapist by the continuity that exists between most structures lying between the base of the skull and the pelvic floor.

Extremity and trunk differences in deep fascia

The deeper fasciae of the extremities differ significantly from that of the trunk. Deep fascia associated with muscles in the limbs slides freely, whereas in the trunk, muscles are more adherent to the deeper fascia.

The deep fasciae of the limbs not only envelop muscles. Evidence shows they comprise two or three dense layers or sheets with undulating arrangements of parallel collagen bundles that may include some elastic fibers. Deep, dense, fascial layers are usually separated by thin layers of loose connective tissue that cushion and allow the deeper layers to slide on each other, so providing frictionless mechanical adaptability.

Where hard and soft tissues meet, where fascia connects to bone, there are local areas of concentrated tensional stress-fibers, in which collagen links to, and anchors, layers of deep connective tissue to each other, or consolidates these into a retinaculum (stabilizing bands around tendons) or fibrocartilage (particularly string-cartilage, such as the meniscus of the knee). The thin, sheet-like, layers of deep, dense fascia are oriented, in relation to each other, at approximately 78°. This orientation apparently allows reduced friction as fascial sheets slide over underlying layers, improving fascia's ability to take up strain.

If a myofascial load is exerted onto muscle, force is automatically transmitted onto the intramuscular connective tissue via the layer of fascia that wraps the muscle (epimysium). For this force to be transmitted adequately, the connections need to be firm, not lax. Huijing and Langevin (2009) argue that since some fascial structures that are not dense are capable of transmitting some muscular force, *'the term "loose connective tissue" for such structures is inadequate and the term 'areolar' is preferred'* (see Fig. 1.3).

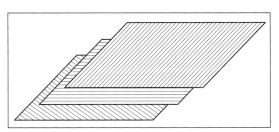

FIGURE 1.3 Schematic image of the deep fasciae of the limbs, showing the composition and fiber direction in three different layers. *Adapted from Figure 1.5.2 from Stecco C, Stecco A 2012 Deep fascia of the lower limbs. In: Schleip R et al. (eds): Fascia: the tensional network of the human body. Churchill Livingstone Elsevier, Edinburgh, Ch. 1, p. 34.*

> **Key Point**
>
> The clinical significance of the different orientations of fascial planes should be taken into account – for example – to achieve optimal applications of directions of load during manual treatment methods that target perceived restriction barriers.

Muscle fascia (Fig. 1.4)

- Every muscle is wrapped by a layer of connective tissue – the **epimysium** – that links it to bone via the tendons
- The muscle itself is separated into smaller units of muscular bundles, or fascicles, by a fascial network – **the perimysium**
- Fascicles are further separated into muscle fibers by the **endomysium**
- **Intramuscular septa** are tough fascial sheets that separate extremity compartments and muscles – for example, anterior and posterior crural septa; lateral and medial femoral septa; and the lateral and medial humeral septa.

These structures facilitate load sharing and load transfer, so that a continuous functional mechanical, three-dimensional network can operate.

Force transmission, load transfer and fascia

Schleip (2003a, 2003b) has described fascia as: *'...the dense irregular connective tissue that surrounds and connects every muscle, even the tiniest myofibril, and every single organ of the body forming continuity throughout the body'.*

How might this accurate summary of fascia's ubiquitous presence change the way we understand movement and locomotion? One key element involves relearning the way that force is transmitted. We have been taught to think of specific muscles contracting with force then being transferred in a linear manner by means of, for example, aponeuroses and tendons, thereby producing joint movement.

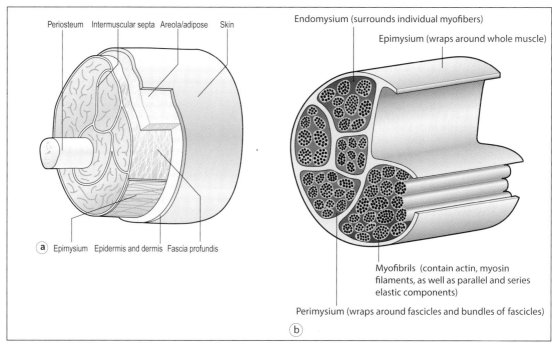

FIGURE 1.4 (a) Muscular fascia layers. (b) Skeletal muscular fascia layers.

Illustrations of muscular activity in standard anatomical atlases usually involve removal of fascial elements to reveal what is commonly and inaccurately presented as the primary mechanical feature of movement – specific muscles – so ignoring vital fascial connective continuities in which force is transmitted in multiple directions simultaneously: sometimes laterally, sometimes obliquely, and sometimes linearly. For example, structures normally described as the muscles of the hip, pelvis, and leg interact with arm and spinal muscles via the thoracolumbar fascia, which allows effective load transfer between the spine, pelvis, legs, and arms in an integrated system (see Fig. 1.5).

The lumbar interfascial triangle (LIFT) (Willard et al. 2012)

As noted above, the TLF integrates forces deriving from passive connective tissues as well as numerous active muscular structures, including aponeurotic and fascial layers that separate paraspinal muscles from the muscles of the posterior abdominal wall.

- The superficial posterior layer of the TLF is mainly an aponeuroses of latissimus dorsi and serratus posterior inferior, while deep to this is retinacular sheath that encapsulates the paraspinal muscles that support the lumbosacral spine.

- Where this sheath meets the aponeurosis of transversus abdominis it forms a raphe (a seam-like ridge) – a dense septum. This is the junction of the hypaxial (anterior to the spine) and – epiaxial (posterior to the spine) fascial compartments – where it forms the lumbar interfascial triangle (LIFT).

- This remarkable structure (a 'roundhouse' in Myers terminology – see Ch. 3) helps distribute load from abdominal and extremity muscles into, and from, the TLF.

- All layers of TLF fuse to merge with posterior superior iliac spine and the sacrotuberous ligament, assisting in support of the lower lumbar spine and sacroiliac joint.

- Load reaching the LIFT from the abdominal muscles, latissimus dorsi, the lower extremity, and pelvic muscles are therefore appropriately distributed, in order to assist in stabilizing the spine, trunk and pelvis.

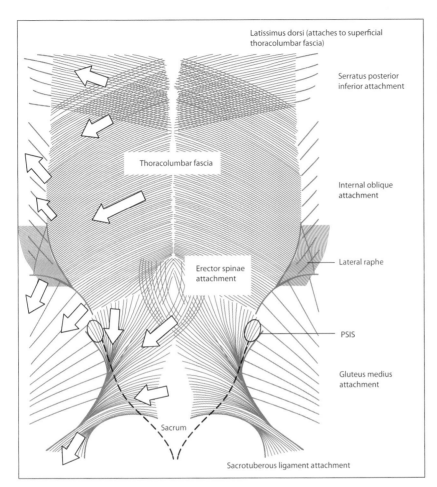

FIGURE 1.5 Deep layer of the thoracolumbar fascia and attachments to gluteus medius and attachments between the deep layer and the erector spinae muscle.

Labels on figure:
Latissimus dorsi (attaches to superficial thoracolumbar fascia)
Serratus posterior inferior attachment
Thoracolumbar fascia
Internal oblique attachment
Erector spinae attachment
Lateral raphe
PSIS
Gluteus medius attachment
Sacrum
Sacrotuberous ligament attachment

Scalenes and the thorax

Because of the fascial sheets and membranes that envelop and connect them, the scalene muscles are continuous with thoracic structures – ranging from the pectoral muscles, to the pericardium. It is therefore unwise to conceive of scalene dysfunction without taking account of what they are connected to – via fascia – anatomically and functionally.

Stecco and Stecco (2012) note that: '*intermuscular and epimysial fasciae serve as areas of insertion for muscle fibers that [...] can mechanically reach a skeletal element without necessarily being attached directly to the bone.*' This is apparently also true for connections to the superficial fasciae (such as fascia cruris and fascia antebrachii), which provide broad insertion areas for muscle fibers (see Fig. 1.6 and Plate 2).

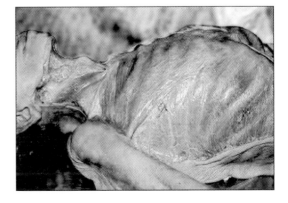

FIGURE 1.6 Epimysial fascia of the pectoralis major and serratus anterior muscles – note the continuity of superficial fascia between these and the cervical fascia. See also Plate 2. Photo courtesy of Carla Stecco.

Shoulder, trunk, cervical fascial continuity

Stecco and Stecco (2012) have reported on the results of their numerous dissections. For example: *'The deep fasciae of the shoulder present characteristics that are similar to both the fasciae of the trunk and of the extremities. In particular, the fasciae of the pectoralis major, deltoid, trapezius, and latissimus dorsi muscles form a unique layer, **enveloping all of these muscles and passing over the serratus anterior**, where it forms a strong fascial lamina.'*

They continue: *'All of these fasciae adhere firmly to their respective muscles due to a series of intramuscular septa that extend from the internal surface of these fasciae, dividing the muscle itself into many bundles.'* It is inconceivable that load on any of these muscles would not directly affect all the others mentioned (see Fig. 1.5). This pattern of 'separate' muscles being bound together by fascial structures is repeated in the limbs, on the back, in the cervical region, etc.

How load from the hamstrings is distributed

Franklyn-Miller et al. (2009) have demonstrated – using micro-strain gauges – that the degree of force used in a hamstring stretch results in a variety of unexpected load transfers:

- 240% of the imposed strain is transferred to the iliotibial (IT) tract
- 145% of the hamstring load is transferred to the ipsilateral lumbar fascia, via the sacrotuberous ligament
- 103% to the lateral crural compartment
- 45% to the contralateral lumbar fascia
- 26% to the plantar fascia.

Strain transmission, via fascial continuities during stretching, can therefore be seen to affect many tissues, other than the muscle to which load is being applied.

The researchers report that, 'strain is distributed through a consistent pattern – [that] – correlates closely with collagen fibre orientation.' This suggests the possibility that apparent muscular restrictions might in fact be fascial in origin, and that the source of such dysfunction may lie at a distance from where it is perceived.

The latissimus dorsi–hip–gluteus maximus connection

Using volunteers, Carvalhais et al. (2013) were able to show that active latissimus dorsi tensioning – for example, when the shoulder was actively adducted and the scapular depressed, using force equivalent to 25% of a maximum voluntary contraction – produced lateral rotation of the contralateral hip, together with increased passive (also contralateral) gluteus maximus (GM) stiffness.

Gluteus maximus and knee pain

Stecco et al. (2013) have also identified a force transmission link from the thoracolumbar fascia, via GM, to the IT tract, and onwards to the knee, suggesting that: *'hypertonicity of gluteus maximus could explain increased tension in the lumbar region, causing low back pain and the lateral region of the knee.*

In all (12) subjects gluteus maximus presented a major insertion into the fascia lata, so large that the iliotibial tract could be considered a tendon of insertion of the gluteus maximus ... [explaining] ... transmission of the forces from the thoraco-lumbar fascia to the knee [and] possibly explaining why hypertonicity of the GM could cause an IT band friction syndrome (IBFS) or, more generally, knee pain.

Resolution of ITBS can only be achieved when the biomechanics of the hip are properly addressed.'

Superficial back line connections validated by electromyography

The muscular associations connected to myofascial kinematic chain, known as the superficial back line (Myers 2009; see details later in this chapter and more fully in Ch. 3, particularly Fig. 3.2b), have been tested using electromyography (Weisman et al. 2014).

The findings of this study, which aimed to '*map the association of muscle activations along the superficial back line (SBL) using separate conditions of active range of motion with and without resistance and passive range of motion,'* were of clinical relevance:

- During maximum isometric contraction of the right gastrocnemius there were strong activation signals recorded at the electrodes placed on: right hamstrings, posterior superior iliac spine (PSIS), left and right 12th thoracic segment (T12), and right upper trapezius
- During maximal isometric cervical extension (prone) there were strong activation signals recorded at the electrodes placed on the upper trapezius, T6, T12, PSIS, with moderate but significant activation in the hamstrings.

Clinical implications and considerations

We can see, for example, that knee pain might emerge from GM dysfunction and that GM (and the hip) may be strongly influenced by contralateral latissimus dorsi activity, via the thoracolumbar fascia.

Data from Stecco studies – described above – have shown the direct connection between latissimus dorsi, upper trapezius, the scalenes and the pectoral muscles. Could knee pain reflect fascial, or other, restrictions involving any of these muscles...or could dysfunction in any of them relate to influences from the knee?

We can also see links between gastrocnemius function and, for example, the ipsilateral upper trapezius muscle; and the cervical muscles and the hamstrings.

These examples highlight the need to revise previously held ideas as to how the body works biomechanically. This revision of previously held concepts is a necessary process in order to appreciate advances in understanding fascial function – as is the need to learn the topography, the geography, the connections and the architecture of the soft tissues, *including fascia – not excluding it,* as happens in many anatomy texts. We need to know where, as well as how, fascia influences function.

Stated simply, fascia integrates and organizes both posture and movement.

Key point

The clinical relevance that is becoming apparent from these studies relates to the need for therapists to become aware – as evidence emerges – of the pathways of force transmission in different areas of the body.

The example described above of the knee–hamstring–GM–hip–TLF–latissimus etc. connections suggests that influences at a distance need to be considered when seeking both the etiological and the maintaining features of pain and restriction.

Muscle chains

This section does not aim to provide a comprehensive list of the many attempts made to catalogue the connections that make up myofascial load sharing.

- Richter (2012) describes a number of different models in which myofascial links, slings etc. form the basis for understanding biomechanical function. He explains: *'Even if these models are sometimes very different, they all have one thing in common: they show the locomotor system and the myofascial tissues as being one unit that always functions as a whole.'*
- Probably the most widely employed model is Myers' (2009) 'Anatomy Trains' in which lines, tracks and junctions etc. are used metaphorically to describe the multiple connections that make up the *'global, geodesic tension complexes'* of the locomotor system, *'that simultaneously stabilize and allow adjustments within the skeletal frame.'* A functional separation of structures within this network can be described as involving the 600+ muscles of the body, and the multiple, more deeply situated force-transmission systems, including ligaments, tendons, capsules etc. Myers acknowledges that the Anatomy Trains model is one that will develop, but that it provides a 'design argument' that matches tensegrity and load-transfer research, and therefore has clinical relevance – as he describes in the context of assessment in Chapter 3.

The 'tracks' that Myers (2009) has described are listed below (and more fully in Ch. 3). When reflecting on these connections catalogued by Myers, bear in mind van der Wal's observation (2009) that no muscle attaches to bone anywhere in the body, and that osseous connections are always made via the intervening connective tissue structures:

1. **Superficial Front Line:** toe extensors, anterior crural compartment, quadriceps, rectus abdominis and abdominal fasciae, sternalis and sternal fascia, sternocleidomastoid.
2. **Superficial Back Line:** short toe flexors and plantar aponeurosis, triceps surae, hamstrings, sacrotuberous ligament, sacrolumbar fascia, erector spinae, epicranial fascia
3. **Lateral Line:** fibularis muscles, lateral crural compartment, IT tract, hip abductors, lateral abdominal obliques, internal and external intercostals, sternocleidomastoid, and splenii
4. **Spiral Line:** splenii, (contralateral) rhomboids, serratus anterior, external oblique, (contralateral) internal oblique, tensor fasciae latae, anterior IT tract, tibialis anterior, fibularis longus, biceps femoris, sacrotuberous ligament, erector spinae
5. **Superficial Back Arm Line:** trapezius, deltoid, lateral intermuscular septum, extensor group
6. **Deep Back Arm Line:** rhomboids, levator scapulae, rotator cuff, triceps, fascia along ulna, ulnar collateral ligaments, hypothenar muscles
7. **Superficial Front Arm Line:** pectoralis major, latissimus dorsi, medial intermuscular septum, flexor group, carpal tunnel
8. **Deep Front Arm Line:** pectoralis minor, clavipectoral fascia, biceps, radial fascia, radial collateral ligaments, thenar muscles
9. **Front Functional Line:** pectoralis major (lower edge), semilunar line, pyramidalis, anterior adductors (longus, brevis, and pectineus)
10. **Back Functional Line:** latissimus, lumbosacral fascia, GM, vastus lateralis (see Fig. 1.5)
11. **Ipsilateral Functional Line:** latissimus-dorsi (outer edge), external abdominal oblique, sartorius
12. **Deep Front Line:** tibialis posterior, long toe flexors, deep posterior compartment, popliteus, posterior knee capsule, adductor group, pelvic floor, anterior longitudinal ligament, psoas, iliacus, quadratus lumborum, diaphragm, mediastinum, longus muscles, hyoid complex, floor of mouth, jaw muscles.

These 'anatomy trains lines' are discussed more thoroughly in Chapter 3.

As mentioned, many different models exist that interpret the chains and connections that fascia provides. As an example, see the discussions in Chapter 9 on Fascial Manipulation®, in which local areas of coordination – and perception – are identified in relation to myofascial sequences.

> ### Key Point
>
> The clinical relevance of an awareness of muscular chains and links (whether the Anatomy Trains model, or one of the many others that have been described) cannot be overstated. Understanding load sharing and the reciprocal function of myofascial continuities widens clinical choices in relation to manual and exercise, treatment and rehabilitation approaches.

How fascial problems start

The multiple ways in which fascial dysfunction can manifest are explored in Chapter 2. As with most musculoskeletal dysfunction the 'causes' tend to be easily summarized as overuse, misuse, disuse and abuse.

Fascial dysfunction may result from slowly evolving trauma (disuse, overuse and misuse) or sudden injury (abuse) leading to inflammation and inadequate remodeling (such as excessive scarring or development of fibrosis):

- 'Densification' may occur involving distortion of myofascial relationships, reducing sliding facilities and altering muscle balance and proprioception (Stecco & Stecco 2009). As a result of such changes, chronic tissue loading forms *'global soft tissue holding patterns'* (Myers 2009).
- *'When fascia is excessively mechanically stressed, inflamed or immobile, collagen and matrix deposition becomes disorganized, resulting in fibrosis and adhesions'* (Langevin 2008).
- Densification and loss of fascial sliding function have been clearly demonstrated

by Langevin et al. (2011b). Individuals with chronic low back pain showed a 25% greater thickness of the TLF than individuals without low back pain. The gliding potential between fascial layers was also shown to be significantly reduced in these individuals.

- Stecco et al. (2013) suggests that a combination of irritation, inflammation, acidification and densification of loose connective tissue may lead to myofascial pain as a result of *'free nerve endings becoming hyperactivated'* resulting in local inflammation, pain and sensitization. These changes can be reversed by manual therapy interventions that reduce stiffness, density and viscosity – and improve pH; all potentially possible via manual therapies.

Fascia is also greatly affected by the aging process (and inactivity that is possibly related to illness or concurrent pain):

- As we age skin changes, characterized by the evolution of wrinkles, which reflects the reduction in superficial fibroblast and collagen cells.
- Collagen fibers gradually become less organized, more tangled, and tissues lose their defined shape (i.e. they sag) and elastic recoil potentials.
- A part of that inevitable – but variable – process involves loss of elastin, so that from around the third decade of life this process is measurable (Kirk & Chieffi 1962)
- At the same time there is an atrophy of fat cells, so that *'quantitative and qualitative characteristics of the fibro-adipose connective system are changed and its viscoelastic properties become reduced.'* Additionally, the skin and underlying superficial fascia stretch and relax, leading to ptosis of the soft tissues, as well as altered shape involving fat deposition and cellulite (Macchi et al. 2010)

Therapeutic options relative to such changes are explored in Chapter 5 and throughout Section 2, where there are separate chapters on 15 different modalities that target fascial dysfunction.

References

Barral J-P, Mercier P 2004 Lehrbuch der Visceralen Osteopathie; Band 1, 2. Auflage. Urban and Fischer, Munich

Benjamin M 2009 The fascia of the limbs and back – a review. J Anat 214:1–18

Binkley JM, Peat M 1986 The effects of immobilization on the ultrastructure and mechanical properties of the medial collateral ligament of rats. Clin Orthop Relat Res 203:301–308

Bouffard N et al 2009 Tissue stretch decreases procollagen-1 and TGF-β1 in mouse subcutaneous fascia. Abstract. 2nd Fascia Research Congress. Free University of Amsterdam, Amsterdam

Cantu R, Grodin A 2001 Myofascial manipulation, 2nd edn. Aspen Publishing, Gaithersburg, MD

Carano A, Siciliani G 1996 Effects of continuous and intermittent forces on human fibroblasts in vitro. Eur J Orthod 18(1):19–26

Carvalhais V et al 2013 Myofascial force transmission between the latissimus dorsi and gluteus maximus muscles: an in vivo experiment. J Biomech 46:1003–1007

Chen C, Ingber D 2007 Tensegrity and mechanoregulation: from skeleton to cytoskeleton. In: Findley T, Schleip R (eds) Fascia research. Elsevier, Oxford, pp 20–32

Comeaux Z 2002 Robert Fulford DO and the philosopher physician. Eastland Press, Seattle

Doubal S, Klemera P 2002 Visco-elastic response of human skin and aging. J Amer Aging Assoc 3:115–117

Drake RL, Vogl AW, Mitchell, AWM 2010 Gray's anatomy for students, 2nd edn. Churchill Livingstone Elsevier, Philadelphia

Fourie W 2009 The fascia lata of the thigh – more than a stocking. In: Huijing PA et al (eds) Fascial research II: basic science and implications for conventional and complementary health care. Elsevier GmbH, Munich

Franklyn-Miller A et al 2009 The strain patterns of the deep fascia of the lower limb. In: Huijing PA et al (eds) Fascial research II: basic science and implications for conventional and complementary health care. Elsevier GmbH, Munich

Fryer G, Fossum C 2009 Therapeutic mechanisms underlying muscle energy approaches. In: Physical therapy for tension type and cervicogenic headache. Fernandez-de-las-Peñas C et al (eds) Jones & Bartlett, Boston

Greenman P 1996 Principles of manual medicine. Williams and Wilkins, Baltimore

Guimberteau JC, Bakhach J 2006 Subcutaneous tissue function: the multimicrovacuolar absorbing sliding system in hand and plastic surgery. In: Siemionow MZ (ed) Tissue surgery. New techniques in surgery. Springer, London, Ch 4, pp 41–54

Guimberteau JC 2012 The subcutaneous and epitendinous tissue behavior of the multimicrovacuolar sliding system. In: Schleip R, Findley T, Chaitow L, Huijing P (eds) Fascia: the tensional network of the human body. Churchill Livingstone Elsevier, Edinburgh, pp143–146

Hicks MR et al 2012 Mechanical strain applied to human fibroblasts differentially regulates skeletal myoblast differentiation. J Appl Physiol 113(3):465–472

Hocking D et al 2009 Extracellular matrix fibronectin mechanically couples skeletal muscle contraction with local vasodilation. In: Huijing PA et al (eds) Fascia research II: basic science and implications for conventional and complementary health care. Elsevier Urban and Fischer, Munich, pp 129–137

Huijing PA 2007 Epimuscular myofascial force transmission between antagonistic and synergistic muscles can explain movement limitation in spastic paresis. J Electromyogr Kinesiol Dec 17(6):708–24

Huijing P, Langevin H 2009 Communicating about fascia: history, pitfalls and recommendations. In: Huijing PA, et al (eds) Fascia research II. Basic science and implications, for conventional and complementary health care. Elsevier, Munich

Ingber DE 1993 Cellular tensegrity: defining new rules of biological design that govern the cytoskeleton. J Cell Sci 104 (pt 3):613–627

Kapandji I 2007 The physiology of the joints, 6th edn. Vol 1–3. Churchill Livingstone, Edinburgh

Kirk JE, Chieffi M 1962 Variation with age in elasticity of skin and subcutaneous tissue in human individuals. J Gerontol 17:373–380

Kjaer M et al 2009 From mechanical loading to collagen synthesis, structural changes and function in human tendon. Scand J Med Sci Sports19 (4):500–510

Klingler W, Schleip R, Zorn A 2004 European Fascia Research Project Report. 5th World Congress Low Back and Pelvic Pain, Melbourne

Kumka M, Bonar B 2012 Fascia: a morphological description and classification system based on a literature review. Can Chiropr Assoc 56(3):1–13

Langevin HM 2006 Connective tissue: a body-wide signaling network? Med Hypotheses 66: 1074–1077

Langevin HM 2008. In: Audette JF, ailey A (eds) Integrative pain medicine. Humana Press, New York

Langevin HM 2010 Tissue stretch induces nuclear remodeling in connective tissue fibroblasts. Histochem Cell Biol 133: 405–415

Langevin HM 2013 The Science of Stretch The Scientist Magazine®, 1 May. Available online at http://www.the-scientist.com/?articles.view/articleNo/35301/title/The-Science-of-Stretch/. Accessed 11 February 2014

Langevin HM, Huijing PA 2009 Communicating about fascia: history, pitfalls, and recommendations. Int J Ther Massage Bodywork 2:3–8

Langevin HM et al 2005 Dynamic fibroblast cytoskeletal response to subcutaneous tissue stretch ex vivo and in vivo. Am J Physiol Cell Physiol 288:C747–C756

Langevin HM et al 2009 Ultrasound evidence of altered lumbar connective tissue structure in human subjects with chronic low back pain. Presentation, 2nd Fascia Research Congress, Amsterdam

Langevin HM et al 2011a Fibroblast cytoskeletal remodeling contributes to connective tissue tension. J Cell Physiol 226(5):1166–1175

Langevin HM et al 2011b. Reduced thoracolumbar fascia shear strain in human chronic low back pain. BMC Musculoskeletal Disorders 12:203

Levin S Martin D 2012 Biotensegrity the mechanics of fascia. In: Schleip R, Findley T, Chaitow L, Huijing P (eds) Fascia: the tensional network of the human body. Churchill Livingstone Elsevier, Edinburgh, pp 137–142

Lock JG et al 2008 Cell-matrix adhesion complexes: master control machinery of cell migration. Semin Cancer Biol 18(1):65–76

Macchi V et al 2010. Histotopographic study of fibroadipose connective cheek system. Cells Tissues Organs 191(1):47–56

Meert G 2012 Fluid dynamics in fascial tissues. In: Schleip R, Findley T, Chaitow L, Huijing P (eds) Fascia: the tensional network of the human body. Churchill Livingstone, Edinburgh, pp 177–182

Mitchell JH, Schmidt RF 1977 In: Shepherd JT et al (eds). Handbook of physiology, Sect. 2, Vol. III, Part 2. American Physiological Society, Bethesda, pp 623–658

Myers T 2009 Anatomy trains, 2nd edn. Churchill Livingstone, Edinburgh

Myers T 2012 Anatomy trains and force transmission. In: Schleip R, Findley T, Chaitow L, Huijing P (eds) Fascia: the tensional network of the human body. Churchill Livingstone Elsevier, pp 131–136

Olson M, Solomonow M 2009 Viscoelastic tissue compliance and lumbar muscles activation during passive cyclic flexion-extension. J Electromyogr Kinesiol 19 (1):30–38

Purslow P, Delage J-P 2012 General anatomy of the muscle fasciae. In: Schleip R, Findley T, Chaitow L, Huijing P (eds) Fascia: the tensional network of the human body. Churchill Livingstone Elsevier, Edinburgh

Reed RK, Lidén A, Rubin K 2010 Edema and fluid dynamics in connective tissue remodelling. J Mol Cell Cardiol 48(3):518–523

Richter P 2012 Myofascial chains. In: Schleip R, Findley T, Chaitow L, Huijing P (eds) Fascia: the tensional network of the human body. Churchill Livingstone Elsevier, Edinburgh, pp 123–130

Roman M et al. 2013 Mathematical analysis of the flow of hyaluronic acid around fascia during manual therapy motions. J Am Osteopath Assoc 113:600–610, doi:10.7556/jaoa.2013.021 Available online at http://www.jaoa.org/content/113/8/600. abstract.html. Accessed 11 February 2014

Ross M, Pawlina W 2011 Histology, 6e. Lippincott Williams & Wilkins, Baltimore, p 218

Schleip R 2003a Fascial plasticity: a new neurobiological explanation. Part 1. J Bodyw Mov Ther 7(1)11–19; 7 (2):104–116

Schleip R 2003b Fascial plasticity: a new neurobiological explanation. Part 2. J Bodyw Mov Ther 7 (2):104–116

Schleip R 2011 Fascia as a sensory organ. In: Dalton E (ed) Dynamic body®, Exploring Form, Expanding Function. Freedom from Pain Institute, Oklahoma City pp 137–163

Schleip R, Jäger H, Klingler W 2012a What is 'fascia'? A review of different nomenclatures. J Bodyw Mov Ther 16 (4): 496–502

Schleip R, Findley T, Chaitow L, Huijing P 2012b Fascia: the tensional network of the human body. Churchill Livingstone Elsevier, Edinburgh

Standring S 2008 (ed) Gray's anatomy – the anatomical basis of clinical practice, 40th edn. Elsevier, Edinburgh

Stecco L, Stecco C 2009 Fascial manipulation: Practical Part. Piccin, Padova

Stecco A et al 2013 The anatomical and functional relation between gluteus maximus and fascia lata. J Bodyw Mov Ther 17(4):512–7

Stecco C et al 2007 Anatomy of the deep fascia of the upper limb. Second part: study of innervation. Morphologie 91: 38–43

Stecco C, Stecco A 2012 Deep fascia of the shoulder and arm. In: Schleip R, Findley T, Chaitow L, Huijing P (eds) Fascia: the tensional network of the human body. Churchill Livingstone Elsevier, pp 44–48

Swanson RL 2013 Biotensegrity: a unifying theory of biological architecture. J Am Osteopathic Assoc 113(1):34–52

Terminologia Anatomica: international anatomical terminology 1998 Federative Committee of Anatomical Terminology (FCAT). Thieme, New York, pp 1–292

Tesarz J et al 2011 Sensory innervation of the thoracolumbar fascia in rats and humans. Neuroscience, doi: 10.1016/j.neuroscience.2011.07.066

Tortora G et al 2007 Microbiology: an introduction. Pearson Benjamin Cummings, San Francisco

van der Wal J 2009 The architecture of the connective tissue in the musculoskeletal system – an often overlooked functional characteristic of its proprioception in the locomotor apparatus. In: Fascia Research II. Elsevier GmbH, Munich

Weisman M et al 2014 Surface electromyographic recordings after passive and active motion along the posterior myofascial kinematic chain in healthy male subjects. J Bodyw Mov Ther: in press

Willard F 2012a Somatic fascia. In: Schleip R, Findley T, Chaitow L, Huijing P (eds) Fascia: the tensional network of the human body. Churchill Livingstone Elsevier, Edinburgh, pp 30–36

Willard F 2012b Visceral fascia In: Schleip R, Findley T, Chaitow L, Huijing P (eds) Fascia: the tensional network of the human body. Churchill Livingstone Elsevier, Edinburgh, pp 53–56

Willard F, Vleeming A, Schuenke M et al 2012 The thoraco-lumbar fascia: anatomy, function and clinical considerations. J Anat 221(6):507–536

Wipff P J, Hinz B 2009 Myofibroblasts work best under stress. J Bodyw Mov Ther 13:121–127

FASCIAL DYSFUNCTION AND DISEASE: CAUSES, EFFECTS AND POSSIBLE MANUAL THERAPY OPTIONS

Leon Chaitow

This chapter discusses and evaluates the causes and processes involved when fascia becomes dysfunctional – whether this is due to trauma, inflammation, genetics, pathology, poor patterns of use (habitual postural or breathing patterns, for example) or the ageing process.

In addition, evidence-informed indications are offered as to prevention and treatment strategies – where these exist. Where they do not, and experience or anecdotal information is available, this will be mentioned. These distinctions, whether evidence, anecdote or opinion, will be clearly stated.

The primary purpose of this chapter is to focus on explaining and, where possible, identifying validated and/or suggested means of preventing, improving or normalizing fascial dysfunction – even in cases of frank pathology, and even if at times symptomatic relief may realistically be the best possible outcome. It is therefore necessary to give attention to the major forms of fascial dysfunction and pathology – whether acquired or inherited.

Fascial dysfunction and adaptation

Adaptation to: overuse, misuse, disuse and trauma

Leaving aside pathology, which is discussed later in this chapter, the effects of overuse, misuse, disuse, and trauma are the features most likely to be brought to the attention of manual therapists of all schools.

These represent the acute or chronic effects of adaptation, compensation, decompensation and the maladaptive changes that manifest in the musculoskeletal system, commonly involving distress in connective tissue structures. In these the normally well-organized functioning of fascial sheets, planes, bands and fibers – as examples – will have modified their force-transmission/load-transfer functions, along with the reduced sliding potentials, due to the evolution of areas of 'densification', adhesion, restriction, fibrosis or scarring (Langevin 2011).

Klingler (2012) observes that: '*painful contractures and reduced range of motion are frequently associated with rigid collagenous tissue within and surrounding skeletal muscle, as well as other connective tissue involved in force transmission. The fascial function, such as that involving joint capsules, tendons, or epi- and endomysium may be disrupted by trauma and/or inflammation.*'

Such changes may occur locally, or might involve more widespread, sometimes global, postural distortions, associated with redirection of the vectors of mechanical force – potentially leading to musculoskeletal restrictions and pain, as well as modified circulatory and drainage effects.

While non-fascial causes may also be operating in all the signs and symptoms listed below, some major features of fascial dysfunction might involve:

- Modified local or general ranges of motion – potentially involving joints as well as soft-tissue structures
- Reduced local tissue viscoelasticity, resilience
- Loss of sliding potential between tissue surfaces (see notes on superficial fascia, glycosaminoglycans, hyaluronic acid and the *microvacuolar* system, in Ch. 1)
- Impaired coordination and motor control – commonly evident when walking or during performance of normal daily activities.
- Postural deviations and misalignments, frequently involving chain-reactions of adaptation and compensation – as illustrated and discussed in Chapter 3 and also in Chapter 17
- Soft tissue pain – usually perceived on movement
- Myofascial (i.e. trigger point related) pain (see below in this chapter, and in Chs 15 & 20)
- Diminished proprioception – potentially involving impaired equilibrium
- Autonomic imbalance – including sympathetic arousal, or chronic fatigue (see Ch. 7 for further discussion of this topic).

All or any of these (and other) adaptive changes, signs and symptoms might evolve gradually over time; however, they may also appear rapidly, for example soon after inflammation-inducing events.

Opinion: fascial focused therapy and adaptation

It is a truism to say that, with few exceptions – whether through overuse, misuse (poor posture, stressful patterns of use, disordered breathing patterns etc.), abuse (e.g. trauma) or disuse (may occur due to aging) – most of the conditions discussed (apart from frank pathology) are the result of adaptation in progress, or of failed adaptation, where the tissues and systems of the body have responded, as best they can, to biochemical, biomechanical or psychosocial demands. If adaptive load, and the failure to adequately cope with this, lies at the heart of dysfunction, therapeutic choices are reduced to either modifying or eliminating adaptive demands, or improving the ability of the tissues locally, or the body as a whole, to handle these – or offering palliative, symptom-oriented methods.

Once dysfunction is identified, and therapeutic measures introduced, adaptation is once more at the core of what then unfolds. Whether a therapeutic intervention involves manual treatment, surgery, acupuncture, exercise prescription, stress-management, life-style changes etc. – the process is always one of reducing adaptive demands, or of provoking an adaptive response from the body. All treatment therefore involves a search for more functional adaptation.

The art and the science of successful 'treatment' – of anything – requires the appropriate choice of therapeutic input, based on a judgement as to the ability of the individual's homeostatic systems to respond beneficially. Treatment of a given condition would clearly be different depending on the age, functionality, vitality, degree of susceptibility of the individual – as well as of the tissues, structures, organs being addressed – in acute, sub-acute or chronic situations.

> ### Key Point
>
> Understanding adaptation is important – in order to explain the etiology of dysfunction, and in order to help to determine appropriate therapeutic choices.
>
> In order for therapeutic interventions to be clinically effective, particular attention should be given to the evidence relating to the effects of different degrees and types of applied load – as described throughout the book, and in summary form in Chapter 5. Different degrees of applied load have different neurological and biomechanical effects – with potential usefulness in different conditions and situations.

In manual therapy terms, therefore, the choice of type of applied force being delivered (compression, distraction, stretch, shear etc.), the degree (light, heavy, variable etc.), the direction(s) and duration (high velocity, low velocity, sustained for seconds or minutes, for example) are all ways of refining the potential responses of tissues, cells, nerves etc., to the adaptive load/demand.

The second half of this book is devoted to the exploration of 15 different modalities that aim to address the dysfunctional states listed above (and others). Therefore, in this section, only a few pertinent examples of the validated benefits of manual therapy are provided.

Densification and loss of fascial sliding function

An under-explored function of many soft-tissues involves their ability to slide, glide and generally to be able to accommodate the movements of adjacent structures. Loose connective tissue (also known as areolar or superficial fascia), as discussed in Chapter 1, is relatively less structurally organized, as compared with dense connective tissue layers.

Pilat (2011) notes that the processes involved in thickening and densification of the loose connective tissues, and its ECM, appears to correspond to the loss (or reduction) of sliding potential between dense fascial layers and adjacent structures. This view is supported by Stecco et al. (2013a, 2013b), who note: *'Ultrasound indicates that the main alteration in the deep fasciae is increased loose connective tissue between the fibrous sub-layers. It is for this reason that, in indicating fascial alteration, we do not use the term 'fibrosis', which indicates an increase in collagen fibre bundles. We prefer the term 'densification', which suggests a variation in the viscosity of the fascia.'*

Luomala et al. (2014) demonstrate the presence of thicker ('denser') layers of loose connective tissue in both the sternocleidomastoid and scalene muscles in individuals with chronic neck pain, compared with those without neck pain.

Langevin (2011) also confirms that the density of superficial thoracolumbar fascia is markedly increased (25% thicker) in individuals with low back pain, as compared with those without low back pain. The process of thickening, densification appeared – in ultrasound video images – to correspond with a marked reduction in the sliding potential of the deeper layers of the thoracolumbar fascia, in individuals with low back pain. The changes in thickness of the deep fascia was found to correlate with an increase in quantity of loose connective tissue – lying between dense collagen fiber layers – with no increase of the collagen fibre layers themselves (Stecco et al. 2013a,b).

The clinical relevance of these sliding features cannot be over-emphasized. See notes on sliding/gliding etc. in Chapter 1, as well as in Chapter 3.

Fascial element in myofascial ('trigger point') pain

- Simons et al. (1998) have defined a trigger point as: *'a hyperirritable spot in skeletal muscle that is associated with a hypersensitive palpable nodule in a taut band.'*

- Dommerholt (2012) summarizes the background: *'Usually, trigger points develop as a result of local muscle overuse and are frequently associated with other dysfunctions, such as pain diagnoses with peripheral and central sensitization, joint dysfunction, dental or otolaryngic diagnoses, visceral and pelvic diseases and dysfunctions, tension-type headaches and migraines, hypothyroidism, systemic lupus erythematosus (SLE), infectious diseases, parasitic diseases, systemic side effects of medications, and metabolic or nutritional deficiencies or insufficiencies.'*

- Shah et al. (2008) have studied the environment of trigger points and reports that oxygen deficit (hypoxia) is a feature, as is the presence of inflammatory markers, such as substance P and bradykinin. The tissues surrounding trigger points are also excessively acidic.

- LeMoon (2008) proposes a convincing 'fasciagenic' pain model in which prolonged, unremitting fascial thickening and stiffening, seems to be responsible for generating myofascial pain symptoms. Local ischemia appears to be a precursor to such changes in muscles that have been constantly or repetitively overused, possibly involving inflammation, micro-trauma and mechanical strain.

- Stecco et al. (2013a,b) report that reduced sliding function between fascial layers, and coincidental stiffness of the deep fascia, are due to changes in the loose connective tissue layers that separate the dense fascial sheets. They have demonstrated that these changes (stiffness/thickening) are commonly predictors of myofascial pain.
- Gautschi (2012) observes that connective tissue 'shortening' involves crosslinks of intramuscular, as well as muscle fascia and intermuscular collagenic tissue. Local ischemia may then act as a pain stimulus leading to the release of sensitizing substances and subsequent myofascial pain.
- Ball (2012) observes that: 'Fibrotic myofascial change can vary in severity both in terms of area(s) affected and degree of ensuing restriction and dysfunction' – resulting in unrelenting, debilitating myofascial pain – particularly in the flexor muscle groups.

Trigger points: therapeutic options (see also Chs 15 and 20)

Connective tissue massage (see Ch. 7) has been identified as an efficient method for elimination of myofascial trigger points in a multicentre trial (FitzGerald 2009).

- If, as seems probable, trigger point activity is frequently a by-product of overuse or misuse activities (poor posture, repetitive overuse patterns etc.), alteration of these to more normal patterns should reduce or remove the trigger point activity.
- Failing removal of causes a range of manual and other methods have been shown to be capable of – albeit temporarily – reducing myofascial pain – and some examples are listed below.
- A combination of manual modalities, known as Integrated Neuromuscular Inhibition Technique (INIT) – described in Chapter 15 – has been shown in clinical studies to efficiently deactivate trigger points (Nagrale et al. 2010).
- Reviews of modalities in treatment of myofascial pain (Feráññdez-de-las-Penas et al. 2005, Rickards 2006) suggest that the following

methods – individually or in combination – seem capable of reducing myofascial pain: ischemic compression (Chs 15, 19 & 20), trigger point compression combined with active contractions of the involved muscle (Ch. 15), myofascial release techniques (Ch. 14), post-isometric relaxation (Ch. 13), connective tissue and fascial stretches, massage therapy (Ch. 19), spray and stretch, muscle energy techniques (Ch. 13), neuromuscular therapy (Ch. 15), as well as other soft tissue mobilization techniques such as skin rolling (Ch. 7) and strain–counterstrain (Ch. 16) – and dry needling (Ch. 20).

Dommerholt (2012) explains: '*It is obvious that research needs to explore the role of fascia in the etiology, pathophysiology, and management of trigger points. While several non-invasive and invasive treatment options are currently available, with reasonable to good efficacy, there are still many unanswered questions.*'

Key Point

Awareness of the fascial connection with myofascial pain lies in having a greater understanding of the possible mechanisms, and therapeutic options that have been shown to be effective – ranging from extremely light, to invasive – offering a range of choices, depending on the specific setting in which treatment is required.

Fascia and aging

The aging process leads to marked changes in the fascia of the body:

- Creases and wrinkles on the surface relate to reduced numbers of fibroblasts and therefore collagen fibers.
- Elastic fibers also reduce or become frayed or thickened.
- The remaining collagen fibers – particularly in the superficial fascia – gradually become disorganized, tangled, losing shape, and contributing to sagging, ptosis.

- Fat cells in the superficial fascia atrophy and distort in shape – presenting as cellulite. Simultaneously, changes in sebaceous and sweat glands lead to dryness of the skin.
- These changes can be seen from the third decade of life (Macchi et al. 2010) and are accelerated by conditions such as diabetes.
- Age-related changes also affect muscle fascia, with endomysial and perimysial tissues developing tangled cross-linkages – which has clear health implications, as these structures act as *'pathways for myofascial force transmission.'* Reduced soft-tissue mobility is the result (Purslow 2005).
- Proprioceptive functions are inevitably affected – with implications for balance and motor control.
- These degenerative aging processes can be accelerated by a variety of lifestyle factors, ranging from inactivity (lack of exercise), to exposure to tobacco smoke, and poor diet (Avery & Bailey 2008).

Retarding fascial aging

The extent to which these processes can be retarded, or reversed, remains to be established; however, it seems that well-designed forms of exercise may enhance the maintenance of less tangled, more coherent, collagen fibers, and to at least partially restore this state once it has been lost.

Schleip has noted that: *'The fascial tissues of young people show stronger undulations within their collagen fibers, reminiscent of elastic springs, whereas in older people the collagen fibers appear as rather flattened. Research has confirmed ... that proper exercise ... can induce a more youthful collagen architecture – [with] – a more wavy fiber arrangement [and] increased elastic storage capacity.'*

Schleip insists that: *'...only a few minutes of appropriate exercises, performed once or twice per week, is sufficient for collagen remodeling. The related renewal process will take between 6 months and 2 years and will yield a lithe, flexible and resilient collagenous matrix.'*

See Chapter 8 for Schleip's suggested exercise protocols.

> **Key Point**
>
> Age and inactivity have predictable – and inevitable – adaptive outcomes. Appropriate exercise appears to be able to retard and, to a degree, reverse those outcomes, via adaptation to the imposed demands.

Fascial inflammation, wounds, scars, fibrosis and adhesions

Inflammation

Inflammation is the starting point of physiological healing, following tissue damage – whether on a macro or micro scale, and whether the result of trauma or surgery. The most obvious signs of inflammation are heat, swelling, and redness, for without inflammation there can be no adequate healing. Therefore, anything that retards inflammation also retards the healing process. At times there may be good reasons medically for use of anti-inflammatory medication; however, the negative influence on healing of such treatment is well understood (van den Berg 2012, Tortland 2007).

This negative effect is most evident in relation to the healing of tissues that have a relatively poor blood supply (easily recognized because they don't bleed much when damaged), such as tendons, ligaments and fascial attachments. This negative effect on healing also results from analgesic medication, because the individual is likely to be confused by masked pain levels, and so exceeds load on healing tissues – retarding that process.

Wounds, scars and adhesions (see Fig. 2.1)

The three primary phases on wound healing are:

1. Inflammation in which the area is prepared for the subsequent stages by the presence of

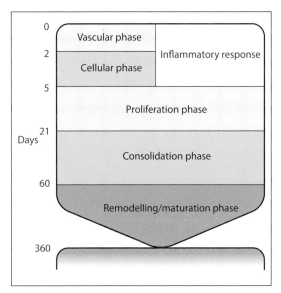

FIGURE 2.1 Wound healing time-scale.

fibroblasts, myofibroblasts, and various mediating substances, such as TGF-β1 – the cytokine, transforming growth factor beta-1, which coordinates much of the initial healing process, while initiating the development of the extracellular matrix (ECM). (See notes on these processes in Ch. 1).

2. The 'rebuilding' fibroplastic phase where an architectural – collagen – scaffolding is created, synthesized by fibroblasts.

3. The remodeling phase where normality is restored as far as is possible.

When tissue damage occurs, dormant fibroblasts (and, to a lesser extent, other local cells) respond to mechanical stress and acquire contractile properties, becoming myofibroblasts.

These form architectural scaffolding by synthesizing the ECM, including various types of collagen (see Ch. 1), in order to support the healing wound. Under normal conditions, as healing continues, these processes slow down and cease.

- Hinz (2013) has summarized the relationship between tissue damage and wound healing: *'Myofibroblasts regulate connective tissue remodeling. During normal tissue repair, such as skin wound healing, controlled and transient activation of myofibroblasts contributes to restoration of tissue integrity by forming a mechanically sound scar.'*

- Quite simply, the success of wound healing depends on the new tissue matrix that the myofibroblasts create, including the collagen they produce.

- Among the factors required for this process to proceed smoothly are the adequate presence of TGF-β1 (as described in Ch. 1) – and most importantly from a mechanotransduction perspective – adequate mechanical tissue tension (Desmoulière et al 2005)

- In a landmark study Hinz et al. (2001) showed that: *'mechanical tension is a prerequisite for the development and maintenance of myofibroblast differentiation and hence of granulation tissue contraction. Given the reciprocal relationship between fibroblast contractility and the mechanical state of the matrix, the modulation of extracellular and intracellular tension may help to influence wound healing and development of fibrocontractive diseases.'*

- When the usually well-choreographed process of wound healing goes wrong and becomes excessive: *'beneficial tissue repair turns into the detrimental tissue deformities.'* These may include hypertrophic scarring, fibromatoses and fibrocontractive diseases, as discussed below.

- There is a, possibly surprising, connection between the individual's breathing pattern and how well wounds heal – see Box 2.1.

- Inadequate healing results in the likelihood of adhesion development, reduced flexibility, and excessive scarring – preventing free movement between usually mobile tissues.

- Chapelle and Bove (2013) summarize the process of adhesion formation in the abdominal viscera:

'a. Adhesions form following a number of injuries to the peritoneum, including mechanical trauma, drying, blood clotting, and foreign object implantation.

The inflammation caused by peritoneal trauma from any etiology leads to a disruption of the balance between the fibrin-forming and fibrin-dissolving capacities of the peritoneum, favoring the deposition of a fibrin-rich exudate on the damaged area.

b. If the fibrin is not resolved by the fibrinolytic system within days, adhesions form.
c. Persistent adhesions can prevent the normal sliding of the viscera during peristalsis and movements of the body, such as respiration. Adhesions become both innervated and vascularized.'

- Almost all surgery, even minor 'keyhole' versions, result in adhesion formation with the potential for chronic pain and possible obstruction as a result (Lee et al. 2009).
- Scars have been shown to predispose towards formation of myofascial trigger points in adjacent tissues, with the potential for initiating pain in distant structures – appendectomy scar, for example, causing low back pain (Lewit & Olsanska 2004).
- Cramer et al. (2010) have confirmed – in animal studies – that inactivity and immobilization result in the development of adhesions in the zygapophyseal (facet) joints. They found that the duration of immobility was directly linked ('small, medium, large') to the size and frequency of these spinal adhesions. They hypothesize that such adhesion development may have relevance to higher-velocity spinal manipulation, which could theoretically break up Z-joint intra-articular adhesions.

Enhancing scar healing and remodeling

- Manual therapy enhancement of healing in poorly vascularized tissues, such as tendons, is achievable by several methods, such as carefully applied deep friction, which increases perfusion
- Careful use of mechanical loading of tissues during the remodeling phase can assist in increasing pliability, mobilizing scar tissue, and preventing adhesion with adjacent tissues. Yang and Wang (2005) reported that rhythmic low amplitude movements have a gentle anti-inflammatory influence (potentially useful if inflammation seems excessive), while, in contrast,

larger magnitude stretching induces pro-inflammatory effects.

- For damaged tissue to regain a collagen structure similar to the pre-injury state, the tissues should be confronted with similar physiological load to that faced pre-injury – with the degree of stress increasing slowly in the 4th week post-trauma.
- Studies by Standley et al. (2007) suggest that myofascial and positional release methods can be used to modulate inflammatory processes.
- van den Berg (2012) notes that nutritional factors can modify scar healing – with anything that reduces pH (i.e. increased acidity) having a retarding influence on fibroblast function – reducing the efficiency of healing (see nutrition notes later in this chapter).
- Grinnell (2008) has reported that: *'Physical manipulation of fascia has the potential to change the cell-matrix tension state, influencing localized release of cellular growth factors. Our research on the fibroblast – collagen matrix interactions, demonstrates that such changes can lead to profound and rapid modulation of structural, functional and mechanical interactions between fibroblasts and the extracellular matrix* [contributing] *to the reorganization of fascia that results from bodywork practice.'*
- Compression and frictional methods can effectively modify inappropriate densification of fascia and enhance remodelling. Myofibroblasts help to reconstruct injured tissue by secreting new ECM and by exerting high contractile force. Myofibroblasts perceive load using specialized matrix adhesions (see Ch. 1; Wipff & Hinz 2009).
- The process of repair and remodeling of damaged tissues is enhanced by movement (exercise) and appropriate mechanical forces, such as those applied during manual therapy (Ramage et al. 2009).
- Bove & Chapelle (2013) have demonstrated – in animal models – that visceral mobilization may have a role in the prevention and treatment of postoperative adhesions.

Key Point

It is clinically important to maintain awareness of the value of inflammation and of manual and movement methods that enhance repair and remodeling, as well as poor (diminished or excessive) inflammatory responses. The influence of pH (and breathing) on wound healing is explained in Box 2.1.

Fibrosis and keloids

Chronic inflammation leads to fibrosis, which may occur in soft tissues or organs as a result of excessive build-up of connective tissue (Wynn 2008).

As Fourie (2012) explains: '*Fibrosis represents a pathologic excess of normal tissue repair. Excessive or sustained production of TGF-β1 is a key molecular mediator of tissue fibrosis. It consistently and*

Box 2.1
Breathing pattern disorders, anxiety, pH, wound healing and hypermobility

As noted earlier (Ch. 1), myofibroblasts have an important role to play during wound healing. The transition from fibroblasts, plentifully located in connective tissues, to myofibroblasts, is stimulated by increases in mechanical strain, as well as by the presence of inflammatory markers (such as cytokines).

A further influence appears to be modified pH, in which respiratory function plays a major part in maintaining pH at optimal levels (approximately 7.4).

A variety of psychosocial, biomechanical and biochemical influences – as well as pure habit (Lum 1984) – can promote an accelerated breathing pattern, including the extremes of hyperventilation and panic attack.

This – in the short term – leads to altered pH with a string of largely negative health implications (Thomas & Klingler 2012).

Breathing and wound healing

- Upper chest breathing patterns, with hyperventilation as an extreme, lead to reduced levels of CO_2 in the bloodstream (hypocapnia), resulting in respiratory alkalosis – elevated pH (Foster et al. 2001)
- Respiratory alkalosis leads to smooth muscle cell constriction, potentially resulting in vasoconstriction, and potentially colon spasm and pseudo-angina – *as well as increased fascial tone* (Ford et al. 1995, Ajani 2007)
- Alkalosis retards early wound repair because it encourages fibroblasts from differentiating into myofibroblasts so reducing the efficiency of collagen synthesis and facilitation of 'architectural' wound closure (Jensen et al. 2008).
- Continued over-breathing can therefore be seen to potentially contribute to excessive scarring – although it may be helpful in the early stages of tissue-repair.

Breathing and hypermobility

- Breathing pattern disorders, such as hyperventilation, are much more common in hypermobile individuals, and are often associated with both anxiety and chronic pain syndromes (Martin-Santos et al. 1998)
- Individuals who present with anxiety and panic disorders – where hyperventilation is a common etiological feature – have been shown to suffer significantly more often with prolapse of the mitral valve, also indicating lax connective tissues (Tamam et al. 2000)
- Long-term physiological and metabolic changes result from chronic breathing pattern disorders as the homeostatic rebalancing mechanisms attempt to restore normal pH
- It may be hypothesized that hyperventilation, which potentially increases fascial tone, may be assisting the hypermobile individual's dysfunctional laxity – a functional dysfunction?

For a greater understanding of the complex processes involved in hyperventilation, see Thomas & Klingler 2012, Krapf et al. 1991 or Chaitow et al. 2013.

powerfully acts on cells to encourage the deposition of extracellular matrix. The connective tissue response to the internal (inflammatory mediators and growth factors) and external (motion and directional strain) stresses applied will determine how the scar matures. Thus the scar can become either dense and unyielding or pliable and mobile. Remodeling is not restricted to the injured area only. Neighboring, non-injured tissue also changes its collagen production rate in response to inflammation.'

Apart from fibrosis, over-production of collagen can result in irregularly shaped keloid scars that may progressively enlarge.

Lifestyle, nutrition and inflammation

- Inflammation can be excessive and therefore promote excessive collagen deposition, leading to fibrosis.
- Lifestyle choices can make this more likely – for example, exposure to tobacco smoke and other pollutants (Avery & Bailey 2008).
- Dietary strategies can modulate inflammation, most notably by reducing intake of arachidonic acid-rich products (dairy and meat fats, for example) and increasing eicosapentenoic acid-rich products, Omega-3 oils (e.g. oily fish) and a wide variety of plant-based foods (flax seed, olive oil, walnuts, garlic, deep-colored fruits and vegetables, herbs such as ginger and cinnamon, green tea; Hankinson & Hankinson 2012).

> **Key Point**
>
> Clinicians need to observe – and, where necessary, consider intervention in – the balancing act between optimal beneficial and damagingly excessive levels of inflammation. Safe modulation may be possible via nutrition and manual approaches that ensure optimal tissue tension (as discussed above and in Ch. 1).

Selected fascial pathologies and conditions

Cerebral palsy

In a small osteopathic study involving 57 children with mild to severe spastic cerebral palsy (CP),

Davis et al. (2007) demonstrated a strong relationship between the neurological and muscular symptoms, and both fascial and spinal motion restrictions. The fascial 'diaphragms' of the body were evaluated: tentorium cerebelli, cervicothoracic junction, respiratory diaphragm, and the pelvic floor. The most implicated restriction in the study was the pelvic diaphragm.

- The spinal regions were assessed for restriction and the most implicated in this study were: upper cervical (C1-C2), upper thoracic (T1-T4) and lower thoracic (T9-T12).
- Davis and colleagues report that: 'indicators of fascial and spinal restriction predict an external measure of impairment, manifesting as muscle spasticity'.
- They further note that the results support the concept that, 'a problem in the spine is often associated with a problem in the fascia and vice versa.'

Note: Davis et al. (2007) suggest that the findings in the CP children may be applicable to other pathological conditions, noting that: *'We have replicated the factorial analyses in a second [unpublished] study, designed to investigate similar factors [fascial and spinal restrictions] in young children with recurrent ear infections. While the sample size in both studies was small, the results from our otitis media study also provide evidence for the factorial validity of the fascial and spinal motion restriction factors.'*

> **Key Point**
>
> This information may have clinical relevance – if, for example, it can be demonstrated in cases of CP that objective improvements in spinal and fascial restrictions are accompanied by enhanced functionality. Further research is needed to validate this possibility.
>
> Note that similar fascial and spinal findings, in other conditions, may also be relevant – as suggested by Zink and Lawson (1979). See Chapter 4 for more on this topic.

Myofascial structural integration options for cerebral palsy (CP)

- Hansen et al. (2012) report that there is increasing evidence suggesting that: *'structural changes within muscle and surrounding tissues are associated with creating and/or increasing muscle stiffness and resistance to stretch, in spastic cerebral palsy.'*

- In a randomized crossover study, motor function was assessed – measured at the start and after the treatment, involving eight children with spastic cerebral palsy, aged 2–7 years.
- The treatment method employed was myofascial structural integration – a deep-tissue manipulation technique *'designed to reorganize muscle and surrounding soft tissue.'*
- All children received 10 weekly 60–90 minute sessions of myofascial structural integration, as well as 10 weekly sessions of a control intervention (play). *'Half of the children underwent play followed by myofascial structural integration and the other half in the reverse order.'*
- Results showed that there were major improvements in six children after the therapy, while three of the children also showed improvements following the control (play) phase, suggesting that: *'myofascial structural integration holds promise as a novel complementary treatment for spastic cerebral palsy.'* See Chapter 17 for information on Structural Integration.

> ### Key Point
> The clinical relevance of the Hansen study, and many anecdotal reports, suggests that it may be possible to modify some of the effects of CP – at least in children.

Fibrocontractive diseases

- **Dupuytren's disease:** appears to be a largely inherited condition, primarily (but not totally) affecting middle-aged males of Northern European origin. It is characterized by a contracture of the protective connective tissue sheet that forms the palmar aponeurosis, covering the flexor tendons of the hand. The initial feature of the subsequent contracture involves changes in the vertically oriented fibers that connect the aponeurosis to the skin. As these shorten they form 'pits' on the palmar surface. Progression – which can be rapid or slow – involves connective tissue proliferation (including fibroblasts, myofibroblasts and contractile smooth muscle cells) resulting in formation of nodules on the aponeurosis that may adhere to the skin. These may form dense, gritty connective tissue meshes. As the condition progresses longitudinal tension is exerted, affecting the ability of the metacarpophalangeal joints to extend. By that time cord-like structures may be noted on the palmar surface of the hand. Surgical and drug interventions have had varying – but limited – degrees of success.
- **Lederhosen's disease:** this is a similar condition to Dupuytren's disease – involving the plantar aponeurosis of the arch of the foot. Surgery has had limited success in treating the resulting deformity.
- **Peyronie's disease:** plaque-like connective tissue changes – involving myofibroblasts – that affect the penis; this is even less understood than Dupuytren's disease, with surgery and medication having poor treatment records.

> ### Key Point
> There are no reports of clinical benefit deriving from manual therapy interventions in these fibrocontractive diseases.

Frozen shoulder (Schultheis et al. 2012)

There are three overlapping phases in this condition that can be summarized as:

- *Freezing:* gradual loss of both active and passive ranges of motion at the shoulder joint, often associated with extreme pain, most evident at night. This phase is characterized by synovitis and capsulitis – i.e. inflammation is active.
- *Frozen:* reduced pain but severe loss of range of motion in all directions, with abduction and lateral rotation most limited. This phase is characterized by capsular fibrosis with a dramatic increase in levels of fibroblasts and myofibroblasts – see Chapter 1 for the relevance of this.
- *Thawing:* a gradual restoration of full range of motion. This phase is characterized by a dissolving of the fibrosis and restoration of – more or less – normal ranges of motion.

The process may last months or years, with the length of each phase being unpredictable, but unlikely to be less than 4 months for each stage.

The condition may arise as a secondary feature of earlier trauma, immobilization or arthritic changes, or it may emerge as a primary frozen shoulder (FS), without any obvious triggering factor. People with diabetes are more prone to the primary form.

No physical treatment is advisable during the first stage of primary (inflammatory) FS; however, mobilization and exercise may be helpful in stage 2. When this is unsuccessful surgical intervention is frequently attempted (for example: arthroscopy with distension, debridement, release, and manipulation under anesthetic) with some evidence of success (Chen et al. 2002).

Secondary FS may be treated from the outset by means of physical therapy, with attention to etiological features, and to mobility.

Manual therapy and exercise options

Standard medical treatment methods in care of FS, including anti-inflammatory medication, suprascapular nerve blocks, arthroscopic surgery and manipulation under anesthetic, are mainly symptom-focused. There is very little evidence that these result in reduction of the overall duration of the condition.

There are only few studies that support manual approaches to FS:

- D'Amato and Rogers (2012) confirm what is generally acknowledged, that there is *'insufficient evidence to draw firm conclusions about the effectiveness of treatments commonly used to manage a frozen shoulder.'* They nevertheless recommend a range of osteopathic soft tissue and manipulative measures (counterstrain, muscle energy, mobilization etc.) – without offering research evidence to support use of the listed methods in FS – with selection largely dependent on the current stage of the FS process, i.e. particularly avoiding exacerbation during the early 'freezing' phase.
- Celik (2010) reported on a comparison of two exercise protocols that accompanied standard medical care (transcutaneous electrical nerve stimulation, cold pack, and non-steroidal anti-inflammatory drugs). Twenty-nine individuals in the second ('frozen') stage of FS participated in 30 supervised physiotherapy sessions of glenohumeral range of motion exercises, alone or combined with scapulothoracic exercises, over a 6-week period. The outcomes showed that all patients, following both protocols, achieved significant reduction in pain and increased range of motion, with the group following the combined exercise approach demonstrating significantly better outcomes at 12-week follow-up.

- Ho et al. (2009) have demonstrated that therapeutic exercise appears to be as effective as either acupuncture or manual therapy in treatment of FS.
- Buchbinder et al. (2009) similarly showed that medium- and long-term outcomes after therapeutic exercise for adhesive capsulitis are similar to those after more expensive treatments, including arthrographic distension and corticosteroid injection.
- When pendular exercises (gentle circular movements with arm positioned as a pendulum) were compared with either 1) intraarticular steroid injections; 2) mobilization; 3) ice therapy; 4) no treatment, there was very little difference or long-term benefit noted, apart from short-term reduction in pain and some increase in range of motion following steroid injections (Bulgen et al. 1984).
- Vermeulen et al. (2006) found that high-grade mobilization (i.e. firm but within patient pain tolerance, to produce no more than a dull ache) is superior to low-grade mobilization (lighter, painless).
- Carter (2001) reported on the effects of Bowen Technique (see Ch. 6) in treatment of FS. Twenty patients with FS received five Bowen Therapy treatments over a period of 3 months. Median 'worst pain' pre-therapy score reduced from 7 (mean 7, range 1–10) to a median 'worst pain' score of 1 (mean 1.45, range 0–5) post-therapy. All participants experienced improvement in their daily activities. It was concluded that Bowen Technique demonstrated an improvement

for participants, even with longstanding history of FS.

- Gerwin (1997) offers his informed opinion that: *'From a clinical standpoint, much of the limitation of motion associated with a frozen shoulder can be explained by **myofascial trigger points** in the shoulder region muscles'* and that: *'Examination and treatment of all affected muscles of the shoulder region must be undertaken, resisting the temptation to treat just one or two of the most obviously painful muscles. The subscapularis, in particular, must be examined in all cases of "frozen shoulder" since trigger points in it and in the latissimus dorsi greatly restrict abduction and external rotation of the arm and prevent elevation of the arm above the shoulder.'* See Chapters 15 and 20 for more on trigger points.

- Neil-Asher (in Chemeris et al. 2004) offers a degree of evidence in support of Gerwin's perspective, noting the positive outcomes of a 2003 pilot study that compared various physiotherapy modalities and a placebo, with his protocol, in management of FS. He reports employing a neuromuscular approach involving *'a specific sequence of soft tissue manipulations, joint articulations (within the pain-free range) and inhibition through various trigger points.'* A summary of outcomes demonstrated marked difference in favor of the **neuromuscular methods**, compared with either physiotherapy or placebo, in both range of abduction increase (52° compared with 24° and 0.8°), as well as pain and disability.

> ### Key Point
>
> Caution is advised in manual treatment of FS. Evidence seems to favor exercise and possibly manual therapy – such as specific myofascial trigger point deactivation, and methods such as Bowen Therapy or strain–counterstrain – but only once the active inflammatory stage is over.

Hypermobility

There are a number of inherited conditions with joint hypermobility as a major symptom (Beighton et al. 1999, Grahame 2009). These are clustered together under the title, *heritable disorders of connective tissue* (HDCT):

- Marfan syndrome (MFS) (also affecting eyes, skin and organs)
- Ehlers–Danlos syndrome (EDS)
- Osteogenesis imperfecta (OI)
- A 'mixed' variety, with characteristics of the three above, is joint hypermobility syndrome (JHS).

These all have joint hypermobility as a common feature, with various symptoms being more prevalent in the different variants of HDCT. As Simmonds (2012) points out: *'Although the cardinal features of EDS, MFS and OI include hyperextensible skin, marfanoid body shape, and brittle bones, respectively, these features are not pathognomonic to each condition.'*

Ethnicity

Simmonds (2012) notes that approximately 12% of individuals have some degree of joint hypermobility; however, hypermobility levels vary widely between different ethnic groups. The largest population percentages are found in individuals from Africa, Arab countries, South Asia and South America.

Hypermobility is more common in:

- Females – ratio of approximately 3:1
- Children – hypermobility tends to reduce with age
- Certain ethnic groups:
  o   Caucasians, Northern Europeans: ~5%.
  o   Non-Caucasians in a West London rheumatology clinic: females 58%, males 29% (Clark & Simmonds 2011).

Remvig et al. (2007) reports evidence that suggests an underlying feature of HDCT relates to the degree of myofibroblast density in muscular fasciae. Certainly, different collagen types are noted in the ECM of affected individuals. A further characteristic of HDCT involves slow wound healing.

Among assessment tools is the Beighton Scale (see Box 2.2), which indicates the degree of severity of an individual's hypermobility. (Note: there are other assessment criteria, including those where

Box 2.2

Nine Point Beighton hypermobility score*

Individuals are scored on their ability to:

1. Passively dorsiflex the 5th metacarpophalangeal joint to 90°
2. Oppose the thumb to the volar aspect of the ipsilateral forearm
3. Hyperextend the elbow to 10°
4. Hyperextend the knee to 10°
5. Place hands flat on the floor without bending the knees.

Total: 1 point is gained for each side, for each maneuver, 1–4, with a total possible score of 9 points.

The major hypermobility diagnostic criteria are:

- Having a Beighton score of 4 or more, either currently or in the past
- Having joint pain for longer than 3 months, in four or more joints.

*Beighton & Horan 1969.

---

the Beighton scale is accompanied by enquiries regarding symptoms.)

Associated conditions of hypermobility

- Individuals with generally increased degrees of connectivetissue laxity are more prone to joint dislocation (Hakim & Grahame 2003)
- Additionally, hypermobile individuals demonstrate an increased tendency to hyperventilation – and associated increased levels of anxiety (Martin-Santos et al. 1998; see Box 2.1)
- Vascular connective tissue laxity may lead to cardiac valve prolapse or varicosities (Tamam et al. 2000)
- Osteoarthritis and osteoporosis are both more common in individuals who are hypermobile (Gulbahar et al. 2005, Bird et al. 1978)
- Both fibromyalgia and chronic fatigue syndrome are common accompanying diagnoses (Simmonds 2012).

Therapeutic options

There appear to be two contrasting positions regarding where to commence therapeutic intervention in patients with chronic hypermobility syndromes. The ingredients appear to be the same; however, the initial emphasis and sequencing are different:

1. A rehabilitation, exercise, and re-education approach with a view to increased joint stability, where local dysfunctional areas are addressed peripherally as they crop up (Simmonds 2012).

2. A focused attempt at reducing myofascial pain in particular, prior to, or synchronous with, exercise-reeducation protocols (Dommerholt, personal communication 2012).

Whichever model is selected, because of the wide range of variations in symptoms of JHS and the many areas affected, therapeutic measures must be individualized:

1. Simmonds and Keer (2007) offer clear indications as to the areas where they believe attention is required:

   o Minimization of joint pain, hypermobile joints, reduced proprioception, altered motor control, weak muscles and reduced stamina – all of which can profoundly affect gait.

   o Where pain is a major feature they advocate pain-management strategies including cognitive behavioral therapy, followed (when pain is reduced) by reeducation regarding body awareness, proprioception and methods to enhance joint stability. They report achieving pain reduction and stability following use of a *graduated exercise program combined with education, behavioral and lifestyle advice.*

2. Myofascial pain is a common feature of individuals with JHS, and Dommerholt (personal communication, 2012) poses a question that challenges the sequencing suggested by Simmonds & Keer (2007): *'Joint pain experienced*

by patients with EDS may actually represent referred pain from trigger points and therefore, an excessive focus on joint stability should not be the main focus of management programs. The mechanisms of TrP referred pain have been described in detail and involve an expansion of the receptive fields of spinal neurons and sensitization (Mense 2010). Many patients with EDS have severe allodynia and hyperalgesia. Could rehabilitation or functional training be counterproductive in the presence of allodynia and hyperalgesia? In other words, is pushing patients with EDS through their pain advisable or would this constitute a threatening input and as such no longer be therapeutic (Moseley 2003)?'

Dommerholt notes that: '*...clinical experience does suggest that manual therapy, including resolution of taut bands and trigger points, prior to initiating rehabilitation programs, allows patients with EDS to exercise relatively pain free and achieve their goals of pain reduction and joint stability.'*

Cautions

- Care is suggested regarding deactivation of myofascial trigger points in individuals with hypermobile joints, since it is conceivable that patients with variants on JHS are likely to develop contractures in local muscles in order to better stabilize unstable joints (Chaitow & DeLany 2003). In such cases attention to these pain generating entities might both reduce joint pain as well as allowing more effective, less uncomfortable, subsequent exercise and reeducation strategies.
- Stretching type modalities, or exercises, are contraindicated, with therapeutic efforts ideally focused on enhanced tone, strength, endurance, balance and posture.
- Reeducation of breathing patterns is likely to be useful, based on the known link between hypermobility and hyperventilation. However, caution is suggested because of the influence of respiration on pH on fibroblast activity as discussed in Box 2.1. It is possible that enhanced breathing would remove the potentially useful stabilizing effect of increased pH (Thomas & Klingler 2012).

- Areas of soft-tissue dysfunction and pain may benefit from use of supportive taping and hydrotherapy-based exercises. Additionally, prolotherapy (also known as sclerotherapy) may be considered, as mentioned in Chapter 5.

> **Key Point**
>
> Therapeutic options: personal preferences, particular skills, clinical evidence, and the needs of the individual are the mix from which choices will be made. Hopefully the opinions and evidence above will assist in that process.

Plantar fasciitis/fasciosis (PF)

Whilst usually termed plantar fasciitis (PF), research indicating a degenerative rather than an inflammatory nature of this painful condition, suggests that plantar fasciosis should be used as a descriptor instead (Lemont et al. 2003). PF involves a painful condition of the shock-absorbing fascial sheet that supports the arch of the foot. It is characterized by increased collagen deposition and thickening; however, this feature may also occur in asymptomatic individuals.

There is also no strong evidence that excessive physiological loading is sufficient to produce PF in healthy tissues. The shape of the longitudinal arch, midfoot loading, and reduced energy-dissipating features (but not the thickness) of the heel pad, all seem to be pain-accentuating features, rather than etiological factors. Wearing et al. (2009) in an ultrasound study of PF, noted that, along with the degree of imposed stress, and the shape of the arch: '*the thickness of the plantar fascia is positively related to the severity of heel pain.'* They found that the fascia thickness at the heel was approximately 50% greater on the symptomatic side. There is some evidence that age, diabetes and obesity may be contributory features (Wearing et al. 2007). It is suggested that as yet unidentified neuromuscular deficits, combined with reduced tolerance to normal compression, bending and shear forces, possibly associated with unaccustomed overuse, leads to degenerative collagenous changes and consequent pain.

Manual therapeutic options for PF

Strain–counterstrain

Strain–counterstrain (SCS; see also Ch. 16) has been shown to beneficially influence PF. *'Clinical improvement occurs in subjects with plantar fasciitis in response to counterstrain treatment [SCS]. The clinical response is accompanied by mechanical, but not electrical, changes in the reflex responses of the calf muscles'* (Wynne et al. 2006; see Fig. 2.2).

SCS (which is fully explained in Ch. 16) involves slow positioning of tender tissues, until sensitivity reduces by around 70%. Urse (2012) has described the method as follows for treatment of PF: *'The supine patient's ipsilateral knee is flexed, and a plantar tender point [an area of local hypersensitivity] is identified where the fascia inserts onto the calcaneus. One thumb is used to monitor the tender point... [while] ...the opposite hand plantar flexes the toes and ankle curving around the tender point. Additional adjustment to the tension may be accomplished by supination or pronation of the foot, until there is*

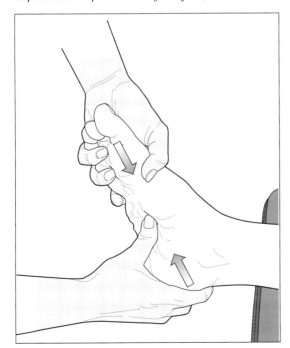

FIGURE 2.2 Strain–counterstrain (SCS) of foot. Redrawn from Urse 2012 – with thanks.

symptomatic relief of the tenderness underlying the monitoring thumb.'

This position-of-ease is maintained for up to 90 seconds, before a slow return to neutral and reassessment.

Instrument assisted soft-tissue mobilization for PF

Looney et al. (2011) have reported on a case series in which 10 individuals with plantar fasciitis were treated with soft tissue mobilization methods, involving use of Graston® instruments (see Ch. 12). The protocol was as follows:

1. Patients received a maximum of 8 treatments over 3–8 weeks, with 1– 2 sessions weekly
2. Focus was on the triceps surae, soleus, plantar fascia, and medial calcaneal tubercle, which were assessed in order to identify local fibrous adhesions
3. Deeper pressure – using the Graston instruments – was then applied for 1–2 minutes to these areas
4. Static stretching of the triceps surae, soleus, and plantar fascia, for 30 seconds each was repeated twice
5. Ice was applied to the plantar region for 15–20 minutes
6. Home stretching was recommended 3× daily.

Seventy percent of the patients experienced statistically significant and clinically meaningful improvements in pain and function.

Stretching methods and PF (see also Chs 13 and 15)

A number of studies have reported on benefits deriving from different forms of stretching in treatment of PF:

1. DiGiovanni et al. (2003) treated 101 patients with PF of at least 10 months' duration. All received soft insoles. Half of the patients were taught *non-weight-bearing self-stretching of the plantar fascia,* and the other half were taught *stretching of the Achilles tendon/ calf.* Outcomes after 8 weeks indicated major benefits for the fascia stretching group. At a 2-year follow-up (DiGiovanni et al. 2007), it was found that there had been continued im-

provement for the plantar fascia-stretching group, where calf muscle stretching had also been employed – with 92% reporting total satisfaction or satisfaction with minor reservations.; and 77% reporting no limitation in their recreational activities. The protocol for plantar self-stretching involved the patient seated, knee flexed, and palpating with a thumb to locate areas of *plantar tension*. With the thumb in contact with a 'tight' area, the patient was required to dorsiflex the foot to produce *'a sense of stretch,'* for 10 seconds, repeated 10 times, three times daily. The protocol for calf/Achilles self-stretching involved the patient standing, knee extended, and introducing a mild stretch to the calf for 10 seconds, 10 times, 3 times daily.

2. Porter et al. (2002) noted that there was the same degree of benefit to patients with PF, in use of *sustained Achilles tendon stretches* (3 minutes, three times daily), when compared with *intermittent Achilles tendon stretches* (5 sets of 20 seconds, twice daily). Both methods increased tendon flexibility which correlated with reduction in pain symptoms.

3. Sweeting (2011) conducted a systematic review of manual stretching and plantar heel pain (PF). And noted that: *'there is some evidence that plantar fascia stretching may be more effective than Achilles tendon stretching alone in the short-term.'*

Key Point

Clinical outcomes following manual therapy interventions involving PF, point to benefit deriving from stretching local plantar fascia, in addition to calf and Achilles areas. Local soft-tissue mobilization methods (instrument assisted) were also found to be helpful, as was the positional release method, strain–counterstrain

---

Scleroderma disorders

Ball (2012) notes that: *'Scleroderma denotes a condition presenting as thickening, hardening, and scarring of the skin. Systemic refers to an autoimmune condition that affects the internal organs, as well as the skin and superficial (subcutaneous and 'deep investing') fascia layers.'*

Scleroderma is associated with a wide range of connective tissue diseases with similar features but different causes, including:

- Raynaud's syndrome (subdivided into primary and secondary Raynaud's phenomenon)
- Systemic sclerosis
- Diffuse systemic sclerosis (dSSc)
- Systemic lupus erythematosus (SLE)
- Mixed connective tissue disease
- Sjögren's disease
- Rheumatoid arthritis.

Readers are advised to investigate these conditions individually for more detail; however, the following generalized summary of some of these female-dominated (8:1) chronic inflammatory conditions may offer insights:

- **Etiologies:** where these are known – are multifactorial, ranging from genetic predisposition to environmental, biochemical, biomechanical and psychological involvement, resulting in autoimmune outcomes.

- **Symptoms:** include pain, fatigue and the effects of organ-related conditions including gut, renal, circulatory and cardio-respiratory distress.

- **Locations:** the fascial structures of the body are commonly affected, with fibrotic changes and excessive collagen production, particularly involving dermal and vascular structures, flexor muscles and joints. *'Ensuing adverse tissue changes include thickening, shortening, hardening, and scarring, which in turn result in reduced range of motion (RoM), vascular, lymphatic, neural, joint, and visceral compression and constriction'* (Ball 2012).

Therapeutic option

No curative methods exist as yet; however, palliative medical approaches may lead to modification or temporary easing of symptoms – see below.

Case reports: structural integration and SLE

Ball (2011) employed Structural Integration (Rolfing®)methods (see Ch. 17 for details of Structural

Integration), described in two detailed case reports involving SLE. She describes the assessment and initial therapeutic objectives as follows: *'The process ... involves accurate 'body reading' to identify departures from tensegrity due to areas of shortened, congested* [connective tissue], *compensated by over-stretched, lengthened fascia elsewhere. 'Interactive' manual manipulative techniques – involving active client participation – are then applied according to a structured treatment strategy devised by sound clinical reasoning.'*

The manual methods used involve: *'applying appropriate softening, releasing, spreading, and/or lengthening techniques'... such as myofascial release* (see Ch. 14) *and ...'neuro-vascular-fascial*

decompression' ...supported by self-applied rehabilitation methods. The two patients received eight or nine treatments of 1-hour duration, spread over 14 and 18 weeks, respectively. The following symptomatic benefits followed manual therapy:
1. Reduced pain and stiffness, swelling and use of analgesics
2. Fewer and reduced duration of episodes of exhaustion and GI tract distress. Additionally functional mobility and range of motion were improved.

Ball (2012) notes that: *'While "spontaneous recovery" cannot be ruled out in the absence of control subjects, these anecdotal outcomes suggest*

Case Example
Myofascial release and dSSc

Martin (2009) describes use of myofascial release (MFR; see Ch. 14) in treatment of diffuse systemic sclerosis, involving 20 treatment sessions spread over 1 year. The objectives were *'To improve breathing and functionality of the temporomandibular joint (TMJ) and hands, by increasing the range of motion (ROM), and to reduce the level of pain.'*

Martin's description of the MFR approach, which she describes as *'negotiation between the pressure of the therapist's hand and the patient's nervous system,'* is as follows – involving her personal interpretation of what she understands to be taking place during the process (see Ch. 14 for details of myofascial induction – as *MFR* is known in some settings):
1. *'The initial load placed on it is the therapist's touch, from which the biochemical and mechanical responses are expected.'* [See notes on mechanotransduction in Ch. 1.]
2. *'The therapist is able to feel a flexible resistance (elastic limit) -* [which] *- is slowly elongated by maintaining pressure until a firm barrier is reached.*
3. *This* [represents] *the beginning of the deformation of the collagen component.*

4. *This barrier should not be forced –* [as this would not give] *– the molecules and collagen fibrils enough time to reorganize.*
5. *Therefore, a proportional pressure to the perceived resistance should be maintained –* [and] *– it is expected that the release will occur within the tissue.*
6. *When this pressure is applied for a long period, respecting that limit which keeps the integrity of the tissue, affects the viscosity of the underlying substance in which the collagen fibers are immersed, increasing hydration at the site.*
7. *As the collagen fibers are released, they reorganize and remodel themselves (Kisner and Colby, 1998).*
8. *The time is determined by the therapist's tactile perception of this change'* (Martin 2009).

The outcomes reported – with photographic evidence provided – include:
1. Chest: expansion increased by 3.5 cm and pain was eliminated from a biopsy scar
2. TMJ: 8 mm increase in mouth opening together with elimination of associated pain
3. Hands and fingers: range of motion of all joints increased in all finger and wrist joints, with total reduction in ulcerations, and restoration of nail growth.

FRT efficacy, alongside ongoing medical management, in alleviating specific symptoms and/or effects of scleroderma-type auto-immune diseases, notably SLE'.

Key Point

There exists some evidence – mainly case reports – that manual therapies may offer symptomatic and functional relief for individuals affected by these autoimmune conditions.

References

Ajani A 2007 The mystery of coronary artery spasm. Heart Lung Circ 16:10–15

Avery N, Bailey A 2008 Restraining cross–links responsible for the mechanical properties of collagen fibers; natural and artificial. In: Fratzl P (ed)-Collagen: structure and mechanics vertebrates. Springer, NY, 81–110

Ball TM 2011 Structural integration based fascial release efficacy in alleviating specific symptoms in systemic lupus erythematosus (SLE): two case studies. J Bodyw Mov Ther 15(2): 217–225

Ball T 2012 Scleroderma and related conditions. In: Schleip R, Findley TW, Chaitow L, Huijing PA (eds)-Fascia: the tensional network of the human body. Churchill Livingstone Elsevier, pp 225–232

Beighton P et al 1999 Hypermobility of joints, 3rd edn. Springer-Verlag, Berlin

Beighton P, Horan F 1969 Orthopedic aspects of the Ehlers-Danlos syndrome. J Bone Joint Surg [Br] 51: 444–453

Bird H et al 1978 Joint hypermobility leading to osteoarthritis and chondrocalcinosis. Ann Rheum Dis 37:203–211

Buchbinder R et al 2008 Arthrographic distension for adhesive capsulitis. Cochrane Database Syst Rev (1):p.CD007005

Bulgen, D et al 1984 Frozen shoulder: prospective clinical study with an evaluation of three treatment regimens. Annals of the Rheumatic Diseases 43(3):353–360

Carter B 2001 A pilot study to evaluate the effectiveness of Bowen Technique in the management of clients with frozen shoulder. Complementary Therapies in Medicine 9(4):208–215

Celik D (2010) Comparison of the outcomes of two different exercise programs on frozen shoulder. Acta Orthopaedica et Traumatologica Turcica 44(4):285–92

Chaitow L, Bradley D, Gilbert C 2013 Recognizing and treating breathing disorders: a multidisciplinary approach, 2nd edn. Churchill Livingstone Elsevier, Edinburgh

Chaitow L, DeLany J 2003 Neuromuscular techniques in orthopedics. Techniques in Orthopedics 18: 74–86

Chapelle S, Bove G 2013 Visceral massage reduces postoperative ileus in a rat model J Bodyw Mov Ther 17(1):83–88

Chemeris I et al 2004 A presentation of stiff and commentary painful shoulder – a case based commentary. JOM 7 (1): 41–47

Chen S et al. 2002 Idiopathic frozen shoulder treated by arthroscopic brisement. Kaohsiung J Med Sci 18 (6): 289–294

Clark C, Simmonds J 2011 An exploration of the prevalence of hypermobility and joint hypermobility syndrome in Omani women attending a hospital physiotherapy service. Musculoskeletal Care 9(1):1–10

Cramer GD, Henderson CN, Little JW, et al 2010 Zygapophyseal joint adhesions after induced hypomobility. J Manipulative Physiol Ther 33: 508–518

Davis M et al 2007 Confirmatory factor analysis in osteopathic medicine: fascial and spinal motion restrictions as correlates of muscle spasticity in children with cerebral palsy. JAOA 107(6):226–232

D'Amato K Rogers M 2012 'Frozen shoulder'– a difficult clinical problem review. Article Osteopathic Family Physician 4(3):72–80

Desmoulière A et al 2005 Tissue repair, contraction, and the myofibroblast. Wound Repair Regen 13(1):7–12

DiGiovanni B, Benedict F, et al 2003 Tissue-specific plantar fascia-stretching exercise enhances outcomes in patients with chronic heel pain: a prospective, randomized study. J Bone Joint Surg 85(7):1270–1277

DiGiovanni B et al 2007 Plantar fascia-specific stretching exercise improves outcomes in patients with chronic plantar fasciitis. J Bone Joint Surg 88(8):1775–1781

Dommerholt J 2012 Trigger point therapy. In: Schleip R, Findley TW, Chaitow L, Huijing PA (eds)-Fascia: the tensional network of the human body. Churchill Livingstone Elsevier, Edinburgh pp 297–302

Fernández-de-las-Penas, C et al 2005 Manual therapies in myofascial trigger point treatment: a systematic review. J Bodyw Mov Ther 9:27–34

FitzGerald MP et al 2009 Randomized multicenter feasibility trial of myofascial physical therapy for the treatment of urological chronic pelvic pain syndromes. J Urol 182(2):570–580

Ford M et al 1995 Hyperventilation, central autonomic control, and colonic tone in humans. Gut 37:499–504

Foster G et al 2001 Respiratory alkalosis. Respir Care 46:384–91

Fourie WJ 2012 Surgery and scarring In: Schleip R, Findley TW, Chaitow L, Huijing PA (eds)-Fascia: the tensional network of the human body. Churchill Livingstone Elsevier, Edinburgh, pp 233–244

Gautschi R et al 2012 Trigger points as a fascia-related disorder In: Schleip R, Findley TW, Chaitow L, Huijing PA (eds)- Fascia: the tensional network of the human body. Churchill Livingstone Elsevier, Edinburgh, pp 233–244

Gerwin R 1997 Myofascial pain syndromes in the upper extremity. Original Research Article. Journal of Hand Therapy 10(2):130–136

Grahame R 2009 Joint hypermobility syndrome pain. Curr Pain Headache Rep 13: 427–433

Grinnell F 2008 Fibroblast mechanics in three-dimensional collagen matrices. J Bodyw Mov Ther 12(3):191–193

Gulbahar S et al 2005 Hypermobility syndrome increases the risk for low bone mass. Clin Rheumatol 26:1–4

Hakim A, Grahame R 2003 A simple questionnaire to detect hypermobility: an adjunct to the assessment of patients with diffuse musculoskeletal pain. Int J Clin Pract 57:163–166

Hankinson M Hankinson E 2012 Nutrition model to reduce inflammation in musculoskeletal and joint diseases In: Schleip R, Findley TW, Chaitow L, Huijing PA (eds)-Fascia: the tensional network of the human body. Churchill Livingstone Elsevier, Edinburgh, pp 457–464

Hansen A et al 2012 Myofascial structural integration: a promising complementary therapy for young children with spastic cerebral palsy. J Evid Based Complementary Altern Med 17(2):131–135

Hinz B et al 2001 Mechanical tension controls granulation tissue, contractile activity and myofibroblast differentiation. Am J Pathol 159(3):1009–1020

Hinz B 2013 Wound healing and the extracellular matrix. Presentation: Touro College of Osteopathic Medicine, August 18

Ho C et al 2009 The effectiveness of manual therapy in the management of musculoskeletal disorders of the shoulder: a systematic review. Man Ther 14:463–474

Jensen D et al 2008 Physiological mechanisms of hyperventilation during human pregnancy. Respir Physiol Neurobiol 161(1):76–78

Klingler W 2012 Temperature effects on fascia In: Schleip R, Findley TW, Chaitow L, Huijing PA (eds)-Fascia: the tensional network of the human body. Churchill Livingstone Elsevier, Edinburgh, pp 421–424

Krapf, R et al 1991 Chronic respiratory alkalosis. The effect of sustained hyperventilation on renal regulation of acid-base equilibrium. N Engl J Med 324 (20):1394–1401.

Langevin et al 2011 Reduced thoracolumbar fascia shear strain in human chronic low back pain. BMC Musculoskeletal Disorders 12:203

Lee T et al 2009 Prognosis of the upper limb following surgery and radiation for breast cancer. Breast Cancer Res Treat 110:19–37

Lemont H et al 2003 Plantar fasciitis: a degenerative process (fasciosis) without inflammation. J Am Podiatr Med Assoc 93:234–237

LeMoon 2008 Clinical reasoning in massage therapy. Int J Therap Massage Bodyw 1(1):12–18

Lewit K, Olsanska S 2004. Clinical importance of active scars: abnormal scars as a cause of myofascial pain. J Manipulative Physiol Ther 27:399–402

Looney B et al 2011 Graston instrument soft tissue mobilization and home stretching for the management of plantar heel pain: a case series. J Manipulative Physiol Ther 34:138–142

Lum L 1984 Editorial: Hyperventilation and anxiety states. J R Soc Med January 1–4

Luomala T, Pihlman M, Heiskanen J et al 2014 Case study: Could ultrasound and elastography visualize densified areas inside the deep fascia? J Bodyw Mov Ther: 18(3) 462-468

Macchi, V et al., 2010. Histotopographic study of fibroadipose connective cheek system. Cells Tissues Organs 191(1):47–56

Martin MM 2009 Effects of myofascial release in diffuse systemic sclerosis. J Biochem Mol Toxicol 13(4):320e327

Martin-Santos R et al 1998 Association between joint hypermobility syndrome and panic disorder. Am J Psychiatry 155 (11):1578–1583

Mense S 2010 How do muscle lesions such as latent and active trigger points influence central nociceptive neurons? J Musculoskelet Pain 18: 348–353

Moseley L 2003 Unraveling the barriers to reconceptualization of the problem in chronic pain: the actual and perceived ability of patients and health professionals to understand the neurophysiology. J Pain 4:184–189

Nagrale A et al 2010 The efficacy of an integrated neuromuscular inhibition technique on upper trapezius trigger points in subjects with non-specific neck pain: a randomized controlled trial. J Man Manip Therap 18(1):38

Pilat A 2011 Myofascial induction. In: Chaitow et al (eds)-Practical physical medicine approaches to chronic pelvic pain (CPP) and dysfunction. Elsevier, Edinburgh

Porter D et al 2002 The effects of duration and frequency of Achilles tendon stretching on dorsiflexion and outcome in painful heel syndrome. Foot Ankle Int 23(7):619–624

Purslow PP 2005 Intramuscular connective tissue and its role in meat quality. Meat Sci 70: 435–447

Ramage L et al 2009 Signaling cascades in mechanotransduction: cell-matrix interactions and mechanical loading. Scand J Med Sci Sports 19:457–469

Remvig L, Jensen DV, Ward RC 2007 Are diagnostic criteria for general joint hypermobility and benign joint hypermobility syndrome based on reproducible and valid tests? A review of the literature. J Rheumatol 34:798–803

Rickards LD 2006 The effectiveness of non-invasive treatments for active myofascial trigger point pain: a systematic review of the literature. Int J Osteopathic Med 9: 120–136

Schultheis A et al 2012 Frozen shoulder. In: Schleip R, Findley TW, Chaitow L, Huijing PA (eds)-Fascia: the tensional network of the human body. Churchill Livingstone Elsevier, Edinburgh, pp 199–206

Shah JP et al 2008 Biochemicals associated with pain and inflammation are elevated in sites near to, and remote from active myofascial trigger points. Arch Phys Med Rehabil 89:16–23

Simons DG et al 1998 Travell & Simons' Myofascial pain and dysfunction: the trigger point manual. Williams & Wilkins, Baltimore

Simmonds J 2012 Hypermobility and the hypermobility syndrome. Assessment and management. In: Schleip R, Findley TW, Chaitow L, Huijing PA (eds)-Fascia: the tensional network of the human body. Churchill Livingstone Elsevier, Edinburgh, pp 279–289

Simmonds JV, Keer R 2007 Hypermobility and the hypermobility syndrome. Masterclass. Man Ther 13:492–495

Standley P 2007 Biomechanical strain regulation of human fibroblast cytokine expression: an in vitro model for myofascial release? Presentation at Fascia Research Congress, Boston

Stecco A et al 2013a Ultrasonography in myofascial neck pain: randomized clinical trial for diagnosis and follow-up. Surg Radiol Anat doi: 10.1007/s00276-013-1185-2

Stecco A et al 2013b Fascial components of the myofascial pain syndrome. Curr Pain Headache Rep 17:352

Sweeting D et al 2011 The effectiveness of manual stretching in the treatment of plantar heel pain: a systematic review. J Foot Ankle Res 4:19

Tamam et al 2000 Association between idiopathic mitral valve prolapse and panic disorder. Croat Med J 41 (4): 410–416

Thomas J, Klingler W 2012 The influence of pH and other metabolic factors on fascial properties. In: Schleip R, Findley TW, Chaitow L, Huijing PA (eds)-Fascia: the tensional network of the human body. Churchill Livingstone Elsevier, Edinburgh, pp171–176

Tortland PD 2007 Sports injuries and nonsteroidal anti-inflammatory drug (NSAID) use. Connecticut Sportsmed Winter, 1–4

Urse GN 2012 Plantar fasciitis: a review. Osteopathic Family Physician 4:68–71

van den Berg F 2012 The physiology of fascia In: Schleip R, Findley TW, Chaitow L, Huijing PA (eds)-Fascia: the tensional network of the human body. Churchill Livingstone Elsevier, Edinburgh, pp 149–155

Vermeulen H et al 2006 Comparison of high-grade and low-grade mobilization techniques in the management of adhesive capsulitis of the shoulder: randomized controlled trial. Phys Ther 86:355-368.

Wearing S et al 2007 Plantar fasciitis: are pain and fascial thickness associated with arch shape and loading? Phys Ther 87 (8):1002–1008

Wearing C et al 2009 Are local mechanical factors related to plantar fascial thickness? J Bodyw Mov Ther 13(1):89

Wipff PJ, Hinz B 2009 Myofibroblasts work best under stress. J Bodyw Mov Ther 13:121–127

Wynne M et al 2006 Effect of counterstrain on stretch reflexes, Hoffmann reflexes, and clinical outcomes in subjects with plantar fasciitis J Am Osteopathic Assoc 106(9):547–556

Wynn TA 2008 Cellular and molecular mechanisms of fibrosis. J Pathol 214(2):199–210

Yang G, Im HJ, Wang JH 2005 Repetitive mechanical stretching modulates IL-1beta induced COX-2, MMP-1 expression, and PGE2 production in human patellar tendon fibroblasts. Gene 19: 166–172

Zink JG, Lawson WB 1979 An osteopathic structural examination and functional interpretation of the soma. Osteopath Ann 7(12):433-440

Chapter 3

GLOBAL POSTURAL ASSESSMENT

Thomas W Myers

This chapter focuses largely on the global postural assessment of compensation patterns in the neuromyofascial web, using the map of 'myofascial meridians' known as the Anatomy Trains® (Myers 2014).

Chapter 4 has additional global, as well as a number of local, palpation and assessment methods that complement the content of this chapter.

Fascial versus neurological patterns

Since this book is about fascial dysfunction, we should first address the question of the degree to which postural patterns are neuromotor patterns versus actual patterning within the fascial tissues. The answer depends primarily on how long they have been established and whether they are sequelae from trauma or simply ingrained habits.

Every movement begins as an experiment, a novel expression of neuromotor firing. Any parent who has been with their 6-month-old when he or she first turns over knows that the child is just as surprised at this accomplishment as the parent.

To our knowledge there is no specific program for 'turning over' in the human brain. There is, however, a very strong program for 'keeping track of Mom and other moving things'. As the eyes track Mom, the reflexive rotation and extension of the neck initiates the spinal rotation and extension, and the rest of the rolling over movement. When the strength of the muscles and bones and the proportion of the head to torso allow it, (remember we are still in the period of *ex utero* gestation and initial ossification), the child does indeed roll over. It may take a few weeks before they can organize turning back the other way by themselves, but in the meantime they are delighted to have you help them come back, so that they can turn from back to belly again and again and again.

This repetition of the movement presumably carves some sort of 'engram' or trace in the brain, so that the motion is easier to repeat (Berthoz 2000). Repeated enough, the sequence of firing becomes fixed as a habit – easily called up, but less subject to change.

If you were to lie on the floor now and roll from back to front, first to the right and then to the left, you would find that you have a preference, that one side is easier and more 'natural' then the other. (Before you put down the book to try this experiment for yourself, which you are encouraged to do, keep in mind the following two elements:

1) Initiate the movement from your eyes, imagining you are tracking something to that side and up, letting your body follow the motion, and 2) be aware of performing it the same way to both the right and left side – you will see you cannot. Subtle, or glaring, differences in the two sides abound.)

Based on hundreds of iterations of this test with many people, this one-sided preference is not related to your dominant handedness or a dominant eye. It is more likely an expression of which way you were commonly laid in the crib, or the accidental side your mother or the family pet passed you to create the initial stimulus - but in the author's experience, everyone has a predilection – a preferred side to which to roll. (**Editor's note:** Consider the information on the Zink common compensatory fascial pattern, as outlined in Ch. 4.)

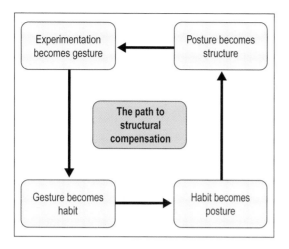

FIGURE 3.1 The Path to Structural Compensation. Every movement begins as an experiment. An experiment repeated becomes a familiar gesture. Repeat a gesture and it becomes ingrained as a habit. Each habit requires a posture. All of these are neural patterns. Hold a posture for long enough and the fascia takes the pattern. At that point, every new experiment arises from that fascial pattern. In reversing the process, both the fascial patterning and the deep postural habit need to be addressed.

Habits, once firmly established, require a posture to maintain them (Fig. 3.1). The preference just outlined will be written visibly into your posture, as well as your movement choices, i.e. which shoulder to look over when you back up your car. Such postural 'sets' are maintained in the cerebellum and brainstem,

and are thus that much less amenable to 'voluntary' control (even though the muscles that these patterns use are all so-called voluntary muscles).

To test this, abduct your arm to horizontal or nearly so and place your forearm on a dresser (or someone else's shoulder, if you have someone available; see Fig. 3.2). Press down with your forearm – some combination of the pectorals, latissimus dorsi, teres major, and coracobrachialis will be the active prime movers in this adduction, while the antagonist deltoid will relax. Reach across with your opposite hand to feel (or have your partner feel) the lateral abdominal obliques on the side you are pressing down. Without doubt, you will feel the lateral part of external and internal oblique contract.

These muscles are, of course, acting to stabilize the rib cage on the pelvis. Here is the experiment: try pressing your arm down *without* contracting those muscles, and keep your other hand or your partner's hand there, to see if you have in fact quelled the tendency to contract these muscles.

If you are like most people – and we have done this experiment with many professional groups in different cultures – the lateral abdominal muscles will pop on automatically when the arm is pressed, and inhibiting this reaction is very difficult. If you are in fact successful in this inhibition, your lower ribs will pull up to the side of the pressing arm (a very 'silly-looking' movement); if the insertion cannot go to the origin, the origin will move toward the insertion.

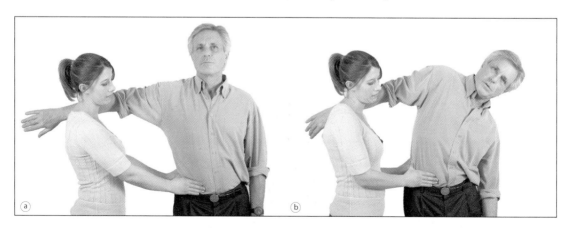

FIGURE 3.2 A simple test for understanding levels of neuromuscular programming involves pressing down against resistance with your arm while attempting to inhibit the side belly wall. If you succeed – which requires a trick of the mind – the result is an unusual and not very 'functional' exercise.

The inability of most people to 'turn off' this re-action speaks to the depth of postural patterns in the nervous system. Once established, such patterns as the 'trunk stabilization program' we just tested become the unconscious substrate of conscious movement. Our 'sitting program' underlies our 'driving program' that underlies our 'this car program' that underlies the consciously controlled move to reach for the turn signal as we approach the intersection.

Most of the important patterns we wish to change in order to improve our patients' biomechanics rest in these deeper regions of postural habitus – the postural set that underlies the habit that underlies this particular gesture that is now painful or limited, for whatever reason. While we need to treat the proximate cause to relieve pain or restore function, we often find ourselves entreating our clients to change the habits that led to the failure of the proximate cause, or we will be seeing them soon again for the same symptom.

These patterns are often body-wide, and therefore somewhat confounding. Supraspinatus tendon inflammation is caused by improper shoulder support caused by a posteriorly tilted rib cage on top of an anteriorly shifted pelvis and so on, down to shortened hamstrings and a chronically dorsiflexed ankle.

Hold these patterns long enough, and the areas under extra strain will produce more fibroblast activity, which creates more collagenous 'strapping' – within or between muscles – to meet the specific strain caused by the repetitive posture (Kjaer et al. 2009).

At this point, we move from a purely neurological pattern to a fascial restriction. From this point on any new experiments, any novel movement the client is learning, will work around that limitation in structure, as opposed to – or more properly, in addition to – a limitation in the neuromotor recruitment.

So, as we look at the common patterns that are outlined below, we cannot know without a physical examination whether we are addressing a 'mere' neural patterning (although we just saw how deeply that can run) versus structural restriction in non-contractile tissues.

We can have more certainty when the problem follows an injury or surgery that fascial adhesions are involved, as fascial 'overdoing' is a common healing response to injury, sustained inflammation, or surgical cutting and sewing (Hyman & Rodeo 2000).

Felt-like adhesions are readily and reliably palpable around old injuries and surgeries in the living, and are often found in dissection in conjunction with surgical intervention or other trauma (Fig. 3.3 and Plate 3).

The best course of treatment will depend on clinical decisions based on our manual and observational assessments. Heavy-handed manual treatment or deep stretching is usually not necessary, or indeed can be detrimental when trying to enhance neuromotor patterning, but seems well-suited to deep tissue dehydration or adhesion, where neural facilitation trigger-point therapies, PNF or muscle-energy style stretches, or Feldenkrais-like decoupling, would likely need to be repeated many times or sustained over long periods of time to have any salutary effect on true fascial restrictions.

When your hand is a hammer, everything looks like a nail. Practitioners tend to see each problem and pattern through the lens of their own training, in terms of the strategic arrows already in their quiver. This is fine as long as we can admit to ourselves when our techniques are not working and change tack or refer out.

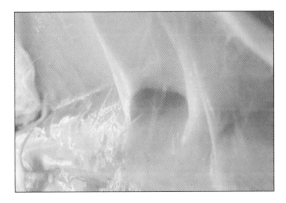

FIGURE 3.3 Fascial adhesion in dissection. Felt-like fascial adhesions are palpable in the living body and visible in the cadaver. See also Plate 3. *Photo courtesy of Robert Schleip.*

Now that we have made this distinction between patterns that are purely held in the neural system versus those that have been there so long (or in response to trauma) that they are now 'written into' the fascial system, we can go on to outline some characteristics of the fascial system.

Fascia as a holistic communicating system

Central to this new Anatomy Trains map is the functional unity of the connective tissue system. There are exactly three networks within the body that if magically extracted intact would show us the shape of the whole body, inside and out: the vascular system, the neural net, and the extracellular fibrous web created by the connective tissue cells.

Large communities of cells need vast infrastructure to maintain their fluid biochemistry in crowded conditions, pressed by gravity, and surrounded by air. It is an astounding feat of engineering that we take for granted every day:

- A community of 70 trillion diverse, humming, and semi-autonomous cells, each built for undersea living, organizes itself to get up, walk around, grab a cup of coffee, and answer email. Most organismic cell-collections, to avoid massive cell death, require a constant exchange of gases, a regular exchange of food and waste, and must find another similar community of cells and go through a complex dance in order to reproduce.

- Simultaneously, our body provides each cell with a mechanically stable environment, oceanic conditions of chemical exchange, and the information it needs to participate meaningfully in the day's work.

- Every living cell needs to be within four cell layers or so of the fluid exchange provided by the vascular system. Without the ability to deliver chemistry and suck away waste, any underserved area becomes stressed, then distressed, and will finally shrivel or burst and die, as happens in necrotic or gangrenous tissue. Secondly, every cell needs to be within reach of the nervous system's signaling to regulate its activity with other cells in other areas of the body. And every cell needs to be structurally held in place (or directed in a flow, in the case of blood and other mobile cells) by the connective tissue net.

Any given single cubic centimeter taken from the body would contain elements of all three of these nets – neural, vascular, and fascial. Seen in such a systemic way, the idea of the body as simply a collection of parts begins to lose its luster. We all survive because we are an interwoven set of systems (Fig. 3.4).

FIGURE 3.4 Vesalius nervous system and circulatory system. Vesalius detailed the neurological and vascular systems in 1548, a miraculous feat of dissection given the methods of the time. We have continued this model more or less unchanged for the ensuing 450 years. *Reprinted courtesy of Dover Publications.*

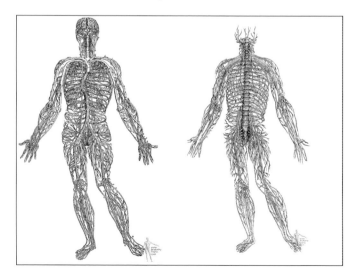

- Each of these nets is networked across the entire body from central organizing structures: from its central spinal cord with the bulbous brain plexus at one end, the nervous system spreads throughout the body in the familiar radiating pattern, to form a sensory simulation of our inner and outer world and a coordinated behavioral response. Dripping through the synapses and interstitia of this system are the messenger molecules of hormones, neurotransmitters, and neuropeptides, regulating neural tone both up and down the system (Pert 1997).
- The circulatory system, from the axis of the aorta and the muscular heart, links the thousands of miles of capillaries and lymphatics in a circle that serves the chemical needs of the cellular community.
- Thirdly, from the central armature of the notochord (the embryological form of the vertebral bodies and discs), connective tissue spreads out to create protective sacs and nets around all the cells, structures, and systems of the body, organizing stable mechanical relationships, allowing certain movements, discouraging others and providing the organization for all movements: voluntary, autonomic, and physiological.

All three networks communicate throughout the body. The nerves carry sensory data in order to construct a second- to-second picture of the world, and send signals out to the muscles and glands, at speeds between 7 and 170 mph (~10–250 kph; Williams 1995). The fluid systems circulate chemistry around the body every few minutes, though many chemical rhythms fluctuate in hourly, daily, or as women know, monthly cycles.

The fibrous system communicates mechanical information – tension and compression – via the intercellular matrix of fascia, tendon, ligament, and bone. This information is a vibration that travels at the speed of sound, about 700 mph – slower than light, but definitely faster than the nervous system. The speed of plastic deformation and remodeling in the connective tissue system, however, is measured in weeks, months, and even years. Thus, the fibrous system is both the fastest (in communicating) and the slowest (in responding) of the three.

Unlike the neural and vascular systems, this connective tissue net has yet to be well-mapped, because it has long been considered to be the 'dead' material that we need to remove to see the 'interesting' neural, vascular, muscular, and other local systems. Because the connective tissue provides the divisions along which the scalpel runs to parse out other systems, the connective tissue has also been studied less as a system than other, more familiar systems.

So, as a thought experiment: what if, instead of dividing the body into individual identifiable structures, we were to dip it into a solvent that stripped away all the cellular material but left the entire extracellular matrix (ECM) intact? (Fig. 3.5) This is being done now in the creation of new artificial organs where the cellular material (of a healthy heart, say) is 'shampoo-ed' out, and the remaining ECM is seeded with cardiac muscle cells to 'grow' a new heart – or kidney, or lung.

The beginning of form

This system of the connective tissue matrix can be seen as our 'organ of form' (Verela & Frenk 1987). From the moment of the first division of the ovum, the intercellular matrix of the connective

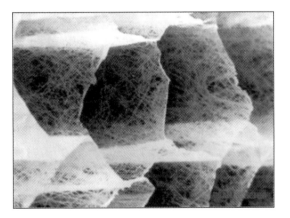

FIGURE 3.5 The endomysium gives us the clearest picture of what a body-wide extraction of the connective tissue matrix would look like. Photo courtesy of Peter Purslow. *Reproduced from Purslow 1994, with kind permission from Springer Science and Business Media.*

tissue exists as a secreted glycosaminoglycans (mucous) gel that acts to glue the cells together (Moore & Persaud 1999). Around the end of the second week of embryological development, the first fibrous version of this net appears; a web of fine reticulin spun by specialized mesodermal cells on either side of the developing notochord (spine).

This net is the origin of our fascial web – our 'metamembrane' – the singular container that shapes our form and directs the flow of all our biochemical processes (Juhan 1987). This ECM, taken as a whole, not only unites the various elements of the body, it unites the many branches of medicine (Snyder 1975).

The ability of the connective tissue cells to alter and mix the three elements of the intercellular space – the water, the fibers, and the gluey groundsubstance gel of glycosaminoglycans – produces on demand the wide spectrum of familiar building materials in the body (Williams 1995). Bone, cartilage, ligament, tendon, areolar, and adipose networks are all examples of this biological fabric. The body's joints, the organ system of movement, are almost entirely composed of ECMs constructed by the various connective tissue cells.

The fiber/gel matrix becomes an immediate part of the environment of every cell, like cellulose in plants, or the coral's limestone 'apartment building'. The animal (and human) ECM, however, is very responsive to change – some in passive response to outside forces, some in active cellular response to damage or need (Schleip et al. 2012). Given that the matrix is a liquid crystal capable of storing and transmitting information, and that it is so intimately married to the lives of our cells, it can be seen as a living part of the body, not a dead packing material (Pirschinger 2007).

Fascial signaling and remodeling is part of our adaptive response to the needs of practical continuance; it is possibly part of the underlying substrate of our consciousness (Koob 2009).

Before we veer any farther into the realm of speculation, let us return to view the development of this network that supports the cellular community in a dynamically upright position.

Whole systems engineering

Thinking in 'wholes', attractive as it is to contemporary therapists, must in the end lead to useful maps. While 'everything is connected to everything else' as a philosophy is technically accurate, it leaves the practitioner adrift in a sea of connections, unsure as to whether that frozen shoulder will respond to work in the elbow, the contralateral hip, or to a reflex point on the ipsilateral foot. While any of these might work, useful maps are necessary to organize our therapeutic choices into a better strategy than 'press and pray'.

The idea 'body as assembled machine', inherited from Descartes and Newton, is so pervasive, and maps based on the 'origin-insertion' isolation of single muscles working as levers around fulcrums are so easily understood and useful, that it is difficult to think outside these parameters.

What can we learn when we shift from a 'symptom-oriented' view of the body to a 'system-oriented' one?

From the initial blastosphere, we see the involution of gastrulation and the subsequent lateral and sagittal folds are followed by literally thousands of others. This developmental origami takes the original simple three-dimensional spider's web of surrounding and investing fascia and folds it into more than a thousand compartments and divisions that we subsequently cut out and identify as separate 'parts'. Initial folds create the dorsal cavity for the brain and ventral cavity for the organs and the coelomic bags surround each organ with a double-layered fascial sac.

One of the final folds brings the two halves of the palate together, which explains why a cleft palate is such a common birth defect.

With this image, we can get away from the shibboleth that there are some 600 muscles in the body. There is, in fact, only one muscle. One mind, and one muscle – contractile tissue is just folded into 600 pockets within the unitary fascial bag. We are so thoroughly imbued with the idea of origins, insertions, and actions of each individual muscle, and it is a mental struggle to rise above this concept, but the view from the mountain of wholeness is breathtaking.

One other holistic image useful in jumping out of this 'machine made out of parts' image so ingrained in our systems, is tensegrity geometry. The normal geometric picture of our anatomy is that the skeleton is a continuous compression framework, like a crane's frame, or a stack of blocks, from which the muscles hang like cables.

This leads to the single muscle theory again – the skeleton is stable but moveable, and we parse out what each muscle does to that framework on its own, adding them together to analyze functional movement. A little thought, however, soon puts this idea out to pasture. Take the muscles away, and the long skeleton on tiny feet is anything but stable; take all the soft-tissue away and the bones would clatter to the floor, as they do not stack in any kind of locked way.

If we can get away from the idea that bones are like girders, and muscles are the cables that move the girders, we are led to a class of structures called 'tensegrity' (a portmanteau signifying that the structural integrity lies in the balance of continuous tension). Originated by Kenneth Snelson and developed by Buckminster Fuller, tensegrity geometry more closely approximates the body as we live and feel it than does the old 'crane' model (Heartney 2009, Fuller 1975).

In the dance of stability and mobility that is a human moving, the bones and cartilage are clearly compression-resisting struts that push outward against the myofascial net. The net, in turn, is always tensional, always trying to pull inward toward the center. Both elements are necessary for stability, and both contribute to practical mobility.

In this new orthopedic model, the bony struts 'float' within the sea of tension provided by the soft tissues (Fig. 3.6). The position of the bones is thus dependent on the tensional balance among these soft-tissue elements. This model is of great importance in seeing the larger potential of soft-tissue approaches to structure, in that bony position and posture is far more dependent on soft-tissue balance than on any high-velocity thrusting of bones back into 'alignment'.

The tendency for these structures to store energy, to 'give' and then restore themselves in an elastic way is very different from the rigidity of the

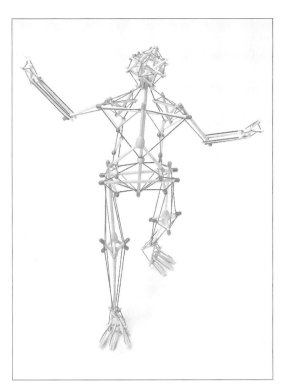

FIGURE 3.6 The tensegrity models created by Intension Designs mimic biological movement in a way that fulcrum and lever models do not. The interplay of tension and compression gives 'proportional stability' in a way that rigid structures cannot accommodate. *Photo courtesy of Tom Flemons*. (For descriptions, short films, and the models themselves, contact designer Tom Flemons at intensiondesigns.com.)

levers and fulcrums model. This property commends them as a model of the body, which also gives and returns in this elastic way. When the shoulder is pressed to the wheel, the shoulder gives, the rib cage adjusts and the spine bends, the pelvis rotates, the legs set – there are a thousand small adaptive reactions all over the body, not a single setting of a rigidly locked system. Although difficult to show on a printed page, tensegrities show this kind of behavior, just like bodies.

These patterns of slight 'give' in multiple segments are, when held into the posture over a long period of time, the very constellation we need to see to make an effective fascial release treatment that will make structural sense to both the mind and the joints. Research supports the idea of tensegrity geometry, ruling mechanical transmission from the cellular level upwards, and macro-level models are becoming more anatomically accurate with each passing year (Turvey & Fonseca, 2014).

How we move and are moved during our lives shapes this web, and the shape of the web, in turn, helps to determine our experience of living in our bodies.

Introduction to the Anatomy Trains

The Anatomy Trains' myofascial meridians map the global lines of tension that traverse the body's muscular surface, acting to keep the skeleton in shape, guide the available tracks for movement, and coordinate global postural patterns (Fig. 3.7 and Plate 4).

Anatomy Trains describes an intermediate level between these overarching global considerations and useful detailed anatomy. These 'myofascial meridians' provide a practical transition between the individual parts and the whole of a human being – the gestalt of physics, physiology, stored experience, and current awareness that often defies mapping. The Anatomy Trains view of the body's locomotor fabric opens new avenues to treatment consideration, particularly for stubborn chronic conditions and global postural effects.

At its simplest, myofascial meridians simply track the warp and weft through the parietal 'myofascialature'. The basic rule is to follow muscular and fascial fibers in a relatively straight line without abrupt changes in depth or intervening fascial walls.

Where does this webbing run continuously in straight lines – lines that can transmit tensional forces that travel out from their local areas to create global effects via the interconnectedness of this overall network? The answer to this question provides a map for tracking myofascial strain transmission and the slight 'give' that allows this system to adapt as a whole.

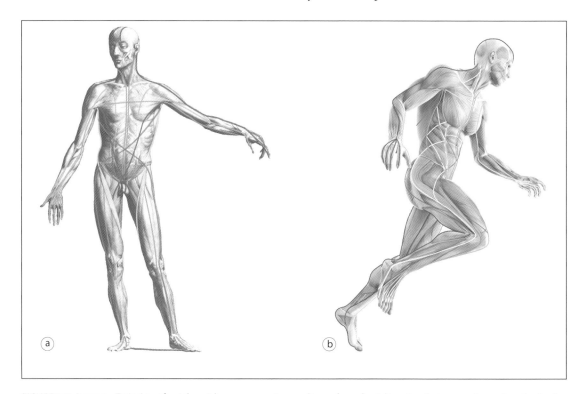

FIGURE 3.7 Anatomy Trains' myofascial meridians map continuous lines of myofascial tension that generally run longitudinally along the body's musculature. See also Plate 4.

Let us introduce the *dramatis personae* of the Anatomy Trains before going on to analyze some common postural compensations. Those already familiar with the system can proceed to the 'BodyReading' section that follows. For a more in-depth exploration of these concepts and their application, see the book *Anatomy Trains* (Elsevier 2001, 2009, 2013), or visit the site at www.AnatomyTrains.com.

Anatomy Trains provides a traceable basis for effective treatment at some distance from the site of dysfunction or pain. This new view of structural patterning has far-reaching implications for treatment strategies, especially for longstanding postural imbalances, unsound body usage, and sequelae from injury or insult.

The concept is very simple: if we follow the grain of the fascial fabric, we can see where muscles link up longitudinally. When this is done, there are 12 or so major myofascial meridians that appear, forming clear lines, or tracks, that traverse the body. A few rules and terminological considerations apply to their construction:

1. **Myofascial continuities must run in straight lines.** Since an Anatomy Train is a line of tensional pull, not compressional push, it must therefore travel in a mostly straight line. So, the first and major rule is that the fibers in adjacent myofascial structures must 'line up' in the fascia, without major changes of direction or depth. While the hamstrings and gluteus maximus might be functionally connected in running or climbing stairs, the change in direction and change of level between the two prevent them from being a fascial continuity. The hamstrings and erector spinae, however, are clearly connected in a mostly straight line via the sacrotuberous ligament.

2. **Fascia is continuous, while muscles are discrete – 'tracks' and 'stations'.** The stripes of muscles and fasciae are termed 'tracks', and what are commonly known as muscle attachments are termed 'stations' to emphasize the continuous nature of the fascial fabric. Muscles themselves may be discrete, but the fascia that contains them is continuous and communicates to the next structure up or down the line. The external oblique muscle and the serratus anterior muscle may be separate and have separate functions, but the sinew that envelops each of them is part of the same fascial plane, which communicates across their attachment points and beyond, in an overall functional continuity called the Spiral Line.

3. **Fascial planes can divide or blend – 'switches' and 'roundhouses'.** Fascial planes sometime split into two planes or, conversely, two planes blend into one. We call these dividing places 'switches', and the physics of the situation will determine which plane takes how much of the force involved. The rhomboids thus communicate fascially with both the serratus anterior and the rotator cuff. Which line is employed will depend on the position, load, and orientation of these and surrounding structures. Places where many muscles meet and provide competitive directions for where a bony structure might be pulled – the ASIS, for instance, or the scapula – are termed 'roundhouses'. See notes on another 'roundhouse' – the LIFT (lumbar interfascial triangle) – in Chapter 1.

4. **Deeper, single-joint muscles hold posture – 'expresses' and 'locals'.** Monoarticular, or one-joint, muscles are termed 'locals', whereas multiarticular muscles are termed 'expresses'. Posture is more often held in the deeper single-joint locals, not in the coordinating expresses that often overlie them. Thus, one looks to relieve a chronically flexed hip via the iliacus or pectineus myofascia, more often than the rectus femoris or sartorius, both of which also cross the knee and are therefore not capable of maintaining an angle in any one joint.

5. **When the rules get bent – 'derailments'.** And finally, we sometimes encounter 'derailments', where the myofascial meridian does not utterly conform to the above rules, but works under particular conditions or positions. For instance, the line of fascia along the back of the body is a continuous string of fascia when the knee is straight, but 'de-links' into two pieces – one above and one below

– when the knee is significantly flexed. This explains why nearly every classic yoga stretch for the Superficial Back Line, as we term it, has the knees in the extended position, and why it is easier to pick up your dropped keys with even slightly flexed knees than with straight legs.

Anatomy Trains lines

Each of these individual myofascial meridians can be viewed as:

1. One-dimensional tensional lines that pass from attachment point to attachment point, from one end to the other
2. Two-dimensional fascial planes that encompass larger areas of superficial fasciae, or
3. Three-dimensional sets of muscles and connective tissues, which taken together comprise the entire volume of the musculoskeletal system.

Superficial Front Line

The Superficial Front Line (SFL – Fig. 3.8) runs on both the right and left sides of the body from the top of the foot to the skull, including the muscles and associated fascia of the anterior compartment of the shin, the quadriceps, the rectus abdominis, sternal fascia, and sternocleidomastoideus muscle up onto the galea aponeurotica of the skull. In terms of muscles and tensional forces, the SFL runs in two pieces – toes to pelvis, and pelvis to head, which function as one piece when the hip is extended, as in standing.

In the SFL, fast-twitch muscle fibers predominate. The SFL functions in movement to flex the trunk and hips, to extend the knee, and to dorsiflex the foot. In standing posture, the SFL flexes the lower neck but hyperextends the upper neck. Posturally, the SFL also maintains knee and ankle extension, protects the soft organs of the ventral cavity, and provides tensile support to lift those parts of the skeleton that extend forward of the gravity line – the pubis, the ribcage, and the face. And, of course, it provides a balance to the pull of the superficial back line.

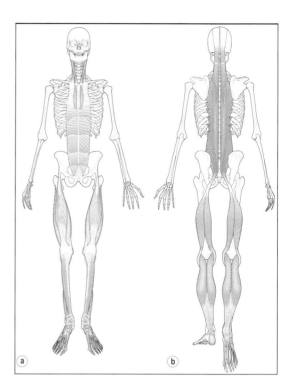

FIGURE 3.8 Two of the Anatomy Trains' myofascial meridians, the Superficial Front Line and Superficial Back Line, counterbalance each other on either side of the skeleton. *Reproduced with the kind permission of Lotus Books.*

A common human response to shock or attack, the startle response, can be seen as a shortening of the SFL. Chronic contraction of this line – so very common after many traumas or childhood – creates many postural pain patterns, pulling the front down, the head forward, and consequently straining the back.

Superficial Back Line

The Superficial Back Line (SBL – Fig 3.8) runs from the bottom of the toes around the heel and up the back of the body, crossing over the head to its terminus at the frontal ridge at the eyebrows. Like the SFL, it also has two pieces, toes to knees and knees to head, which function as one when the knee is extended. It includes the plantar tissues, the triceps surae, the hamstrings and sacrotuberous ligament, lumbosacral fascia, the erector spinae, and the epicranial fascia.

The SBL functions in movement to extend the spine and hips, but also to flex the knee and ankle. The SBL lifts the baby's eyes from primary embryological flexion, progressively lifting the body to standing. In psychomotor terms, dysfunction in the SBL is often linked to difficulties in attaining full maturity.

Posturally, the SBL maintains the body in standing, spanning the series of primary and secondary curves of the skeleton (including the cranium and heel in the catalogue of primary curves, and knee and foot arches in the list of secondary curves). In very basic terms, that primary curves – heel, sacrum, mid-back, and occiput – are designed to align over each other, and the secondary curves – neck, low back, knees, and arches – should align over each other.

Because of its 'all-day' postural function, the SBL is a more densely fascial line than the SFL, with strong fascial bands along its length, and a predominance of slow-twitch fibers in the muscular portion.

Lateral Line

The Lateral Line (LL – Fig. 3.9) traverses each side of the body from the medial and lateral midpoints of the foot around the fibular malleolus and up the lateral aspects of the leg and thigh, passing along the trunk in a woven pattern that extends to the skull's mastoid process.

In movement, the LL creates lateral flexion in the spine, abduction at the hip, and eversion at the foot, and operates as an adjustable 'brake' for lateral and rotational movements of the trunk.

The LL acts posturally like guy-wires of a tent, to balance the left and right sides of the body. In this way, the LL restrains more movement than it creates in the human, maintaining a stable base for the flexion–extension that characterizes our direction through the world, restricting side-to-side movement that would otherwise be energetically wasteful.

Many of our side-to-side asymmetries are held in the LL, so that complementary parts of the LL can maintain the compensation. In the short leg pattern, for instance, the LL will be held short from hip to ankle on the short leg side, but held short hip to shoulder on the contralateral side.

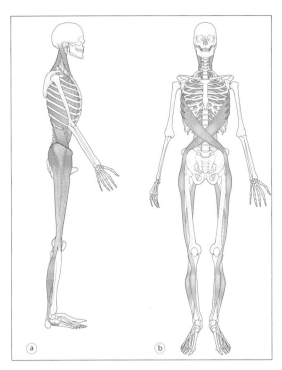

FIGURE 3.9 Lateral and Spiral Line. The Lateral Line runs from the outer arch to the ear up the lateral side of the body and acts primarily to stabilize movement. The Spiral Line acts to create or stabilize rotational and oblique motions. *Reproduced with the kind permission of Lotus Books.*

Spiral Line

The Spiral Line (SL – Fig. 3.9) winds through the three cardinal lines, looping around the trunk in a helix, with another loop in the legs from hip to arch and back again. It joins one side of the skull across the midline of the back to the opposite shoulder, and then returns to the side we started on, running across the front of the torso to the hip, knee, and arch of the foot. The line then returns up the back of the body to the head.

In movement, the SL creates and mediates rotations and oblique movements in the body. The SL interacts with the other cardinal lines in a multiplicity of functions from the watchspring-like rotations of walking to the multiple spirals of a golf swing.

In posture, the SL wraps the torso in a double helix that helps to maintain spinal length and balance in all planes. The SL connects the foot arches with tracking of the knee and pelvic position. The

SL often compensates for deeper rotations in the spine or pelvic core.

Since side bends are almost always accompanied by spinal rotations, any strong side-to-side asymmetries will involve compensation in the SL, and will often look a bit 'wonky' as they move out of these compensatory patterns toward health.

Arm Lines

The four Arm Lines (AL – Fig. 3.10) run from the front and back of the axial torso to the tips of the fingers. They are named for their planar relation in the composition of the shoulder, and they are roughly parallel to the four lines in the leg. These lines connect seamlessly into the other lines, particularly the Lateral, Functional, Spiral, and Superficial Front Lines.

In movement, the AL place the hand in appropriate positions for the tasks before us – examining, manipulating, or responding to the environment. The AL act across 10 or so joint levels in the arm to bring things to us or to push them away; to push, pull, or stabilize our own bodies; or simply to hold some part of the world still for our perusal or modification.

The AL affect posture indirectly, since they are not part of the structural column. Given the weight of the shoulder and arm assembly, however, displacement of the shoulders in posture or

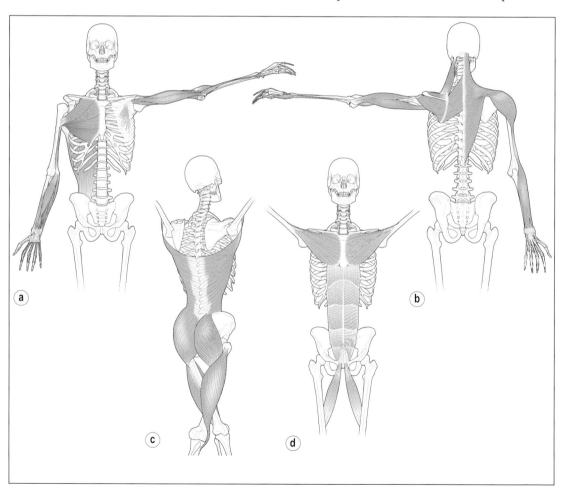

FIGURE 3.10 Arm Lines and Functional Lines. The four Arm Lines go to the four corners of the hands from the axial skeleton. The Functional Lines extend the arm lines to the contralateral hip. Reproduced with the kind permission of Lotus Books.

in a movement strategy will affect other lines. Conversely, structural displacement of the trunk in turn affects the arms' effectiveness in specific tasks and may predispose them to injury.

Functional Lines

The two Functional Lines (FL – Fig. 3.10) join the contralateral girdles across the front and back of the body, running from one humerus to the opposite femur and vice versa.

The FL are used in innumerable active movements, from walking to the most extreme sports. They act to extend the levers of the arms to the opposite leg, as in a kayak paddle, a baseball throw, or a cricket pitch (or leg to opposite shoulder in the case of a football kick). Like the SL, the FL are helical, and thus help create strong rotational movement. Their postural function is minimal; their role in coordinating limb movements to the trunk is invaluable.

Deep Front Line

The Deep Front Line (DFL – Fig. 3.11 and see Plate 5) forms a complex core volume from the inner arch of the foot, up the inseam of the leg, into the pelvis before and behind the hip, and up the front of the spine to the bottom of the skull and the jaw. This 'core' line lies between the Front and Back Lines in the sagittal plane, between the two LL coronally, and is wrapped circumferentially by the Spiral and Functional Lines. This line contains many of the more obscure supporting muscles of our anatomy, and because of its internal position, it has a strong fascial density around the muscular tissue.

Structurally, this line has an intimate connection with the arches, the hip joint, lumbar support, and neck balance. Functionally, it connects the ebb and flow of breathing, dictated by the diaphragm, to the rhythm of walking, organized by the psoas. In the trunk, the DFL is intimately linked with the front of the spine and the autonomic ganglia, and thus uniquely involved in the sympathetic/parasympathetic balance between our neuromotor 'chassis' and the ancient organs of cell-support in the ventral cavity.

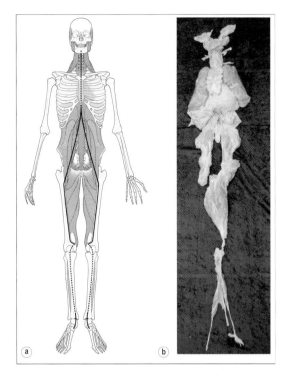

FIGURE 3.11 Deep Front Line. (a) The Deep Front Line forms the body's core, from the inner arch to the inner hip, up around the ventral cavity to the skull. (b) The Deep Front Line dissected as one myofascial meridian (at least for the left leg) including the hyoid and jaw bone as 'sesamoids' within the line.

The importance of the DFL to posture, movement, and attitude cannot be over-emphasized. A dimensional understanding of the DFL is necessary for successful application of nearly any method of manual or movement therapy. Because many of the movement functions of the DFL are redundant to the superficial lines, lack of participation in the DFL can be barely visible in the outset, but these small dysfunctions will gradually lead to larger problems. Restoration of proper DFL functioning is by far the best preventive and treatment-sustaining measure for structural and movement therapies.

BodyReading the lines

In order to describe the anomalies in the lines and the relationships among them, we will use a simple set of four terms that describe skeletal relationships. These readily understandable terms can be used to create a sketch of the generalized body pattern (which is what we will be doing here), but they can also bear the weight of a detailed intersegmental analysis or argument.

Tilt describes simple deviations from vertical or horizontal, in other words, a body part or skeletal element that is higher on one side than on another. We are using this word with its readily understood common meaning.

The term is modified by the direction to which the top of the structure is tilted. Thus:

- In a left side tilt of the shoulder girdle, the client's right acromion would be higher than the left, and the clavicles would lean to the client's left
- A posterior tilt of the rib cage would involve the upper ribs going back relative to the lower
- In a right side tilt of the head, the left ear would be higher than the right, and the planes of the face would tilt to the right
- In a posterior tilt of the head, the eyes would look up, the back of the head approaches the spinous processes of the neck, and the top of the head moves posteriorly.

For clarity in communication and accuracy in translating this language into soft-tissue strategy, it is very important to understand 'relative to what': an 'anterior pelvic tilt relative to the femur' is a useful observation, a simple 'anterior pelvic tilt' opens the door to confusion – to the floor? To the femur? To the rib cage?

Bend is a series of tilts resulting in a curve, usually applied to the spine. The normal lumbar curve thus has a back bend, and the normal thoracic spine a forward bend. If the lumbar spine is side bent, this could be described as a series of tilts between each of the lumbar vertebrae, which we usually summarize as a bend, which can, again, be to either side, forward, or back, and is named for where the top of the bend is pointing relative to the bottom.

Ergo, in the common situation where the hips are tilted to the left, and the lumbars correct that tilt with a bend so that the rib cage can be straight up, those lumbars have a right bend, as the top lumbar points to the right compared to the lower.

Tilts and bends are modified by left, right, anterior, or posterior.

Rotation occurs around a vertical axis in the horizontal plane, and thus often applies to the femur, tibia, pelvis, spine, head, humerus, or rib cage.

Rotation is named for the direction in which the front of the named structure is pointing – right or left. For instance, in a right rotation of the head (relative to the rib cage), the nose or chin would face to the right of the sternum. Notice that, if the rib cage were left rotated relative to the pelvis, the head could be right rotated relative to the rib cage and still be neutral relative to the pelvis or feet. *Thus relativity is very important in assessing postural rotations.*

In paired structures, we use medial or lateral rotation. While this is in common use as regards femoral or humeral rotation, we extend this vocabulary to all structures. What is commonly called a 'protracted' scapula would, in our vocabulary, be a 'laterally shifted and medially rotated' scapula, since the anterior surface of the scapula turns to face the midline.

Shift (translate, shunt) is an additional useful term for displacements (right–left, anterior–posterior, or superior–inferior) of the center of gravity of one structure relative to another. Balinese dance involves a lot of head shifting – side-to-side movement while the eyes stay horizontal. The rib cage of fashion models is commonly shifted posteriorly while staying relatively vertical relative to the ground.

Such shifts, of course, commonly co-occur with tilts, bends, and rotations. We can use the terminology to specify these particular relationships when called for, but using 'left side shifted rib cage' or 'head shifted to the right relative to the pelvis' is a useful shorthand when making an initial evaluation.

The mobile scapula is commonly shifted in any of the six modifying directions. The pelvis is commonly described as being anteriorly or posteriorly shifted relative to the malleoli, with the understanding that some tilts must occur along the way for that to happen.

We may employ these terms and the Anatomy Trains lines to understand global postural patterning. The following examples are designed to demonstrate common postural problems. The reader is advised to see them in terms of fascial patterning and myofascial meridians, and to outline strategies for creating sturdier, self-sustaining structural balance.

Head forward posture and front–back balance

No one is typical but the woman in **Figure 3.12** typifies a very common posture in both the Western and Asian world, and serves as a point of discussion about the fascial fabric relations between the Superficial Back, Superficial Front, and Deep Front Lines.

In terms of the language just outlined, this person demonstrates a number of tilts and shifts:

- The femur is anteriorly tilted relative to the tibia, a common correlate of posteriorly shifted (hyperextended) knees.
- The pelvis is posteriorly tilted relative to the femur.
- The rib cage is posteriorly tilted relative to the pelvis.
- The lower cervicals are anteriorly tilted relative to the rib cage.
- The mid-cervicals have a posterior bend that allows the head to be horizontal.
- The head is anteriorly shifted relative to the upper ribs and shoulders, and the pelvis has shifted forward over the forefeet. The result is that the SBL is acting like a bowstring from shoulder to ankle. (In this case, since the knees are shifted back into hyperextension, the SBL is more accurately short here between T6 and the knee.)
- The tightening of the SBL puts much of the SFL under eccentric strain, which often shows up, naturally enough, in the abdomen/anterior lumbar area. This eccentric loading does not, however, extend to the whole line. The top and bottom portion of the SFL are often both concentrically shortened in this pattern.
- The lowest track of the SFL, the anterior crural compartment of the tibialis anterior and long toe extensors, will be held short and often pinned down the retinacula and tibia along the way. *Freedom and de-adhesion for this compartment is crucial to undoing the pattern above.*

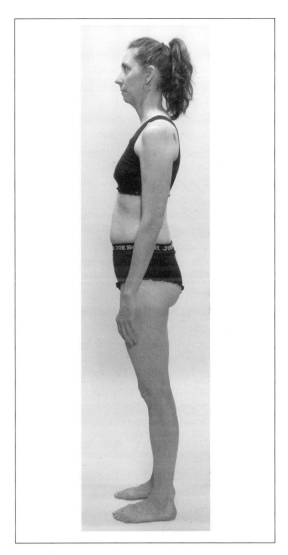

FIGURE 3.12

- At the top, the section of the line from the mastoid process to the mid-sternum is also shortened and will need to be lengthened. Under the general rule of 'lengthen the short before strengthening the weak', toning the abdomen will make no sense and may have either little positive, or an actual negative, effect until 1) the middle part of the SBL is lengthened; and 2) both ends of the SFL are eased.
- In the legs as a whole, we have a very common situation whose solution requires the unique perspective of the fascial fabric. Regardless of

the tonus of the various individual muscles, the superficial, profundis, and myofascial tissue layers all along the front of the leg need to be lifted (allowing them to de-adhere and 'glide' on underlying layers), and the corresponding layers along the back of the leg need to be de-adhered and dropped toward the heel.

- We manual therapists so often think in terms of 'what's short?'. In this case, we need to think about the relationship between these fascial planes, and, by freeing fascial glide among layers, 'redrape the toga' of the myofascia as a whole over the skeleton beneath so that it hangs properly. We have found no other strategy that so reliably and sustainably allows the client to recenter the pelvis over the ankle and (in this case) allow the locked knees to ease.

- The LL will be part of the treatment plan here, where they are pulled down into the mid ribs by the internal intercostals and internal oblique. Because of the hyperextended knees, the lowest track of the LL, the fibulari muscles, will be locked to maintain plantarflexion against the pull of the iliotibial tract above.

- Any of the strategies outlined above will be for naught if the DFL is not also included in the treatment plan. Although obscured by the outer lines in this photo, the adductor section of the DFL will be rotated forward, putting most of the adductor magnus in concentric loading, like the hamstrings, and the anterior adductors into eccentric strain, like the hip flexors.

- Although this woman will likely report her hip flexors as 'tight', the last thing she needs is lengthening in the psoas complex (pectineus, psoas, iliacus). As the mid-SBL eases in the back and the pelvis can ease posteriorly to center over the ankles, she will be able to 'gather' and balance her hip flexors. Central to this change will be an ease in the deep lateral rotators (which in this case are actin g as 'short hip extensors', helping to keep the pelvis simultaneously pushed forward and held into posterior tilt on the femur).

- Once the upper SFL is freed from sternum to mastoid, the final, and essential, part of the DFL that needs to be released runs up the visceral cavity from the diaphragm to about C4. This will definitely involve the anterior scalene and attendant fascia, and possibly the cupola of the lungs as well. In this case, the transversus thoracis and pericardium can be approached with visceral or osteopathic indirect manipulation.

- Unhooking this deep downward pull in the DFL is crucial to correcting the head forward posture and restoring a sturdy and free front–back balance. Despite its centrality, freeing these tissues (in the author's experience) should follow the strategies outlined above for the more superficial lines; it is not advisable to go directly to this primary problem without freeing the outer fascial pieces of the puzzle first.

- Although individuals vary, here are a few common palpation and strategy tips for these pattern-types:
  - In hyperextended knees, palpate all the plantar flexors to see which one(s) are holding the ankle into plantarflexion. Often the fibularii of the LL or the deep posterior compartment (DFL) will be the culprits, although the deeper part of the soleus is involved in the stronger patterns.
  - With the anterior shift/posterior tilt of the pelvis so common in today's 'gym-trained' people, the hip flexors will palpate as very 'tight', but this will be eccentric tension, and will not respond to stretching or manipulation until the 'short hip extensors' (the deep lateral rotators) are functionally lengthened.
  - The lower ribs are held forward and will palpate as sluggish or unmoving in the breath movement. Any number of fascial release, trigger point or facilitated stretching techniques will help their buried ribs to participate in breathing again.
  - Corresponding to the lower ribs, palpate the anterior scalene under the clavicular head of the sternocleidomastoid to find a steel strap linking the lower neck to the upper ribs.

The girl shown in Figure 3.13 presents a similar pattern, so we will point only to the instructive differences.

The SBL bowstring goes all the way from shoulder to ankle here, so the ankle is plantarflexed rather than dorsiflexed under hyperextended knees, as in the previous example. Thus, the tilt that brings the pelvis over the forefoot involves the whole leg. The strategy of 'up the front, down the back,' in terms of tissue relation, still applies. Look at the knee – can you see how the front of the knee tissue is down relative to the tissue behind the knee?

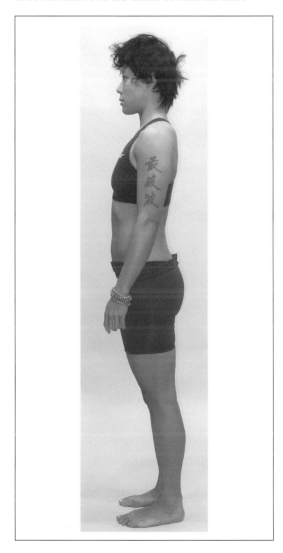

FIGURE 3.13

The pelvis is more anteriorly tilted in this case, and we can imagine that will find a good amount of tension in both the hip flexors (the lower fibers of the psoas) and the hip extensors, the deep lateral rotators, which will show a combination of concentrically and eccentrically loaded tissue in this pattern. The rib cage is not as collapsed onto the pelvis; the 'core' of the DFL is more intact.

This neck does not have such a strong posterior bend, but nevertheless the lower neck is similarly pulled into the upper ribs and chest cavity. The lower ribs are shoved forward to lift the head above the body in what looks to be an 'I am strong' attitude. Opening up the posterior portion of the lower ribs and that portion of the erectors is insufficient to the task, as it will leave her with her head jutting forward in a way that will make no sense to her. The complementary compensation requires opening up the deep front of the neck and first two ribs for the body to find a new stability that 'makes sense' kinesthetically.

The last of our front–back comparisons (Fig. 3.14) presents other variations on this common theme. In this case:

- The anterior tilt that creates the (milder, here) anterior shift of the pelvis occurs in the tibia, creating dorsiflexed ankles but a vertical femur. The knees are flexed, not locked back.
- The pelvis is anteriorly tilted relative to both the femur and the rib cage.
- The rib cage is more posteriorly shifted than tilted. There is a bit of posterior tilt, somewhat disguised by the protraction (medial rotation in the language outlined above) of the scapulae.
- The head forward posture is more evident as exactly that – the center of the head is literally forward of any other gravitational center other than the lower arm.

Strategically, this posture has commonalities with the others, but to add another element that would be of help when we see this 'slumped' pattern: the SL are both slack to allow this pattern. The SLs cross between the shoulder blades in back and across the umbilicus in front. By toning the SLs – boxing or kayaking are both excellent ways to do this – the belly would be brought back and the mid-back and medial scapulae supported for-

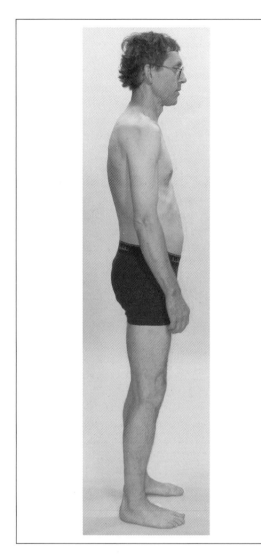

FIGURE 3.14

front or back views. The LL differences will be most obvious, of course, though these are often underpinned by differences in the DFL sandwiched between the two LLs as it is sandwiched sagittally between the SBL and SFL.

The practical reality of human postural compensation is that side-to-side differences most often involve rotations as well, though these are difficult to parse in two-dimensional photographs.

The lady photographed in Figure 3.15 presents some clear differences from right to left. Her right Lateral Line is shorter from hip to lateral arch than its complement on the left. The left LL is shorter between hip and shoulder than the right, and then it switches again in the neck, where the right is shorter. This alternation between upper and lower LLs is a common compensation pattern.

Strategically, lengthening the shorter myofascial lines is a good preparation for training tone in the antagonist eccentrically-loaded portions. As stated, this type of pattern when released in this way will almost certainly reveal some rotations, which we can see in nascent form here: the pubis points to her left, the shoulder girdle comparatively to the right, and the neck around to the left again. The prominent sternocleidomastoid on the left is a giveaway here, required to give head stability when this posture goes into motion.

Her right SL, from the right side of the head around the left shoulder to the right hip, is significantly shorter than its left complement, which is another cue to the involvement of rotations in this apparent side-to-side compensatory pattern.

In this case, the DFL is maintaining its integrity pretty well, despite the multiple compensations going on around it. The core support on the inner line of the leg and up the front of the spine is fairly well intact.

In cases where right–left differences predominate, palpation of both sides to notice differences is essential to precise treatment. In this model, you would find the right splenii and scalenes shorter and denser on her right, the quadratus lumborum shorter on the left, and fascial density differences between the hip abductors on either side.

ward, correcting much of the low-energy stance we see here.

Aside from points mentioned above, palpate the line between the pectoralis major and the rectus abdominis along the 6th and 7th ribs, to find a fascial strap that extends horizontally from slips of the serratus anterior across the front of the chest. Creating 'glide' between the planes of this fascial 'bra line' will be key to adaptive structural change in this client.

Now we turn our attention to right–left differences, which can be most easily seen from the

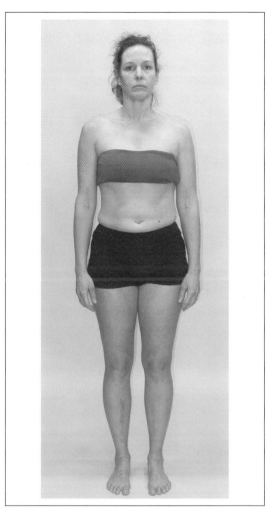

FIGURE 3.15

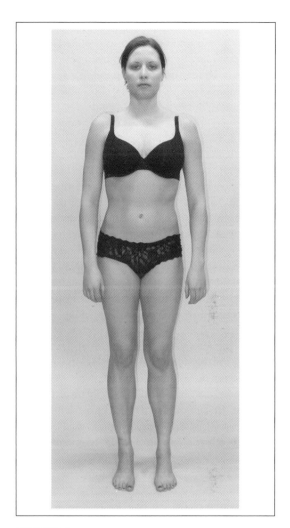

FIGURE 3.16

The trained dancer photographed in Figure 3.16 shows us another common Lateral and Spiral Line pattern. The most evident aspect of this pattern is that the rib cage is shifted to her left relative to the pelvis. To take this measure quickly in practice, measure the horizontal difference between the waist and the greater trochanter. (Using the space between the arms and the body is an unreliable measure.) If it is significantly different on the two sides, as it clearly is here, then look for a lateral shift of the ribs.

In this case, the left upper Spiral Line is shorter than the right, pulling the ribs into a right rotation.

This woman, despite the length in her waist, will have a very complex pattern in the DFL, quadratus lumborum and surrounding thoracolumbar fascia, as well as psoas major, which will present differing challenges on each side. The spine will have a significant two-bend pattern between the sacrum and mid-thoracic region. The head is following the ribs in being shifted to the left, so we can surmise that the neck is less strained than in the previous model.

In this case, however, much of the weight of the upper body falls on the left leg, which is compensated in the lower SL. The right anterior SL in the left leg is pulled or collapsed down into the inner arch, and the corresponding posterior line - the fibularis longus and biceps femoris pulled upward to the sacroiliac joint. The short head of the biceps appears to be maintaining a lateral rotation of the tibia on the femur. Her right leg shows hints of the same pattern but to a much lesser degree.

Although myofascial tonus in this young dancer is likely to be quite even across her body, we could benefit from checking the two sides of the quadratus lumborum and psoas, which will be used quite differently with the lateral rib shift and rotation.

It would also be instructive to palpate the inside and outside of the knee on both sides, to feel how the 'toga' of the fascia profundis (fascia lata above, crural fascia below) is being pulled up on the outside and down on the inside of her left knee, compared to the right.

The gentleman shown in Figure 3.17 presents a different set of challenges. The collapse of the entire upper body into the right arch is very dramatic – perhaps a true anatomical leg-length difference. The inner line of the right leg – the DFL – is pulling from the arch to the groin.

The pelvis, rib cage, and shoulders are all tilted to the right. The neck must perforce have a left bend to retain the eyes and vestibular system on a horizontal plane, albeit shifted to his right compared with the rest of the body. The amount of strain in the left side of the neck must be considerable.

The entire right LL requires a lift, and concomitant lowering of the left LL. The DFL on the right side needs to be lifted and stabilized through the groin. The left SL is shorter than the right, drawing him around into a left thoracic rotation.

- Palpation of the two sides of the neck would be very instructive here, as all the deeper muscles would be arranged quite differently
- The left upper shoulder muscles will palpate as tight and thick, as they are attempting to hold his head on
- Palpation of the hip flexors on both sides would be instructive to see exactly where the hip joint is positioned on both sides.

The young lady illustrated in Figure 3.18 presents an odd pattern, variants of which can nevertheless be seen fairly often. Like the dancer shown in Figure

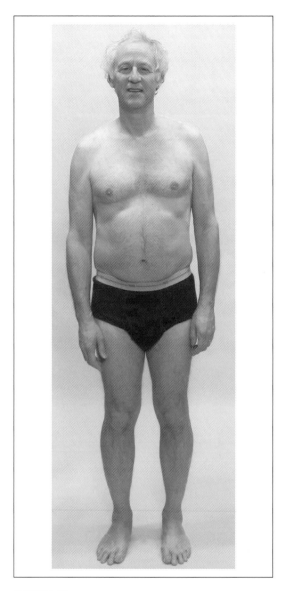

FIGURE 3.17

3.16, we can see the significant left shift of the rib cage as evidenced by the waist-to-trochanter horizontal measurement. The hips and legs themselves have very little compensation (as of yet, she is young).

The rib cage is, however, also tilted to the right, so that the shoulder girdle is tilted to the right along with it. Resist the temptation to fault the shoulder girdle; many people look first at the shoulders and

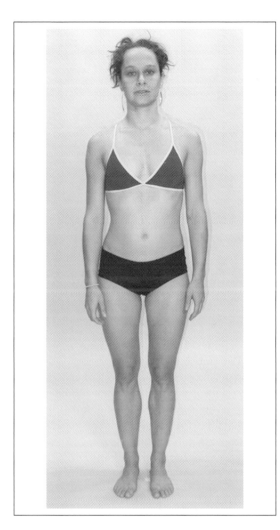

FIGURE 3.18

left side and imagine it doubled over; then do the same with the right. The left side is square, a swimmer's upper body, whereas the right is sloped and less assertive.

Specifically, palpate the LLs and SBLs to feel the fascial tonus differences between the left and right support for the trunk.

Like the last gentleman, this woman will probably have dense, solid upper shoulder muscles on her left but the solution is not to work on those muscles, but on the shortness on her right side. Relieve that shortness and the shoulder muscles will soften of their own accord.

The woman photographed in Figure 3.19, seen from behind, shows the same kind of displacement of the ribs over the hips as seen in Figure 3.18 and in the dancer (Fig. 3.16), this time to the right, using the waist-to-trochanter measure.

For this model, we include a picture from the 'breathing down her neck' perspective; a position we recommend the practitioner observe, as it foreshortens the spine and makes the assessment of spinal rotations easier. Below, there is an obvious rotation to the right between the pelvis and the feet, which we can assess by drawing a line from heel to heel, and comparing it to the line from posterior superior iliac spine (PSIS) to PSIS – clearly a turn to the right. This will be held, in our experience, primarily in the muscles and intermuscular septa of the adductors, with the

start working. The shoulders are not at fault; they are doing the best they can with the rib cage they have to sit on.

Interestingly, both the neck and the head continue the rightward tilt, instead of leveling out like the gentleman in Figure 3.17.

Like the dancer in Figure 3.16, she will have complex tissue disposition on both sides of the lumbar spine – quadratus lumborum and psoas – which will need to be approached differently on each side.

The young woman looks oddly different on her left and right sides in the upper body, despite the symmetry in her lower body. Obscure the upper

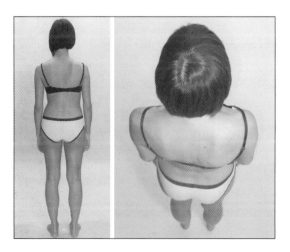

FIGURE 3.19

compartment drawn back on the right and forward on the left.

Note that the two hips, when seen from above, are resting at markedly different states of rotation, with the left hip in lateral rotation and the right in medial rotation. This is not readily discernible in any of the horizontal views, so use this vertical view to assess rotations more easily.

If we compare the line between the two PSISs to the line along the bottom of the scapulae (represented in this photo essentially by the bra line), we can see that there is only a limited amount of additional right rotation between the pelvis and the lower thoracic spine. Above this line, however, the rotation goes to the left, strongly, such that by the top of the ribs the manubrium is essentially facing straight ahead, and only a small additional left rotation is required in the shoulders and neck to face fully forward.

While the right SL is clearly shorter than the left here, it is probably countering a short left psoas complex that is pulling the lumbars forward on the left, and pectineus on the right, which will be pulling the pubis to the right.

The state of the spine in terms of the idiopathic scoliosis is unknown without an X-ray or MRI, so we are limited to this soft-tissue analysis.

- Palpate each psoas to feel a marked difference in fascial tone. Different portions of the psoas will assess short or relaxed in these rotoscoliotic patterns.
- Precise palpation of the spinal muscles is required in every scoliotic pattern, as the soft-tissue patterns are highly individual.

Our final model (Fig. 3.20) demonstrates a common fascial pattern type that is not easily amenable to a myofascial meridian analysis, but is nevertheless commonly seen, useful to notice, and subject to manual correction.

While some of this pattern is similar to models above, the essential characteristic can be expressed as 'cylinders'. The two legs are essentially two cylinders, which can easily be either medially rotated or laterally rotated. Carry that idea up into the trunk, and you can see the two cylinders in the trunk are laterally rotated, while the hips and legs are overall medially rotated. Trouble often occurs

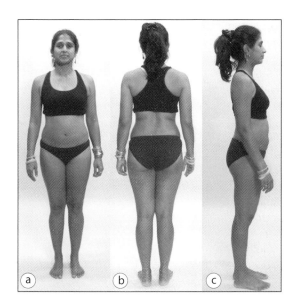

FIGURE 3.20

where cylinders change orientation – in this case around L4 and L5.

If we imagine that this concept of cylinders extended up through the torso to the shoulders, one cylinder on either side of the spine, and further imagine that these cylinders can rotate on each other medially or laterally like the legs, we can arrive at a strategy for the pattern we see here.

Her lower legs are more laterally rotated than her thighs, and the hips follow the medial rotation pattern: she looks narrower in the front across the pubic bone than she does across the ischia at the back of the pelvis. At the lumbar section, however, the situation reverses and the lumbars are narrow at the back and the belly is wide at the front. This pattern of the cylinders – open at the front, closed at the back – continues up her body through the shoulders. (Rarely, and only when the pattern has been strongly held for a long time, this pattern enters the cranium and can be seen or felt in the cranial respiration. Also rarely, and usually only in response to a more extreme trauma or scoliosis, one can find trunk cylinders where one side is rotated medially and the other laterally. This pattern involves significant strain and usually chronic pain in the system.)

Loading this structure significantly with weights or performance stress would not be a good plan. These patterns are especially vulnerable in the place where the medial and lateral rotations interface – in this case at the SI joints or L5-S1. When observed, this pattern calls for fascial opening across the closed parts of the cylinders before attempting a strengthening program.

In this case, this would mean widening the myofascial and fascial tissues along the front of the pelvis, meaning the attachments along the ischiopubic ramus and the pectineus on the iliopectineal ridge. The medial rotators of the hip – the tensor fasciae latae and the anterior gluteus medius and minimus – would also need attention. The deep lateral rotators are most probably 'locked long' in eccentric loading, and would thus require some cross-fiber work to help them reset their tone.

In the lumbars, the cylinders change to a lateral rotation. This takes the lumbars forward, and as the spinous processes move forward they take the fascial planes with them, narrowing the tissue in the back and opening it in the front.

While the widening in the front in the belly will be more amenable to a training-toning-strengthening program, such as Pilates or physical therapy, the tendency of the fascial layers in the back to narrow as the lumbars move forward is best dealt with by strong and specific fascial stretching. Putting the client over a physioball to encourage widening is a good start, but is usually insufficient or requires a great deal of time.

More efficient is a protocol – whether over a ball, seated, or prone with a bolster supporting the belly, in order not to push the lumbars more anterior – of widening the thoracolumbar fascia away from the midline. Because of the number of layers of thoracolumbar fascia and fascially dense erector spinae and multifidus, and the long expanse of this cylinder rotation along her spine, we should not expect this to happen all in one session. Progressive work from layer to layer and section to section is often necessary, along with the educational/homework piece, to effect a sustained change of these ingrained patterns.

- Palpate the anterior adductors – pectineus, brevis, and longus – to find the restraining guy wires that hold the pelvis down.

- Palpate along either side of the lumbar spine about 1" (2 cm) from the midline to find the thick and slick vertical fascial bands running with the erectors and the thoracolumbar fascia. Palpating this tissue will convince you of the necessity for sustained and effective work to change this pattern.

Conclusion

Numerous other examples in clinical application are offered in the book, *Anatomy Trains* (Myers 2014), and its supporting video programs and courses.

Every therapist has seen shoulders drop away from the ears when the feet and legs are worked, low back pain melt away from work in the groin, or a client's breathing open from work on the forearms. The Anatomy Trains map offers one way of understanding and managing these effects in terms of mechanical or energetic communication across our 'sinew channels' of the fascial connections.

Once the relationships within each line are understood, the interactions among the lines open new possibilities for resolving longstanding postural and movement patterns that will not yield to 'single part' attempts to remedy a problem. Progressive work with the lines can create dynamic shifts in these patterns, resulting in the reintroduction of 'poise' – an integral balance and length in body structure.

An additional 'global' assessment protocol, together with a number of local palpation approaches are detailed in Chapter 4 – a companion to the exploration in this chapter of clinical methods of evaluation of fascial function and dysfunction.

References

Berthoz A 2000 The body sense of movement. Harvard University Press, Cambridge, MA

Fuller B 1975 Synergetics. Macmillan, New York, Ch 7

Heartney E 2009 Kenneth Snelson: forces made visible. Hudson Hills, Easthampton, MA

Hyman J, Rodeo SA 2000 Injury and repair of tendons and ligaments. Phys Med Rehabil Clin N Am 11(2):267–268

Juhan D 1987 Job's body. Station Hill Press, Tarrytown, NY

Kjaer M et al 2009 From mechanical loading to collagen synthesis, structural changes and function in human tendon. Scand J Med Sci Sports 19 (4):500–510

Koob A 2009 The root of thought. Pearson Education, Upper Saddle River, NJ

Moore K, Persaud T 1999 The developing human, 6th edn. WB Saunders, London

Myers T 2014 Anatomy Trains, 3rd edn. Churchill Livingstone Elsevier, Edinburgh

Pert C 1997 Molecules of emotion. Scribner, New York

Purslow P 1994 The morphology and mechanical properties of endomysium in series-fibred muscles: variations with muscle length. J Muscle Res Cell Motil 15(3): pp 299–308

Pirschinger A 2007 The extracellular matrix and ground regulation. North Atlantic, Berkeley

Schleip R, Findley T, Chaitow L, Huijing P 2012 Fascia: the tensional network of the human body. Churchill Livingstone Elsevier, Edinburgh

Snyder G 1975 Fasciae: applied anatomy and physiology. Kirksville College of Osteopathy yearbook, Kirksville, MO

Turvey M, Fonseca S 2014 The medium of haptic perception: a tensegrity hypothesis. J Motor Behav 46(3)

Verela F, Frenk S 1987 The organ of form. J Social Biological Structure 10:73–83

Williams PL 1995 Gray's Anatomy, 38th edn. Churchill Livingstone, Edinburgh pp 75, 906

ADDITIONAL GLOBAL AND LOCAL ASSESSMENT APPROACHES

Leon Chaitow

Apart from detailed protocols for both global and local assessment, this chapter contains notes and descriptions that focus on particular skill requirements when seeking to identify fascial (and other) dysfunctional patterns. No skill is more important than being able to identify a safe end-of-range – 'the barrier'– for tissues during either assessment or treatment of dysfunction. Barriers are noted when tissues are extended and also when they are compressed, or moved in different directions – as in twisting, bending, torsional or shear force applications. Identification of barriers is therefore intimately linked to the degree of force/load being applied in any given situation. The barrier topic is also discussed elsewhere, particularly Chapters 13 (Muscle energy technique) and 18 (Scars).

Barriers

The Zink assessment method, described below, requires that the therapist evaluates the directions of preferred rotation of specific junctional regions of the spine. Those evaluations do not seek to identify an end-of-range, merely whether or not rotation is freer (or more restricted) in one direction compared with the other.

However, in many assessment and treatment procedures, end-of-range decisions are required, as tissues are positioned before or during treatment.

Load applied to the body can target superficial, intermediate or deep structures, and clearly varying degrees of compression, stretch etc. will be necessary to achieve the ideal depth, or length. In summary:

- Moving towards the normal physiological end-of-range motion of soft tissues involves a subtle build-up of tension, gradually leading to a recognizable barrier
- If edema, congestion or swelling is causing a reduced range of motion, the end-feel will be 'boggy' and spongy

- If hypertonicity, spasm, or contracture are involved, the end-feel will involve a tight, tugging sensation as the pathological barrier is reached
- If tissues are chronically fibrotic, end-feel will be more rapid and harsh, but with a slight elasticity remaining
- If osseous features are responsible for a reduction in range (arthritis for example), end-feel will be sudden and harsh, without any elasticity
- Where hypermobility is a feature, the end-feel will be loose, with a pliable, unstable, end-of-range
- Pain may lead to a reduced range, with end-feel being noted rapidly as surrounding tissues protect against further movement
- The barrier suggested for most techniques, unless otherwise stated in the guidelines of a particular procedure, are those universally used in MET treatment – the very *'first sign of resistance'* barrier – the *feather-edge* of resistance (see Ch. 13 for more detail).

Defining degrees of pressure

Applied pressure (compression) also engages barriers, with degrees of force potentially graded as light, moderate to firm, firm to deep, and deep (see Ch. 18 for expansion on this theme).

- Pick (2001), discussing palpation assessment pressure, notes that one of three levels might be chosen: 1) touch – quite literally no pressure, merely contact with skin; 2) intermediate, 'working' level, somewhere between touch and a deeper pressure in which the tissues almost 'reject' the contact; and 3) the deep 'rejection' layer – as deep as a palpating contact can go without causing pain.
- In neuromuscular therapy terminology (see Ch. 15) the ideal initial assessment pressure – the same as the 'working' level described above – is described as *'meeting and matching tissue tension'*. This level is variable as it moves through or across tissue, as it comes in contact with denser or more relaxed tissues.
- These palpation levels of compression can turn instantly into treatment approaches, simply by altering the intent from evaluation into one that aims to modify what has been evaluated.

Load/pressure/force can also be defined by descriptors that imply the objective – for example, forces may aim to lengthen, compress, rotate, bend, shear/translate, or combinations of these.

Building on the evaluations of body postures so clearly outlined in Chapter 3, a further consideration looks at a protocol for assessing acquired and inborn fascial compensation patterns, before any exploration of local palpation methods that can be employed in fascial assessment.

Zink and Lawson's Common Compensatory Pattern

In the mid-1970s, osteopathic physicians Zink and Lawson (1979a) examined the structural and functional patterns and characteristics of well over 1000 hospitalized patients, as well as numerous individuals in good health.

Patterns of adaptational changes were identified (see notes on adaptation in Ch. 2), which they termed the Common Compensatory Pattern (CCP). The term was used to describe commonly found patterns of fascial bias – defined as the direction of ease of motion of the superficial and deeper fasciae in particular areas – specifically at transition areas of the spine, where relatively mobile segments meet relatively immobile segments – the atlanto-occipital junction, cervicothoracic junction, thoracolumbar junction, and the lumbosacral junction.

These compensation patterns appear to emerge from a combination of developmentally acquired changes, superimposed on inborn features, resulting in clinically relevant – and identifiable – structural and functional fascial asymmetries (Pope 2003).

It has been suggested that some specific etiological features may involve:

- Asymmetrical position of the fetus in utero during the final trimester (Previc 1991)
- Presentation at birth – with the left occiput anterior (Greenman 1996)
- Postural asymmetries such as anatomical short-leg, small hemipelvis, etc. (Pope 2003)
- Cerebral lateralization – for example leading to right hand and foot dominance
- Traumas and adaptations in early life that accentuate already present features (Zink & Lawson 1979a).

Three broad compensation classifications are described:

1. **Ideal compensation:** Where assessment of rotational preferences at the key junctional sites demonstrate relative balanced and unrestricted ranges of motion. Zink has observed that this 'ideal' pattern is rarely seen in clinical practice (1979b).
2. **Compensated:** Where rotational preferences alternate – seen in approximately 80% of individuals. Suggesting that a good degree of adaptational resilience remains. The commonest pattern, starting at the atlanto-occipital junction, is a left-right-left-right rotational preference (Fig. 4.1a).

3. **Uncompensated:** Where rotational preferences do not alternate, suggesting 'adaptation exhaustion', with a less than optimal ability to compensate. This pattern is the one most likely to be displayed by patients with chronic health and pain issues (Fig. 4.1b).

A logical clinical objective is to restore the uncompensated individual to a more compensated level of functionality so that the musculoskeletal system can more readily tolerate, and adapt to, the stresses and demands of daily life.

Defeo and Hicks (1993) explain: *'Zink and Lawson observed clinically that a significant percentage of the population assumes a consistently predictable postural adaptation, arising from non-specific mechanical forces, such as gravity, gross and micro-trauma, and other physiological stressors. These forces appear to have their greatest impact on the articular facets in the transitional areas of the vertebral column.'*

In their hospital-based study, involving over 1000 patients, Zink and Lawson also observed that approximately 20% of people whose compensatory pattern did not alternate in the CCP manner had poor health histories, low levels of 'wellness' and had poor stress-coping abilities. This observation has been confirmed by more recent clinical evidence, highlighting the potential value of assessing the levels of adaptation present in the physical structures of the body.

As detailed in Chapter 2, Davis et al. (2007) confirmed precisely these myofascial compensation patterns in the most dysfunctional individuals amongst juvenile patient groups with cerebral palsy and recurrent ear infections. They note that *'indicators of fascial and spinal restriction predict an external measure of impairment, manifesting as muscle spasticity.'*

Ascending or descending adaptation patterns (Figs 4.1a & b)

A prominent German osteopath/author, Torsten Liem (2004), has suggested that if the rotational preferences, alternate (L-R-L-R) when supine, and

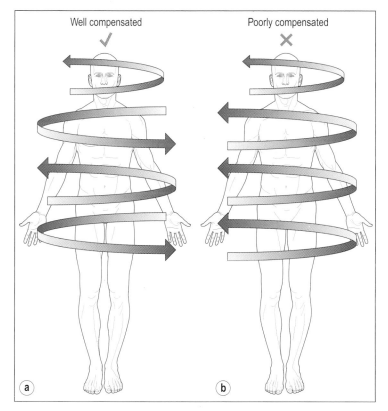

Well compensated ✓   Poorly compensated ✗

a   b

FIGURE 4.1 (a) Appropriate/minimal adaptive compensation – capable of absorbing, adapting to, additional stresses and change. (b) Poorly compensated pattern, reduced adaptive capacity, unlikely to easily accept additional load and change. Please see explanations in the text that explain the background to compensated (a) and poorly compensated (b) patterns of adaptation.

FIGURE 4.2 Palpation of the atlanto-occipital junction.

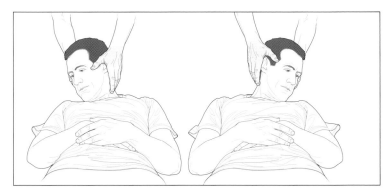

display a greater tendency to not alternate (i.e. they rotate in the same directions – for example, L-L-L-R or L-L-R-L or R-R-R-R, or some other variation on a non-alternating pattern) when standing, a dysfunctional adaptation pattern that is 'ascending' is more likely, i.e. the major dysfunctional influences lie in the lower body, pelvis or lower extremities.

However, if the rotational pattern remains the same when supine and standing, this suggests that the adaptation pattern is primarily 'descending', i.e. the major dysfunctional influences lie in the upper body, cranium or jaw.

Assessment

Zink and Lawson (1979a) described methods for testing tissue preference – rotation and side-flexion – in these transitional levels of the spine where fascial and other tensions and restrictions can most easily be noted. These junctional sites may be tested for rotation and side-flexion preferences, as described below (See Figs 4.2 – 4.5).

Palpation of the atlanto-occipital junction. With the patient supine the therapist is seated or standing at the head of the table. Both hands are used to take the neck into maximal unstressed flexion (to lock the segments below C2) and the rotational preference to an easy end of range – not a forced one, is assessed. Is rotation more free left or right (Fig. 4.2)?

Palpation of the cervicothoracic (CT) area. The patient is supine and the therapist's hands are placed so that they lie, palms upward, be- neath the scapulae. The therapist's forearms and elbows should be in touch with the table surface. Leverage can be introduced by one arm at a time as the therapist's weight is introduced toward the floor, through one elbow, and then the other, easing the patient's scapulae anteriorly. This allows a safe and relatively stress-free assessment to be made of the freedom with which one side, and then the other, moves, producing a rotation at the cervicothoracic junction. Rotational preference can easily be ascertained. Is rotation more free left or right (Fig. 4.3)?

Thoracolumbar (TL) area: the patient is supine or prone. The therapist stands at waist level facing cephalad and places the hands over the lower thoracic structures, fingers along lower rib (7–10) shafts laterally. Treating the structure being palpated as a cylinder, the hands test the preference for the lower thorax to rotate around its central axis, testing one way and then the other. Is rotation more free left or right? The preferred TL rotation direction should be compared with those of OA and CT test results. Alternation in these should be observed if a healthy adaptive process is occurring (See Fig. 4.4).

Lumbosacral (LS) area: the patient is supine. The therapist stands below waist level facing cephalad and places the hands on the anterior pelvic structures, using the contact as a 'steering wheel' to evaluate tissue preference as the pelvis is rotated around its central axis, seeking information as to its 'tightness/looseness' preferences. Is rotation more free left or right? Alternation with previously-assessed preferences should be observed if a healthy adaptive process is occurring (See Fig. 4.5).

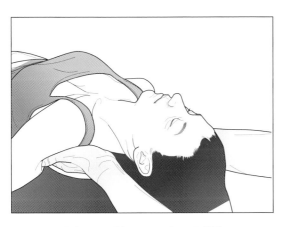

FIGURE 4.3 Palpation of the cervicothoracic (CT) area.

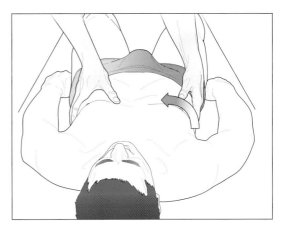

FIGURE 4.4 Palpation of the thoracolumbar (TL) area.

Zink assessment protocol

Restoration of relative symmetry in rotational preferences at these transitional junctions is a legitimate clinical objective, utilizing manual, rehabilitation and exercise methods such as those described in subsequent chapters.

Janda and Lewit's postural patterns

As compensation occurs to overuse, misuse and disuse of muscles of the spine and pelvis, some muscles become overworked, shortened and restricted, with others becoming inhibited and weak, and body-wide postural changes take place that have been characterized as 'crossed syndromes' (Janda 1968, Lewit 1999) (Figs 4.6 & 4.7)

These crossed patterns demonstrate imbalances that occur as antagonists become inhibited due to the overactivity of specific postural muscles. One of the main tasks in rehabilitation is to normalize these imbalances, and while joint and muscular features obviously require attention – underlying fascial restrictions will be a part of that process.

Local signs and features of dysfunction

After evaluating global, whole-body patterns it is necessary to look for as many 'minor' signs and

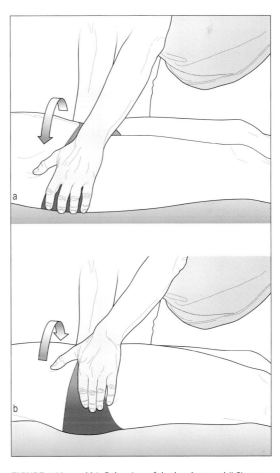

FIGURE 4.5(a and b) Palpation of the lumbosacral (LS) area.

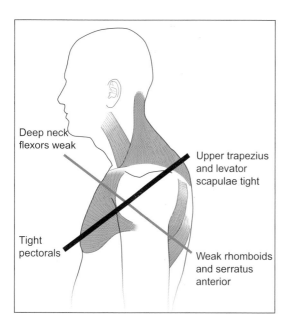

FIGURE 4.6 Upper crossed syndrome. In the upper crossed pattern, we see how the deep neck flexors and the lower fixators of the shoulder (serratus anterior, lower and middle trapezius) have weakened (and possibly lengthened), while their antagonists, the upper trapezius, levator scapula and the pectorals, will have shortened and tightened. Also short and tight are the cervical extensor muscles, the suboccipitals, and the rotator cuff muscles of the shoulder.

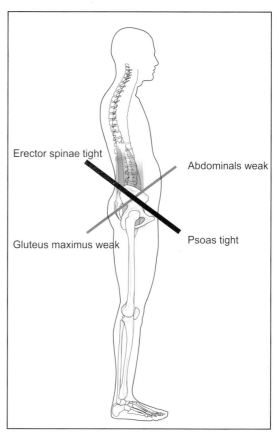

FIGURE 4.7 Lower crossed syndrome. In the lower crossed pattern we see that the abdominal muscles have weakened, as have the gluteals, and at the same time psoas and erector spinae will have shortened and tightened. Also short and tight are tensor fascia lata, piriformis, quadratus lumborum, hamstrings and latissimus dorsi – with the strong likelihood of fascial restrictions as a part of these dysfunctional patterns

features of dysfunction as possible, by observation, palpation and assessment:

- What's short?
- What's tight?
- What's contracted?
- What's restricted?
- What's weak?
- What's out of balance?
- Are firing sequences abnormal?
- What has happened – overuse, misuse, trauma (abuse), disuse – to encourage or maintain dysfunction?
- What is the patient doing, or not doing, that aggravates these changes?
- What can be done to help these changes to normalize?

Our task then is to reduce the adaptive burden that is making demands on the structures of the body, while simultaneously attempting to enhance functional integrity so that the struc-tures and tissues involved can better handle the abuses and misuses to which they are routinely subjected.

Osteopathic STAR palpation

Most practitioners who employ manual means of treatment will have experienced the phenomenon of palpating soft tissues that appear to be more densely indurated, less pliable, than would be anticipated, relative to the age and physical status of the individual.

In osteopathic medicine this experience is clustered, together with several other indicators, to suggest an area of what has been termed 'somatic dysfunction' (Rumney 1979).

Somatic dysfunction is defined as *'impaired or altered function of related components of the somatic (body framework) system: skeletal, arthrodial, and myofascial structures, and related vascular, lymphatic, and neural elements'* Ward et al. 1997).

The osteopathic model of somatic dysfunction, which attempts to make sense of such a finding, has been summarized by the acronym STAR (Dowling 1998). This includes:

- **S** = sensitivity (abnormal tenderness)
- **T** = tissue texture change such as altered tone, laxity etc.
- **A** = asymmetry (malalignment)
- **R** = range of motion and pliability reduction (e.g. contracture).

The STAR designation offers no diagnosis – only an observation that all may not be well in the tissues being evaluated, demanding further investigation as to causal, aggravating and maintaining features – whether local, global or distant.

Other descriptors in the literature for this phenomenon of tissues that have a perceptibly different (from 'normal') feel include terms such as fibrotic (Purslow 2010), densification (Borgini et al. 2010), indurated (Fritz & Grosenbach 1999).

The STAR palpation model, and its constituent elements, has been partially validated by Fryer et al. (2006), and it is widely employed in osteopathic manual assessment.

Investigation of the possible etiological and maintaining features of somatic dysfunction may include any of a wide range of observational and functional tests. These might involve evaluation of painful features, altered motor control, and/or modified 'end feel' qualities, as tissues are taken towards restriction barriers.

More recently, the degree of normal gliding potential between fascial, visceral, and muscular tissue layers has been recognized as a potentially important form of somatic dysfunction.

Lost or reduced fascial glide potential?

Assessment of changes in the sliding/gliding potential of tissues remains a work-in-progress. Clues are available if it is possible to match symptoms with manually assessed tissue changes (see notes on skin assessment, below), as well as objective signs, such as the presence of depressed, retracted or elevated bands or areas – for example, in the cervical region, the border of the scapulae, lower thoracic, pelvic, sacral and gluteal areas.

The developer of connective tissue massage, Dicke (1954), has suggested that when such raised

Exercise

Palpation of activation using research evidence

In their study of myofascial kinematic chains, Weisman et al. (2014) found (with the individual prone) that isometric contraction of gastrocnemius was strongly registered (electronically) at, for example, the ipsilateral hamstrings, posterior superior iliac spine (PSIS), and at the lumbodorsal junction (T12/L1), as well as at both upper trapezius muscles.

They also found that cervical extension (with the individual prone) resulted in strong activation, paraspinally, at T6 and T12 levels, as well as in both upper trapezius muscles – whether there was resistance (i.e. isometric contraction) or no resistance to cervical extension. When resistance was offered to cervical extension there was strong activation at the PSIS and moderate activation at hamstring levels.

As an exercise: palpate the areas indicated as a model reproduces the contraction variables listed. Can you sense – for example – ipsilateral upper trapezius contraction during an isometric gastrocnemius contraction? Do you feel the same degree of activity in someone with low back pain?

or depressed tissue areas are not amenable to being resolved by means of massage, they may represent chronic reflex viscerosomatic activity, involving altered blood supply and lymph drainage, that has led to colloidal changes in the cells and tissues.

Altered vascular skin reactions, tissue sensitivity, tension and density (see skin evaluations below, and STAR palpation above) as well as possible tissue displacement (retracted, elevated etc.), may offer valuable clinical evidence of underlying fascial dysfunction. Observation of posture and functional motion may offer additional opportunities for identification of restrictions existing between fascial layers (Myers 2013) (see Ch. 3).

Skin's sliding function and underlying fascial restriction

Skin lies directly above a layer of fascia – most usually a loose, superficial, areolar layer, on which skin slides freely – and is easily lifted away from the underlying tissues. Sometimes, however, as on the palmer surface of the hand (or the sole of the foot), skin is firmly anchored to dense connective tissue and cannot easily slide, and cannot easily be lifted away from underlying tissues. As Benjamin (2009) notes, *'The palm of the hand and the sole of the foot contain a tough sheet of dense connective tissue that protects underlying vessels and nerves from the pressure associated with grip or body weight. Both are firmly attached to the thick skin overlying them, to limit movement.'*

Compare also the 'slideability' and lifting potential of – for example – the skin on your anterior thigh, compared with your anterior shin where a layer of tightly adherent crural fascia lies between the slideable skin and the bone.

Lewit's hyperalgesic skin zones

Czech physical medicine pioneer, Karel Lewit (1999), suggests that:
- When skin is moved (slid) on underlying tissues, resistance indicates general locality of

reflexogenic activity, a 'hyperalgesic skin zone' (i.e. hypersensitivity) such as a myofascial trigger point
- Local loss of skin elasticity – for example, if skin is gently stretched to its elastic barrier – can refine identification of the location of underlying dysfunction
- A light stroking of the skin, seeking 'drag' sensation (increased hydrosis), may offer pinpoint accuracy of location of dysfunction – fascial or other. *Drag palpation* as well as alternative palpation methods, such as *neuromuscular technique (NMT)* evaluation, are discussed in Chapter 15.

Objective assessment to confirm subjective findings

The global and local assessment methods, as outlined in this chapter – together with those detailed in subsequent chapters – should provide a foundation for assessment of fascial dysfunction. However, what has become apparent in recent years is the need to back subjective with objective assessment and diagnostic methods.

A variety of instruments have been developed that can assist in this – ranging from the relatively inexpensive to the extremely costly. As technology evolves and market forces come into play, prices are likely to come down dramatically – as they have done, for example, in ultrasound imaging equipment.

Imaging and soft tissue changes

In addition to palpation and functional assessment, imaging (utilizing a range of technologies) is being employed to identify objective soft tissue changes – including use of real-time ultrasound, and its color-coded variant, sonoelastography.

Boon et al. (2012) observe that the *'...monographer has the ability to combine sonopalpation (direct pressure with a transducer over structures of interest) and receive real-time feedback from the patient. The ability to palpate and to be able to visualise*

Exercise

Skin assessment and connective tissue massage assessment (see also Ch. 7; Dicke 1954, Bischof & Elmiger 1960)

The normal ability, in most body areas, of skin to slide on underlying superficial fascia can be used as a means of identifying dysfunction – for example, where skin is less elastic, or slides less easily, and contains excessive levels of water ('increased hydrosis').

- The model/patient is seated or lying prone
- Both hands (or fingerpads), using a flat contact, displace the subcutaneous tissues simultaneously against the fascia with small to-and-fro pushes (Figure 4.8)
- The degree of displacement possible will depend upon the tension of the tissues
- It is important that symmetrical areas (i.e. both sides of the body) are examined simultaneously, to identify asymmetrical behavior
- With your fingers lightly flexed and using only enough pressure to produce adherence between the fingerpads and the skin (do not slide on the skin, instead slide the skin on the underlying fascia), make a series of slow, short, deliberate, pushing motions, simultaneously with both hands, which eases the tissues (skin on fascia) towards the elastic barrier on each side
- The pattern of testing should be performed from inferior to superior, either moving the tissues superiorly or bilaterally in an obliquely diagonal direction toward the spine
- Whether your model/patient is prone or seated, tissues from the buttocks to the shoulders may be tested, always comparing the sides for symmetry
- As a palpation exercise, try to identify local areas where your 'push' of skin on connective tissue reveals restriction as compared with its opposite side

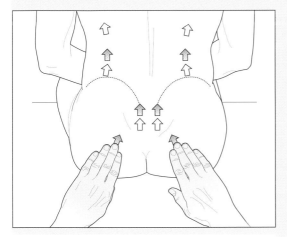

FIGURE 4.8 Skin push. Using a flat contact with both hands (or fingerpads), displace the subcutaneous tissues simultaneously against the fascia with small to-and-fro pushes.

simultaneously – for example during muscle activation – is a unique feature of sonography.'

Such approaches are particularly useful where visualization of scar tissues, or altered tissue-density, is concerned – pre- and post-treatment.

For example, Martínez Rodríguez and Galán del Rio (2013) observe – substantiated by imaging – that myofascial repair processes, following tissue trauma, result in visible (and palpable) connective tissue changes, although in their observation such changes involve fibrosis, rather than densification: 'Fibrosis can be defined as the replacement of the normal struc-tural elements of the tissue by distorted, non-functional and excessive accumulation of fibrotic tissue.'

Imaging caution

Can the way an operator handles an ultrasound transducer (for example) modify the images that result?

While the non-invasive visualization of soft tissue behavior and structure is a compelling clinical and research advance, providing as it does many mechanical attributes and characteristics

Exercise

Different levels of load for glide assessment

- Choose an area of the posterolateral thigh of your model to assess where you can easily move your contact from biceps femoris to the ischial tuberosity, or to the iliotibial band.
- Place fingerpads, or flat of hand (depending on size of area being palpated), on the biceps femoris and take out the slack of the tissue as you apply a light to moderate degree of pressure.
- Slide the skin over the fascia immediately below its surface, feeling for the quality of the easy end-of-range, in different directions.
- Then increase your pressure and test the sliding potential as you try to move the muscle on deeper structures, in different directions. Is movement easier laterally or medially; or moving superiorly or inferiorly? What tissues are involved in this aspect of the exercise?
- Now move your palpating contact to the iliotibial band, and use both light, and slightly deeper pressure, as you again test the directions of glide that are possible under your contact hand, as you move one layer on another. How deeply can you palpate here? How does this differ from when your hand was on biceps femoris?
- Were you able to achieve the same variable levels of compression on these dense fascial structures, as you were on the more muscular biceps femoris?
- Using deeper palpation pressure, perform the same assessment close to where biceps femoris meets the ischial tuberosity. This could be mildly uncomfortable, so move very slowly, as you feel for changes in the tissues, as the muscle nears its attachment site. What lines of force do you feel? What structures can you identify?
- This exercise is designed to assist in discrimination between the glide potential of skin on underlying fascia, and those tissues on underlying muscle, and also on deeper fascial structures; as well as the changes noted as bone is approached.
- By palpating 'normal', as well as dysfunctional tissues, the ability to discriminate between normal glide and restricted glide, and between pliable and fibrotic tissues – as examples, will become easier.

Exercise

Skin lifting ('displacement')

Two different levels of displacement are possible:
- The most superficial displacement occurs between skin and subcutaneous tissues and is easier to observe in children and in old people because the displacement is slight
- The main displacement occurs between the subcutaneous tissue and the fascia

The age of the individual, constitutional state and posture, may all alter findings
- It is easier to displace skin against underlying tissue in slim individuals, with little fatty tissue
- Obese individuals have a higher subcutaneous fat and water content, making displacement more difficult. (See Fig. 4.9.).

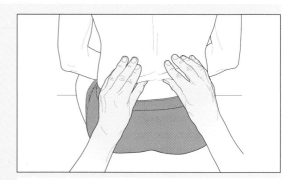

FIGURE 4.9   Skin lift. By lifting and pulling away a skinfold from the fascia, the degree of tissue tension and displacement may be determined.

Compare your findings using this method with those identified by 'skin on fascia pushes' - as described above.

Exercise

Palpation of the superficial fascia of the sacrum

Use the skin palpations described above – or NMT palpation methods described in Chapter 15 – to carry out assessment of the tissues described by Hammer (1999), who suggests that: *'Palpation of the fascia over the sacrum where the superficial and deep TLF fuses often reveals tenderness and restrictions in particular directions which require [appropriate] fascial release to allow the normal transfer of load from, for example, the right lower extremity to the left latissimus dorsi. Any portion of the load transfer mechanism may require a fascial release. In the lumbar region, the deep TLF should be more freely mobile over the back muscles. Palpation may [also] reveal hardening and thickening of this tissue, which would require a [appropriate] fascial release. The deep TLF fuses with the fibers of the serratus posterior inferior muscle, which often requires a release.'*

See Chapter 1, Figure 1.5 for detail of this region.

of both normal and pathological tissues, a caution is required, as the element of operator-bias needs to be highlighted (Konofagou et al. 2003).

Since the operator manually controls the transducer, variations in the compressive pressure, orientation or direction of the ultrasound transducer can all potentially modify the resulting echo-signal images (Drakonaki et al. 2009). However, as new more automated imaging methods evolve, the subjective nature of currently utilized approaches should reduce the risk of inadvertent bias.

Chapter 5 summarizes the evidence regarding manual, instrument assisted and exercise methods that have been shown to influence fascial behaviour clinically.

References

Benjamin M 2009 The fascia of the limbs and back – a review. J Anat 214:1–18

Bischof I, Elmiger G 1960 Connective tissue massage. In: Licht S (ed) Massage, manipulation and traction. Licht, New Haven, CT

Boon AJ, Smith J, Harper CM 2012 Ultrasound applications in electrodiagnosis. PMR 4(1):37-49

Borgini E, Antonio S, Julie Ann D, Stecco C 2010 How much time is required to modify a fascial fibrosis? J Bodyw Mov Ther 14: 318-325

Davis M et al 2007 Confirmatory factor analysis in osteopathic medicine: fascial and spinal motion restrictions as correlates of muscle spasticity in children with cerebral palsy. JAOA 107(6):226-232

Defeo G, Hicks L 1993 A description of the common compensatory pattern in relationship to the osteopathic postural examination. Dynamic Chiropractic 24:11

Dicke E 1954 Meine Bindegewebsmassage. Hippokrates, Stuttgart

Dowling D 1998 S.T.A.R.: a more viable alternative descriptor system of somatic dysfunction. American Academy of Applied Osteopathy Journal 8(2):34–37

Drakonaki EE, Allen GM, Wilson DJ 2009 Real-time ultrasound elastography of the normal Achilles tendon: reproducibility and pattern description. Clin Radiol 64:1196-202

Fritz S, Grosenbach J 1999 Mosby's basic science for soft tissue and movement therapies. Mosby, St Louis

Fryer G, Morris T, Gibbons P et al 2006 The electromyographic activity of thoracic paraspinal muscles identified as abnormal with palpation. J Manipulative Physiol Ther 29(6):437–447

Greenman P 1996 Principles of manual medicine. Williams & Wilkins, Baltimore pp 545-546

Hammer W 1999 Thoracolumbar fascia and back pain. Dynamic Chiropractic 17(16):1-3

Janda V 1968 Postural and phasic muscles in the pathogenesis of low back pain. In: Proceedings of the XIth Congress International Society of Rehabilitation and Disability, Dublin, Ireland, 553–554

Konofagou E, Ophir J, Krouskop TA, Garra BS 2003 Elastography: from theory to clinical applications. Presented at Summer Bioengineering conference, Key Biscayne, FL, June 25-29

Lewit K 1999 Manipulative therapy in rehabilitation of the locomotor system, 3rd edn. Butterworths, London

Liem T 2004 Cranial osteopathy: principles and practice. Churchill Livingstone, Edinburgh, pp 340-342

Martínez Rodríguez R, Galán del Río F 2013 Mechanistic basis of manual therapy in myofascial injuries. Sonoelastographic evolution control. J Bodyw Mov Ther 17(2):221-234

Mosby's Medical Dictionary 2012 9th edn, Elsevier, St Louis

Myers T 2013 Anatomy Trains, 3rd edn. Churchill Livingstone Elsevier, Edinburgh

Pick M 2001 (October) Presentation 'Beyond the neuron'. Integrative bodywork – towards unifying principles. Conference, JBMT/University of Westminster, London

Pope R 2003 The common compensatory pattern. American Academy of Applied Osteopathy (AAO) Journal Winter pp 59-83

Previc F 1991 General theory concerning prenatal origins of cerebral lateralization in humans. Psychol Rev 98(3):299-334

Purslow P 2010 Muscle fascia and force transmission. J Bodyw Mov Ther14 (X):411-417

Rumney IC 1979 The history of the developmental term 'somatic dysfunction'. Osteopath Ann 7(1):26–30

Ward RC 1997 Foundations for osteopathic medicine. Williams & Wilkins, Baltimore

Weisman M et al 2014 Surface electromyographic recordings after passive and active motion along the posterior myofascial kinematic chain in healthy male subjects. J Bodyw Mov Ther; in press

Zink JG, Lawson WB 1979a An osteopathic structural examination and functional interpretation of the soma. Osteopath Ann 7(12):433-440

Zink JG, Lawson WB 1979b Pressure gradients in osteopathic manipulative management of the obstetric patient. Osteopath Ann 7(5):42-49

REMOVING OBSTACLES TO RECOVERY: THERAPEUTIC MECHANISMS AND FASCIA

Leon Chaitow

While evidence is essential when evaluating clinical methods, experience-based opinion is often useful to set the scene – to describe objectives, and to offer a perspective.

Ida Rolf (1977) has offered us her informed opinion regarding where therapeutic attention should be focused, in relation to fascia: *'Our ignorance of the role and significance of fascia is profound. Therefore even in theory it is easy to overlook the possibility that far-reaching changes may be made not only in structural contour, but also in functional manifestation, through better organisation of the layer of superficial fascia which enwraps the body. Experiments demonstrate that beneficial changes may be made in the body, solely by stretching, separating and relaxing superficial fascia in an appropriate manner.'*

The question that arises from this statement – what therapeutic methods are appropriate? Hopefully some (many?) of the answers are provided in this chapter, where you will find summaries of what is currently known about methods and mechanisms that can modify fascial dysfunction. Most notably there is evaluation of methods of load application – compression, stretching, shear force, oscillation etc. – that have been shown to be, or are thought to be, effective in particular settings, based on clinical experience as well as published reports and studies?

General objectives of therapeutic intervention

The model of care emphasized in this text recognizes that to be optimally successful, therapeutic interventions need to focus on achieving one, or all, of the following:

- Enhancement of function, so that the person, system or part, can better adapt and self-regulate in response to the multiple biochemical, psychosocial and biomechanical adaptive demands of life ('stressors')
- Modification *or removal* of adaptive load factors – overuse, misuse, disuse etc. (see adaptation discussions in Ch. 2) that are resulting in, or are maintaining, symptom-producing compensatory changes

- Symptomatic relief, without imposition of unmanageable additional adaptive demands.

Specific fascia-related therapeutic objectives

Within the framework of general objectives, outlined above, lie numerous more specific aims, such as:

- Pain modification – working with fascia, muscles, joints, the nervous system and the brain
- Working with (not against) healthy inflammatory processes; and safely modulating excessive degrees of inflammation
- Restoring function, such as normal fascial gliding/sliding potential, where this has been compromised

- Enhancing kinematic myofascial function, so that distant connections respond to load-transfer (as in the Weisman et al. study (2014) reported in Ch. 1), where gastrocnemius activation is recorded in the ipsilateral upper trapezius muscle
- Restoring normal ranges of joint and muscular motion
- Enhancing resilience, elasticity, mobility and stability
- Preventing and reducing fibrosis, densification, excessive stiffness – possibly including use of controlled micro-trauma and initiation of an inflammatory response – for example, in treatment of chronic fibrosis, so that subsequent remodeling results in more functional tissue behavior (see notes on eccentric stretching later in this chapter, and in Ch. 13)
- Enhancing wound healing and remodeling – post-trauma and post-surgery
- Prevention of post-surgical adhesions
- Improving posture and function (e.g. breathing) via recognition and clinical employment of the links, chains, trains of fascial connections
- ...and undoubtedly more.

Direct or indirect: two possible intervention models

Tozzi (2012) has offered a useful osteopathic definition of the two broad models of soft tissue therapeutic intervention relating to fascial restrictions: direct and indirect – see Box 5.1.

Glimpses of the potential: study of hysteresis

One way to evaluate the potential for manual treatment methods that may influence fascial behavior is to measure the degree of 'tissue stiffness' before and after application of a controlled degree of therapeutic load (stretch, compression etc.). As outlined in Chapter 1, any change – whether an increase or a reduction – in stiffness in tissues following treatment or activity, involves hysteresis.

Barnes et al. (2013) conducted a study to measure hysteresis (fascial stiffness modification) in response to different manual methods. The osteopathic researchers adopted the following protocol:

1. Areas of cervical articular somatic dysfunction (SD) were identified in 240 subjects using carefully controlled palpation assessment

---

Box 5.1
Direct and indirect approaches defined

According to Tozzi (2012):

1. '*Direct Approach to Fascia: requires tissue restrictions to be engaged and maintained until release is gained. Occasionally, as the affected tissue is brought against the functional barrier, a tridimensional compression or traction is applied and held (generally for 60–90 seconds) until tensions melt (Pilat 2011). When the first barrier is released, the procedure is repeated for consecutive barriers, adjusting the compressional force according to each barrier's vectors, up to a point when a release is felt. Pressure is reduced when there is any increase in pain. This is variously known as* myofascial release, or myofascial induction [see Ch. 14].'

2. '*Indirect Approach to Fascia: requires the exaggeration of the pattern of dysfunctional tissues, bringing the restricted fascial tissue into its position of 'ease' (balanced tension), maintaining it until tensional forces relax (Ward 2003).*'

3. A further definition of **indirect methodology** involves disengagement from restriction barriers, allowing self-regulating influences to operate, resulting in a sense of change, or 'release'.

These models will be recognized as various clinical approaches are described in this chapter and throughout the rest of the book.

methods – involving the STAR palpation protocol – as described in Chapter 4. Tissue stiffness was measured prior to treatment (or sham treatment) using an instrument designed for that purpose – a durometer.

2. Four different techniques – balanced ligamentous tension (Ch. 10); muscle energy technique (Ch. 13); high velocity manipulation; strain–counterstrain (Ch. 16); and a sham technique – were randomly applied in a single application to the most severe area of identified somatic dysfunction, after which (10 minutes post-treatment) the 'changes in tissue stiffness' (i.e. hysteresis) was re-measured by a durometer.

3. The durometer measurement of the myofascial structures overlying each cervical segment (pre- and post- intervention) used a single consistent piezoelectric impulse. This quantified four different characteristics – fixation, mobility, frequency and motoricity (described as *'the overall degree of change of a segment'*) – including 'resistance' and range of motion.

4. When baseline – pre-treatment – and post-treatment findings were compared for all restricted (dysfunctional) segments, the results showed that strain–counterstrain (Ch. 16) produced the greatest changes in overall tissue stiffness, as compared with the other methods used, and with sham treatments.

The results of this study suggest that the behavior of myofascial tissues can be rapidly modified (becoming 'less stiff') using *any of the four methods tested – with the greatest effect (albeit short term as the study did not follow-up beyond the study term) being observed following strain–counterstrain.*

As in the study reported above, this book presents, as far as is possible, evidence-informed information. Some of that evidence derives from current interpretation of basic science research, while other evidence is based on clinical experience – and as such, this is clearly stated. See Box 5.2 for a brief discussion of 'what is evidence?'

Box 5.2

What is 'evidence'?

- The expression that *'lack of evidence of benefit is not the same as evidence of lack of benefit'* should be kept in mind
- Above all it is important to recognize that both safety and efficacy are the criteria for selection of any particular therapeutic modality, in any given situation, and that appropriate selection represents both an art and a science.
- Sackett (1996) provided the basic formula that has led to what is known as *'evidence based medicine' –'best practice.'*
- The suggested hierarchy of evidence is listed below, and while systematic reviews of randomized clinical trials may be seen as the best way of establishing both efficacy and safety for any procedure – it is not the only way that evidence can be developed.
- Value is also found in expert opinion based on clinical experience, even if there have been no research trials – as long as there is

no actual evidence of risk or of there being 'no value.'

The evidence hierarchy:

1. Systematic reviews and meta-analyses
2. Randomized controlled trials
3. Cohort studies
4. Case-control studies
5. Cross-sectional studies
6. Case reports
7. Expert opinion
8. Anecdotal.

- Clinical trials are expensive, and many of the methods used in manual therapy have simply not been studied in large-scale research programs. The fact that there is no research-based evidence of usefulness is therefore not evidence that a method is useless – only that no research has yet been carried out to show its value (or lack of value).
- Some assessment and treatment methods, techniques, and concepts are strongly

evidence-based, in that studies have demonstrated their efficacy and safety – when appropriately applied by suitably trained practitioners, in appropriate clinical settings.

- Other assessment and treatment methods, techniques and concepts may have been found to be safe and clinically useful – by individuals or professions. However, these clinical opinions and experiences may have not been validated by research. Any of the methods described in this book that fall into this 'clinically useful but unproven' category will have another important characteristic: they will **not** have been shown to be either unsafe, or ineffective, by research.
- In some instances peer-review literature will have carried reports of cases (case reports, case studies, case-series etc.) where particular methods have been used that have

apparently led to individuals or conditions deriving benefit. If, in addition, there have been no studies that demonstrate potential harm from use of such method – it is safe to say that clinical experience suggests that this is a safe and potentially effective approach.

- In some cases translational evidence may have been used to suggest – *not prove* – the potential value of a particular method. An example of this is the basic science evidence that when cells, such as myofibroblasts, are treated in a certain way, their behavior changes. For example, modeled myofascial release (Ch.14) – or counterstrain (Ch. 16) – have been shown in laboratory settings to modify inflammation (Standley & Meltzer 2008). This may be translated to *suggest* – not *prove* – that these methods might have similar effects when used in treatment settings.

Fascia's potential to reorganize itself

Tozzi (2012) has observed that: *'studies suggest that fascia reorganises itself along the lines of tension imposed or expressed in the body, and in ways that may cause repercussions of fascial restriction that are body-wide. This may potentially create stress on any structures enveloped by fascia itself, with consequent mechanical and physiological effects.'*

Thus the major focus of this chapter is on evaluating proposed and established mechanisms in relation to treatment of fascial dysfunction. If details or discussions of such mechanisms are contained elsewhere in the book, cross-references are given to the appropriate chapter.

Various theoretical models are also discussed, allowing suggestions for deductions, hypotheses and assumptions. A number of modalities and techniques that are not explored in detail in subsequent chapters also receive attention.

Explanations of clinical effects

The wide range of clinical approaches to soft tissue dysfunction in general, and fascial dysfunction in particular, demands explanations for their apparent effects – based on evidence or plausible theory.

Box 5.3 summarizes current selected evidence and opinion.

Box 5.3

Clinical effects and possible mechanisms of manual therapies on fascia: evidence and theory

Neural

Changes in neural input, when dysfunctional tissues are appropriately loaded or unloaded, will influence local receptors (muscle spindles, tendon organs, and others – see Box 1.3), as well as central processes, potentially modifying pain and sympathetic effects (Standley & Meltzer 2008).

Box 5.3 (Continued)

Autonomic effects

Kuchera (2007) has highlighted the potential for manual approaches to modulate sympathetic tone ('hypersympathetonia'), and in so doing to enhance autonomic balance, resulting in processes that would potentially reduce fascial stiffness.

Cellular changes

Mechanotransduction effects (see Ch. 1), described by Harris (Beloussov 2006) as *'geometric homeostasis,'* result from changes in cell shape in response to alterations in load (increased or reduced), with potentially beneficial effects on inflammatory and other processes (Kumka & Bonar 2012).

Collagen deposition

Modified by compression, friction and shear force application (Pohl 2010) – altering superficial fascial density and function (see Ch. 1).

Circulatory changes

Tissue repair following surgery or trauma depends, among other things, on fibroblasts differentiating into myofibroblasts and the production of collagen, as well as appropriate levels of inflammation and tissue repair; all of which processes are more optimal when fluid flow (blood, nutrients and lymph, supply and drainage) is encouraged, as it is following many forms of manual therapy (Hinz et al. 2004, Bhattacharya et al. 2005).

Altered viscosity, stiffness and lubrication

Frictional, vibratory, tangential shear-force and similar forms of load application influence hyaluronic acid production and modify the intercellular matrix tissues – ground substance – from a gel-like state to a more solute one, with consequent palpable softening effects, potentially even on deeper dense fascial layers (Luomala et al. 2014).

Endocannabinoid upregulation

McPartland (2008) has gathered evidence of increased levels of the pain-relieving, euphoria-inducing endocannabinoids in response to many forms of manual therapy – as well as to exercise and acupuncture. Cannabinoids, such as anandamide and N-palmitoylethanolamine, have an effect on fibroblast remodeling, inflammation and pain, possibly accounting for the anecdotal benefits described in many post-manual therapy reports. McPartland points out that: *'The endocannabinoid system alters fibroblast "focal adhesions," by which fibroblasts link the extracellular collagen matrix to their intracellular cytoskeleton—the mechanism of fascial remodeling. Cannabinoids prevent cartilage destruction such as proteoglycan degradation and collagen breakdown.'*

Altered acid–base balance

Nutrition and physiological features, such as the breathing pattern and various pathologies, can modify acid–base balance, commonly represented as the pH of tissues or the blood. See Box 2.1 for more on the fascia-breathing connection. Breathing pattern disorders (BPD) can have far-ranging physiological effects due to depletion of CO_2 and elevated pH, resulting in acute or chronic respiratory alkalosis (Kellum 2007). Alkalosis induces vascular constriction, decreased blood flow, and inhibition of O_2 transfer from hemoglobin to tissue cells (Bohr effect; Jensen 2005). Resulting ischemia may be seen as a precursor to myofascial pain evolution. In addition alkalosis/increased pH is likely to influence early wound repair because it leads to oxygen deficits that severely inhibit collagen synthesis, retarding wound healing (Jensen et al. 2008).

> **Key Point**
>
> Manual and rehabilitation methods profoundly influence multiple aspects of fascial function, from the cellular to the neural, circulatory and biochemical. Attention to breathing patterns can be seen to be of clinical relevance in managing fascial dysfunction.

Therapeutic load

The different ways in which load is applied to the body include:

1. **Pressure/compression** light to moderate, superficial – slow or rapid or oscillating: as used in Bowen therapy (Ch. 6), neuromuscular techniques (NMT; Ch. 15), Rolfing® (Ch. 17), scar tissue release (Ch. 18), massage (Ch. 19), trigger point release (Ch. 20)
2. **Pressure/compression** heavy and/or deep; slow or rapid or oscillating – as used in Fascial Manipulation® (Ch. 9), scar release (Ch. 18), deep tissue massage (Ch. 19), trigger point release (Ch. 20)
3. **Stretching following isometric contraction** – active or passive: as used in muscle energy technique (MET; Ch. 13)
4. **Stretching during contraction (isotonically)** – active or passive: as used in slow eccentric isotonic stretching (SEIS) and isolytic stretching – MET (Ch. 13)
5. **Isometric contractions** – sustained or rhythmically pulsed: as used in MET (Ch. 13)
6. **Shear force:** as used in connective tissue manipulation (Ch. 7), myofascial release (Ch. 14), scar release (Ch. 18), massage (Ch. 19)
7. **Compound movements** (e.g. bending, twisting, pressure and/or vibration): as used in NMT (Ch. 15), Rolfing (Ch. 17), scar release (Ch. 18), massage (Ch. 19)
8. **High velocity manipulation:** discussed in Chapter 2 (in relation to zygapophyseal adhesions), and also in this chapter
9. **Unloading (indirect) methods:** such as fascial unwinding (Ch. 10), balanced ligamentous tension (Ch. 11), positional techniques – including counterstrain (Ch. 16)
10. **Percussive, vibratory, frictional, oscillating methods:** as used in Graston Technique® (Ch. 12), NMT (Ch. 15), Rolfing/Structural Integration (Ch. 17), scar release (Ch. 18), massage (Ch. 19)
11. **Mechanical or instrument assisted methods:** as used in Graston, Gua sha (Ch. 12) acupuncture/dry needling (Ch. 20), foam rolling, which is discussed later in this chapter
12. Note on **Exercise:** this topic is not covered in this chapter but is fully explored in Chapter 8.

The subjects listed above will be mentioned when there is evidence of their potential therapeutic usefulness in relation to conditions, or methods, highlighted in this chapter.

Effects of digital compression (load) applied to soft tissues

It is worth reflecting that when load is applied:

1. Some superficial tissues will lengthen automatically, while a simultaneous compression/crowding of adjacent tissues will occur, together with possibly unappreciated levels of additional load being transmitted tangentially, via fascial septa and other attachments.
2. Circulation will be affected, creating temporarily increased local ischemia, but this will reverse when compression is released – a flushing/pumping process.
3. Cells are influenced via mechanotransduction (see Ch. 1), for example, modifying the behavior of myofibroblasts to potentially reduce inflammatory reactions (Standley et al. 2007, Standley 2008).
4. Local mechanical lengthening of tissues will occur – depending on the degree and directions of load applied.
5. Water extrudes – in a sponge-like manner – making the tissues more pliable for a period up to 30 min (Klingler et al. 2004).
6. A variety of neurological effects occur – either inhibitory or stimulatory – depending on the degree, amplitude, speed, rhythm, direction(s) and duration of force application (Schleip et al. 2003).

A list of neural receptors and their functions is given later in this chapter.

7. As Schleip (2003) has observed in relation to light pressure affecting Ruffini corpuscles, *'applying a slow, extended stretch to the skin can create desirable changes both locally and centrally, decreasing tension in the area where the hands are applied, as well as creating an overall sense of relaxation ... [these] corpuscles respond to lateral skin stretch ... Tangentially, or along the same plane as the tissue below.'*

8. The previous point reminds us that sensations resulting from therapeutic pressure or stroking impact on the brain (cortical body) and may modify the individual's perceptions. Moseley et al. (2012) have proposed the concept of a *cortical body matrix,* a virtual map in the brain. This is conceived as a dynamic neural representation that – among other things – integrates sensory data with homeostatic and motor functions. How therapeutic load, whether compression, manual strokes or stretching, relates to this matrix may be significant therapeutically. Schleip (personal correspondence 2013) notes – in relation to manual treatment – that: *a "gestural" effect (e.g. light strokes in a particular direction on a limb) probably involves short term changes in the cortical body schema, and it can be beautifully tailored towards the specific needs of each client.'*

9. Blyum and Driscoll (2012) demonstrate something that may seem to be counter-intuitive; that is, following application of manual pressure ('stress transfer') outcomes are more significant – *if the load is 'softly' applied.* The results of such loading of tissues on neural influences (see below) may lead to soft-tissue relaxation and/or pain relief. As explained in Chapter 1, these effects are at least partially due to mechanotransduction – the translation of mechanical energy into biochemical and neurological responses – that may also encourage remodeling of the tissues involved. Blyum and Driscoll have shown that when a soft (for example weak/soft foam) is used to apply load to the skin, epidermis and superficial connective tissues, this is more effective in 'stress transfer' than when a more dense foam, or harder material, is used to apply load to tissues. The notes on colloidal behavior in Chapter 1 may offer a partial explanation for this. However, this same trend was not noted in deeper (muscle) tissues. An interpretation of these findings supports a well-known clinical observation (see Myers' quote below), suggesting that slow, gentle 'meeting and matching of tissue tension' is more effective than heavier strategies in achieving beneficial changes in superficial structures, as well as potentially obtaining pain-free access to deeper tissues.

10. Myers observes (personal communication): *'In general, less deformation occurs in connective tissue that is loaded more quickly than the same tissue loaded at a slower rate, suggesting that a slower stretch will be more effective in tissue lengthening than one that is rapidly applied.'*

11. Shear force compression and oscillation influence hyaluronic acid production and behavior, affecting local sliding function (Roman et al. 2013) as well as modifying collagen status. Pohl (2010) shows that shear-force applications – as in skin rolling (see Ch. 7) – leads to *'highly significant differences in the structure of the collagen matrix in the dermis before and after treatment. These changes reflect the differences in tension, softness and regularity, which can be palpated before and after treatment and are thought to be caused by changes in the mechanical forces of fibroblasts and increased microcirculation.'*

12. Sustained combinations of compressive force involving different vectors – for example, pressure, torsion, shear – that engage tension against restriction barriers, deep in soft tissues (adhesions, fibrosis, scarring) have been shown in elastography images to result in relative structural and functional normalization (Martinez Rodriguez et al. 2013, Borgini et al. 2010).

> **Key Point**
>
> Compressive load – either with or without vibration/oscillation or additional stretching – has variable mechanical, proprioceptive and other neurological effects (depending on degree, direction, duration etc. of load); as well as hydraulic and circulatory effects, together with enhanced lubrication (sliding function – a topic that is discussed more thoroughly later in the chapter).
>
> Also significant is the suggestion that lighter contacts may be more effective than heavier ones in many instances, if the objective is to influence superficial mechanoreceptors and to avoid defensive tissue responses. It is possible to increase the depth of digital penetration over time via slow moving, steadily sustained, pressure.

Potential range of load application variables

As noted above, different types, degrees, and durations of load all may have profoundly different effects – hence the need for accurate descriptions of treatment modalities, protocols and methods:

- How firmly should load be applied?
- On how large a surface area?
- Affecting which structures?
- In which direction(s) – i.e. using which vectors?
- Engaging, exaggerating, or disengaging from restriction barriers? (See Box 5.1)
- To what degree/distance (amplitude)?
- At what velocity – slow, medium, high?
- Passive or active or mixed?
- Sustained or variable?
- Static or moving?
- For how long?
- Repeated?

...and possibly other variables, depending on circumstances. See Chapter 19 for additional discussion.

Question: how do these multiple load variations influence mechano- and other neural receptors in the superficial and deeper fascial (and other) tissues?

Fortunately, at least partial explanations are available:

- Schleip (2003) has noted in his extensive fascial research that there are a wide range of proprioceptors – embedded in the extracellular matrix (ECM), that respond variously to stretch, pressure, vibration and shear forces.
- Dutch anatomist, Jaap van der Wal (2009) has identified up to 10 times the number of mechanoreceptors in the ECM (see Ch. 1 for explanation of this important aspect of fascia, 90% of which is collagen) compared with muscle. These receptors are intimately involved in the responses of muscle to both stretching and compression, as outlined below (Moore & Hutton 1980).

Neural influences and fascial structures (see also Ch. 1, Box 1.3)

The class of neural receptors known as **mechanoreceptors** respond in different ways to applied load, and provide proprioceptive information to the brain, concerning movement and position of the body. These are found in different locations, but are commonly located in fascia.

- **Pacinian corpuscles** are found in the deeper skin layers and deeper dense fascia, and respond rapidly to transient, changing – but not sustained – vibration and pressure. They are more responsive to rough textures than smooth ones. Their proprioceptive role is to provide the brain with information regarding the external body surface. After a short period the applied load is adapted to, and no longer stimulates, strong proprioceptive transmission.
- Different mechanoreceptors, **Merkel cells,** found more superficially in the skin, adapt far more slowly and continue to report on sustained load and any tissue displacement. They respond more to localized pressure rather than broad areas of contact, and may continue firing for up to 30 minutes. They are densely present in the fingertips.

- Another receptor found superficially in the skin of the fingertips (and elsewhere) are **Meissner corpuscles.** These are extremely sensitive to light touch and vibration.
- **Golgi receptors** sense changes in muscle tension, and are found in dense fascia, in ligaments **(Golgi end organs),** in joint capsules, as well as around myotendinous junctions **(Golgi tendon organs).** It remains uncertain to what degree manual treatment can influence Golgi responses (Schleip 2003a, 2003b).
- **Ruffini corpuscles** are found below the skin and in dense connective tissue, ligaments and peripheral joints. They register small degrees of mechanical change within joints, and slowly adapt to sensations of continuous pressure, as well as slow rhythmic movements and lateral (tangential) stretch or shear forces, resulting in reduced sympathetic activity.
- There are a variety of types of **free nerve endings** that adapt at different rates, reporting on changes in temperature, mechanical stimuli (touch, pressure, stretch) possibly leading to pain.
- **Interstitial mechanoreceptors** (also known as **interoceptors**) are plentifully located in fascia (for example in the periosteum), responding to rapid pressure or extremely light touch or stretching. Schleip (2003) suggests they have an autonomic influence.

> **Key Point**
>
> There appears to be a strong possibility that normalizing the fascia, where these various mechanoreceptor cells are abundantly located, might be a significant factor in restoring normal muscle coordination, motor control and balance, that depends on accurate proprioceptive information reaching the brain (Stecco & Stecco 2009). Additional influences may include improved sympathetic–parasympathetic balance.

Ligamentous reflexes

Solomonow (2009) notes that ligaments are sensory organs and have significant input to reflexive/synergistic activation of muscles. For example, muscular activity associated with the reflex from the anterior cruciate ligament acts to prevent distraction of the joint, while simultaneously reducing the strain in the ligament. There is also evidence that **ligamentomuscular reflexes** have inhibitory effects on muscles associated with that joint, inhibiting muscles that destabilize the joint or increasing antagonist co-activation to help stabilize the joint. One potential therapeutic use of this ligamentous function is found in positional release methodology (see Ch. 16) in what is known as 'facilitated positional release', where various forms of crowding (compaction) of joints are part of the protocol, with the objective of reducing muscular tone and increasing range of pain-free movement.

> **Key Point**
>
> The ability to modify excessive rigidity surrounding joints by sustained (a minute or more) compression may be a useful strategy on its own; while this approach as part of the facilitated positional release protocol (Ch. 16) may account, at least in part, for the benefits of that treatment method.

Sliding and gliding

As discussed in Chapter 1, fascial planes are frequently designed to slide and glide against each other and other structures (muscles, organs etc.), reducing friction and facilitating movement. When sliding functions are reduced or lost, symptoms of restriction and pain are likely to result. The ability to slide involves the presence of lubricating substance, hyaluronan (also known as hyaluronic acid), which is widely distributed throughout connective and neural tissues.

In 1992, Cantu and Grodin suggested that fascia-related therapeutic approaches should be designed to involve the superficial tissues involving proprioception and autonomic responses, as well as deeper tissues that influence the mechanical components of the musculoskeletal system that determine stability and mobility. Research has now allowed this suggestion to be realized – as discussed below, commonly including vibrational or oscillating modes of treatment.

Helping fascial glide: tangential oscillation and vibration

As discussed in Chapter 2, fascial function (including sliding functions) can change with age, inactivity, inflammation, trauma etc. For example, different parts of the ECM of superficial fascia can 'thicken' (Langevin et al. 2009) or become more 'dense' (Stecco & Stecco 2009), or there may be binding among layers that should glide and slide on each other (Fourie 2009).

The general effect of these changes may result in *'bodywide soft tissue holding patterns'* (Myers 2009).

Roman et al. (2013), in their detailed investigation and mathematical modeling of fascia's gliding processes, note that:

The fluid pressure of hyaluronic acid (HA) increases substantially as fascia is deformed during manual therapies. There is a higher rate of pressure during tangential oscillation and perpendicular vibration than during constant sliding. This variation of pressure caused HA to flow near the edges of the fascial area under manipulation, and this flow results in greater lubrication. The pressure generated in the fluid between the muscle and the fascia during [...] manipulative treatment causes the fluid gap to increase. [...] The presence of a thicker fluid gap can improve the sliding system and permit the muscles to work more efficiently.

Conclusion: *The inclusion of perpendicular vibration and tangential oscillation may increase the action of the treatment in the extracellular matrix, providing additional benefits in manual therapies that currently use only constant sliding motions.*

This suggests that the sliding functions of fascia can be assisted if manual treatment methods incorporate additional elements, such as tangential oscillation, and/or vertically applied vibration.

Some examples include:

- Myofascial release (Ch. 14) - especially if a vibrational element is included.
- Rhythmic, active pulsed MET, or vibratory isolytic MET (Mitchell 1998) - see Chapter 13.
- Deep cross-fiber friction also clearly fits into the group of vibrational/oscillating methods, as does a version of this technique (compression with friction), which is used in Fascial Manipulation® (see Ch. 9), involving deep friction delivered by means of elbow, knuckle or digital contact (Day et al. 2012).
- Similar enhancement of the sliding functions of fascia might be achieved via the shear forces associated with connective tissue manipulation methods, including skin rolling (see Ch.7).
- Fascial self-treatment involving use of a foam roller has been shown to offer some benefits in range of motion enhancement and reduction in arterial stiffness – possibly involving nitric oxide release (Okamoto et al. 2013). For more on foam rolling see Chapter 8.
- A wide range of vibratory treatment methods have been described over the years - for example Fulford's mechanical 'percussion vibrator' (Comeaux 2008) - or manually applied 'harmonic technique' (Lederman 1997).
- Additional methods that combine oscillation and lengthening are to be found in Chapter 15 – Neuromuscular techniques.

> **Key Point**
>
> The sliding potential of fascia can be enhanced by methods that include friction, vibration and shear forces.

Stretching and fascia

It is generally agreed that stretching of deep dense fascia is not possible using manual methods.

Chaudhry (2011) notes that while superficial fascia may be directly amenable to manual treatment (discussed later in the chapter), *'dense tissues of plantar fascia and fascia lata require very large forces—far outside the human physiologic range—to produce even 1% compression and 1% shear'.*

But how does that information correlate with therapist reports that palpable changes emerge from application of compression and shear forces? Chaudhry suggests: *'fascia may be able to respond to mechanostimulation with an altered tonus regulation of its own—myofibroblast-facilitated active tissue contractility.'*

Importantly, Chaudhry and colleagues (2007) note that in order to achieve a viscoelastic deformation (such as stretch) without causing tissue damage, there should be no slow increase in the applied force. Instead, a fairly constant force should be maintained, for up to 60 seconds, in order to allow for a plastic stress–relaxation response of the tissues.

Other explanations may answer the question of what apparently palpable fascial changes actually represent, for example:

- Perceived changes in 'stiffness' of deeper fascial structures following exercise or manual therapies may relate to altered fluid content (Schleip 2012). This is discussed later, under the heading: *Water and stretching.*
- Palpated changes in fascia may be due to reduced load because of relaxation of muscles attaching to, or associated with, the deep fascia. Franklyn-Miller et al. (2009) note that any linear stretch will be converted in the complexities of fibrous connections to bending, shear, or torsion forces in surrounding or 'downline' tissues.
- Palpated change may relate to enhanced sliding facility of associated superficial fascial layers, which had been reduced or lost following inflammation or trauma, as discussed earlier in this chapter.
- Changes in fascial tone might be due to the effects on fascial structures capable of responding to stretch (and isometric contractions), including intrafascial structures – the series elastic and parallel elastic components of muscles – lying inside the muscle's sarcomeres, as discussed below as we consider the effects of isometric contractions on fascial structures.
- Purslow's research (2010) suggests that most of the 'release' felt in myofasciae during manual therapy is due to muscular relaxation rather than actual lengthening of the fascial elements.

Water and stretching

Both compression and stretching reduce the water content of fascia – temporarily – making it more pliable. Klingler and Schleip (2004) examined fresh human fascia and noted that during stretching water is extruded, refilling afterwards. As water levels reduce, temporary relaxation occurs in the longitudinal arrangement of collagen fibers. If the strain is moderate and there are no micro-injuries, water soaks back into the tissue until it swells and, after 20–30 minutes, becomes stiffer than before (Schleip 2012).

> ### Key Point
> Many effects of manual therapy may relate to the sponge-like squeezing and refilling in the semi-liquid ground substance, with its water binding glycosaminoglycans and proteoglycans.

Self-stretching and fascia

The process of stretching after sleep (whether human, cat or dog) is known as pandiculation (Bertolucci 2011). Schleip and Muller (2013) highlight one unique aspect of this form of stretching when they note that this involves relaxation of muscles that are simultaneously lengthening – which they call a 'melting' stretch. They suggest that this involves intramuscular connective tissues as well as extramuscular connections. For more on this topic see Chapter 8.

> ### Key Point
> Sustained stretch may add length or modification to superficial fascia, but not to deeper dense fascia. Those structures may appear more relaxed and less dense following manual treatment but they will not have been lengthened.

Strain transmission during stretching

Stretching of muscles results in widespread load distribution; for example, a hamstring stretch will produce 240% of the resulting strain in the iliotibial tract – and 145% in the ipsilateral lumbar fascia – compared with the hamstrings.

The process of strain transmission that occurs during stretching involves many other tissues beyond the muscle being targeted, largely due to fascial connections, making the use of the word 'isolated' – together with 'stretching' – difficult to justify (Franklyn-Miller et al. 2009). Consider for example the uninterrupted mechanical transmission between the lower extremity, the pelvis and the trunk as load is transferred between the biceps femoris, the sacrotuberous ligament and gluteus maximus, and on to the contralateral latissimus dorsi, by means of tension transmitted via the superficial and deep thoracolumbar fascia (TLF). Transferred load would also influence the erector spinae, internal oblique and serratus posterior inferior muscles. Any dysfunctional situations, in any of these, could alter function of all the others listed, with unpredictable symptoms (Barker & Briggs 1999).

Key Point

This phenomenon applies throughout the body, and the clinical implications are profound. For example, if a hamstring stretch imposes load on the TLF, it should be obvious that perceived or palpated restrictions in the hamstrings or latissimus dorsi, or the other named muscles, might be due to altered function in the TLF.

Contractions and intramuscular fascial lengthening

Proprioceptive neuromuscular facilitation, as well as METs (see Ch. 13), use isometric and isotonic eccentric contractions as part of their methodology. Before considering the evidence for stretching influences on superficial (areolar, loose) connective tissues, we need to consider what happens inside muscles during contractions (isometric and isotonic) and/or stretching.

Fryer and Fossum (2009) report that, apart from the influence of mechanoreceptors on pain via both ascending and descending pathways, the isometric contractions used in MET (Ch. 13) induce mechanical stretching of fibroblasts in vivo that both alter interstitial osmotic pressure and increase blood flow, so reducing concentrations of pro-inflammatory cytokines, thereby reducing sensitization of peripheral pain-receptors.

Parmar et al. (2011) compared isotonic eccentric stretching in postoperative settings (following femur fracture or hip or knee surgery) with passive stretching methods. The objective was to: *'promote orientation of collagen fibers along the lines of stress and direction of movement, limit infiltration of cross bridges between collagen fibers, and prevent excessive collagen deposition.'* Both methods proved successful during postoperative rehabilitation; however, the isotonic eccentric stretching method produced a greater degree of pain reduction and an enhanced tendency towards a greater range of motion. These methods are discussed further in Chapter 13.

Physiology of contraction

Myofibrils are tubular filaments, comprising long protein strands of varying thicknesses – actin, myosin, and titin. Muscular contractions involve a sliding of the actin (thin) and myosin (thick) filaments across each other. Titin (also known as connectin) is a giant protein that functions as a molecular spring, responsible for the passive elasticity of muscle (Minajeva et al. 2001).

Myofibrils repeat along the length of muscles, in sections known as sarcomeres. These contain non-contractile fascial/connective tissue elements known as the *series elastic components* (SEC), and *parallel elastic components* (PEC) (Fig. 5.1)

- SEC store energy when stretched and contribute to the elasticity of muscle fibers. Tendons are examples of SEC, as are the cross bridges between actin and myosin – the sliding elements of the sarcomere

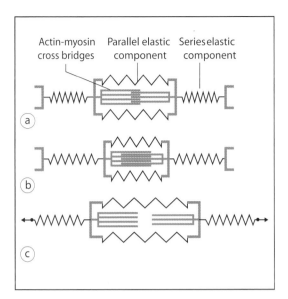

Actin-myosin   Parallel elastic   Series elastic
cross bridges   component   component

(a)

(b)

(c)

FIGURE 5.1 (a) The sarcomere at rest with the main elements–including three actin-myosin cross-bridges, as well as both the series and parallel elastic fascial components – at their resting lengths. (b) The sarcomere contracting isometrically – with actin and myosin sliding across each other as that part of the muscle contracts. The parallel elastic fascial component also shortens. However, because this is an isometric contraction and no overall length change occurs, the series elastic (fascial) component has to lengthen in order to accommodate the shortening of the other components. (c) This shows the changes when passive stretching is introduced. The parallel elastic and the actin-myosin components lengthen, while the stiffer series elastic component does not. (Note: The degree of separation of the actin/myosin components is exaggerated in this diagram).The overall message is that a degree of lengthening of the fascial elements of muscle occurs both during isometric contraction and during stretch. *Adapted, with permission, from Lederman 1997.*

that allow contractions to occur (Huxley & Niedergerke 1954).

- PEC provide resistive tension when passively stretched. They are non-contractile and consist of the muscle membranes (fascia), which lie parallel to the muscle fibers, as shown in Figure 5.1.

During an isometric contraction the SEC lengthens while the PEC shortens, as actin and myosin slide across each other. In this way the muscle does not change length, although elements in the muscle (i.e. within the sarcomeres) are either lengthening or shortening, to accommodate the contraction.

Repeated isometric contractions effectively lengthen the SEC – particularly if additional active or passive stretching is added, after the contraction (Lederman 2005). As Milliken (2003) notes: *'In this way both the active and passive phases of MET can be seen to contribute to muscle elongation.'*

> **Key Point**
>
> Contractions used in MET and other modalities induce lengthening of the fascial structures inside muscles, influencing both tone and pain.

Stretching superficial fascia

Evidence suggests that light degrees of sustained stretching have the most useful effects on superficial connective tissue. Howe et al. (2004) investigated the effect of tissue stretch on mouse subcutaneous tissues. They found that sustained light stretch (no more than 25% of the available elasticity of these tissues), maintained for between 10 minutes and 2 hours, caused a significant increase in fibroblast cell size. Cells were on average 200% larger following stretching. They noted that these dynamic changes in loose connective tissue (superficial, areolar) may be accompanied by important changes in cellular and tissue biochemistry, possibly explaining some of the therapeutic mechanisms involved in physical therapy, massage and acupuncture.

> **Key Point**
>
> *Light,* sustained stretch of superficial fascia, as in myofascial release (Ch. 14), produces lengthening, over time.

Heat and fascia

Heat has a direct effect in the therapeutic range (up to 40ºC) on the regulation of fascial stiffness, leading to relaxation of many fascial contractures associated with myofascial dysfunction (Klingler 2011). The various methods of applying heat include therapeutic ultrasound, diathermy, hot water, transdermal application of pharmaceuticals, etc. (Muraoka et al. 2006).

Mechanical (instrument assisted) load and fascia

Graston Technique® is an example of an instrument-assisted soft tissue assessment and mobilization method, delivering load deformation via stainless steel instruments (Hammer 2007); see Chapter 12 for greater detail on the methods and mechanisms.

Gua sha is a similar – more ancient – modality, deriving from traditional East Asian medicine, in which unidirectional press-stroking with a smooth-edged tool is applied at a lubricated area of the body until petechiae appear (Nielsen et al. 2007).

Nielsen et al. (2007) observe that: *'Hard surface myofascial tools show promising usefulness for a variety of treatment rationales and combination with other manual therapies. They may offer a different type of "access" and produce different clinical effects in muscles, tendons, ligaments, fascia, and the extracellular matrix than using the hands alone.'*

Corey et al. (2011) note : *'Transduction of force and stretch are thought to influence connective tissue rehabilitation.'*

The ECM is influenced by mechanical deformation of the superficial tissues, modulating the synthesis of proteoglycans and collagen by fibroblasts, increasing collagen formation (Sarasa & Chiquet et al. 2005).

> ## Key Point
> Tool-assisted assessment and treatment have been shown to be effective in influencing fascial behavior – as has warming of tissues before or during treatment.

Taping and fascia

Various models of elastic and anelastic adhesive taping have been developed – along with hypothetical models that attempt to explain their apparent efficacy.

Explanations include, variously, proprioceptive, neurological, mechanical, and specific fascial considerations. It appears that while symptomatic and functional benefits result from different forms of taping, the underlying mechanisms remain speculative:

- Gusella et al. (2014) report that kinesiologic-taping produces an increase in the muscle tone of the underlyin+g muscle, in healthy subjects. This study also suggests that tape-induced fascial stimuli can influence distant areas, even contralaterally.
- Chen et al. (2012) have developed and researched the effects of a functional fascial taping (FFT) method, involving anelastic (rigid) tape being applied from painful areas, in directions that relieve pain. Findings suggest that FFT is an easy and rapid pain modifying approach that can be used as an adjunct to exercise prescription in order to encourage individuals to return to normal functional activity.

Prolotherapy: stabilizing unstable structures

Prolotherapy – also known as sclerotherapy, and 'regenerative injection therapy', among others – is an injection-based intervention used to treat chronically unstable ligamentous and other fascial and tendinous tissues. The objective is to stimulate collagen proliferation at fibro-osseous junctions in order to promote repair of damaged or weakened soft tissues. A variety of different substances are injected (such as dextrose) with the aim of assisting in the restoration of stabilizing support for incompetent joints (Yelland et al. 2004, Rabago et al. 2005).

High velocity manipulation and fascia

Cramer et al. (2010) have shown in animal studies that *'hypomobility results in time-dependent adhesion development within the zygapophyseal (Z) joints* [and that] *such adhesion development may have relevance to spinal manipulation, which could theoretically break up Z-joint's intra-articular adhesions'* as joint surfaces are rapidly separated.

Simmonds et al. (2012) observe, however, that the number of receptors around a joint is far outweighed by those in surrounding fascia, so that absolute joint motion may not play a large component in the response to a high-velocity manipulation. This suggests that benefits such as increased range of motion and/or pain reduction may result from reflex neurological effects – rather than purely structural ones.

Key Point

Whether considering taping or high velocity manipulation, a common theme emerges – that clinical benefits are not always open to explanation, with hypothetical models remaining to be clarified, validated or eliminated.

Conclusion

This chapter shows the complexity of possible effects of different forms of therapeutic load applied to the body in general, and to fascial structures in particular – ranging from extremely gentle to fairly heavy frictional compression. Responses to these forms of load are seen to be equally varied, involving as they do hydraulic, circulatory, neurological and mechanical/structural viscoelastic changes.

The next section of the book is divided into 15 chapters, each of which presents a therapeutic model that builds on the mechanisms outlined in this chapter, addressing the dysfunctional patterns described in Chapter 2 that were observed, evaluated, assessed and palpated in Chapter 3.

Underlying all the subsequent information are the foundational aspects of our current knowledge, as summarized in Chapter 1.

Each of the following 15 chapters offers a glimpse of possibilities, a mosaic of methods and ideas, all of which aim to tap into the self-regulating potential of the human body, by removing obstacles to recovery, while enhancing functionality.

References

Barker PJ, Briggs CA 1999 Attachments of the posterior layer of lumbar fascia. Spine 24:1757-1764

Barnes P et al 2013 A comparative study of cervical hysteresis characteristics after various osteopathic manipulative treatment (OMT) modalities. J Bodyw Mov Ther 17:89-94

Bertolucci LF 2011 Pandiculation: nature's way of maintaining the functional integrity of the myofascial system? J Bodyw Mov Ther 5: 268-280

Bhattacharya V et al 2005 Live demonstration of microcirculation in the deep fascia and its implication. Plast Reconstr Surg 115(2):458-463

Blyum L, Driscoll M 2012 Mechanical stress transfer – the fundamental physical basis of all manual therapy techniques. J Bodyw Mov Ther 16: 520-527

Beloussov L 2006 An interview with Albert Harris. Direct physical formation of anatomical structures by cell traction forces. Int J Dev Biol 50: 93-101

Borgini E, Stecco A, Day JA, Stecco C 2010 How much time is required to modify a fascial fibrosis? J Bodyw Mov Ther 14(4): 318-325

Cantu R, Grodin A 1992 Myofascial manipulation. Aspen Publications, Gaithersburg, MD

Chaudhry H et al 2007 Viscoelastic behavior of human fasciae under extension in manual therapy. J Bodyw Mov Ther11:159–167

Chaudhry H 2011 Three-dimensional mathematical model for deformation of human fasciae in manual therapy. JAOA 108(8):379-390

Chen S et al 2012 Effects of functional fascial taping on pain and function in patients with non-specific low back pain: a pilot randomized. Clinical Rehabilitation 26 (10):924-933

Comeaux Z 2008 Harmonic healing – a guide to facilitated oscillatory techniques. North Atlantic Press, Berkeley, CA

Corey SM, et al 2011 Sensory innervation of the nonspecialized connective tissues in the low back of the rat. Cells Tissues and Organs 194: 521-530

Cramer GD et al 2010 Zygapophyseal joint adhesions after induced hypomobility. J Manipulative Physiol Ther 33: 508-518

Day JA, Copetti L, Rucli G 2012 From clinical experience to a model for the human fascial system. J Bodyw Mov Ther 16 (3): 372-380

Fourie W 2009 The fascia lata of the thigh more than a 'stocking'. Fascial Research II: Basic Science and Implications for Conventional and Complementary Health Care. Elsevier GmbH, Munich

Franklyn-Miller A et al 2009 In: Fascial Research II: Basic Science and Implications for Conventional and Complementary Health Care. Elsevier GmbH, Munich

Fryer G, Fossum C 2009 Therapeutic mechanisms underlying muscle energy approaches. In: Fernández-de-las-Peñas C, Arendt-Nielsen L, Gerwin R (eds) Physical therapy for tension type and cervicogenic headache: physical examination, muscle and joint management. Jones & Bartlett Learning, Burlington, MA

Gusella A et al 2014 Kinesiologic taping and muscular activity: a myofascial hypothesis and a randomised, blinded trial on healthy individuals. J Bodyw Mov Ther, in press

Hammer W 2007 Functional soft-tissue examination and treatment by manual methods, 3rd edn. Jones & Bartlett Learning, Burlington, MA, pp 33-161

Hinz B et al 2004 Myofibroblast development is characterized by specific cell-cell adherens junctions. Mol Biol Cell 15(9):4310-4320

Howe A et al 2004 Subcutaneous tissue stretch ex vivo and in vivo. Am J Physiol Cell Physiol 288:C747-C756

Huxley AF, Niedergerke R, 1954 Structural changes in muscle during contraction: interference microscopy of living muscle fibres. Nature 173(4412): 971–973

Jensen et al 2005 Effects of human pregnancy on the ventilatory chemoreflex response to carbon dioxide. Am J Physiol-Regul Integr Comp Physiol 288:R1369–R1375

Jensen D et al 2008 Physiological mechanisms of hyperventilation during human pregnancy. Respir Physiol Neurobiol 161(1):76-78

Kellum J 2007 Disorders of acid-base balance. Crit Care Med. 35(11):2630-2636

Klingler W et al 2004 European Fascia Research Project Report. 5th World Congress Low Back and Pelvic Pain, Melbourne

Klingler W 2011 Stretch response of thoraco-lumbar fascia at different temperatures In: Chaitow L, Lovegrove R (eds) Practical physical medicine approaches to chronic pelvic pain (CPP) and dysfunction. Churchill Livingstone Elsevier, Edinburgh

Kuchera ML 2007 Applying osteopathic principles to formulate treatment for patients with chronic pain. JAOA 107(6): 23-38

Kumka M, Bonar B 2012 Fascia: a morphological description and classification system based on a literature review. Can Chiropr Assoc 56(3):1-13

Langevin HM, Bouffard N, Fox J et al 2009 Fibroblast cytoskeletal remodeling contributes to viscoelastic response of areolar connective tissue under uniaxial tension, as reported in Fascial Research II. Elsevier GmbH, Munich

Lederman E 2005 Harmonic technique. Churchill Livingstone, Edinburgh

Lederman E 1997 Fundamentals of manual therapy. Churchill Livingstone, Edinburgh

Luomala T Pihlman M Heiskanen J et al 2014 Case study: Could ultrasound and elastography visualize densified areas inside the deep fascia? J Bodyw Mov Ther; in press

McPartland J 2008 The endocannabinoid system: an osteopathic perspective. J Am Osteopath Association 108(10):586–600

MacDonald GZ et al 2013 An acute bout of self-myofascial release increases range of motion without a subsequent decrease in muscle activation or force. J Strength Cond Res 27(3):812–821

Martinez Rodriguez R et al 2013 Mechanistic basis of manual therapy in myofascial injuries. Sonoelastographic evolution control. J Bodyw Mov Ther 17:221-234

Milliken K 2003 The effects of muscle energy technique on psoas major length. Unpublished MOst Thesis, Unitec New Zealand, Auckland, New Zealand

Minajeva A, Kulke M, Fernandez JM, Linke WA 2001 Unfolding of titin domains explains the viscoelastic behavior of skeletal myofibrils. Biophys J 80 (3): 442–51

Mitchell F 1998 The muscle energy manual, vol. 2 MET Press, Lansing MI

Moore MA, Hutton RS 1980 EMG investigation of muscle stretching techniques. Med Sci Sports Exerc12 (5): 322–329

Moseley GL, Gallace A, Spence C. 2012 Bodily illusions in health and disease: physiological and clinical perspectives and the concept of a cortical 'body matrix'. Neurosci Biobehav Rev 36(1):34-46.

Muraoka T et al 2006 Passive mechanical properties of human muscle-tendon complex at different temperatures. J of Biomechanics 39(1):S197

Myers T 2009 Anatomy Trains, 2nd edn. Churchill Livingstone, Edinburgh

Nielsen et al 2007 The effect of Gua Sha treatment on the microcirculation of the surface tissue: a pilot study in healthy subjects. Explore 3: 456-466

Okamoto T, Masuhara M, Ikuta K, 2013. Acute effects of self-myofascial release using a foam roller on arterial function. J Strength Cond Res: Epub ahead of print.

Parmar S et al 2011 The effect of isolytic contraction and passive manual stretching on pain and knee range of motion after hip surgery: A prospective double-blinded randomized study. Hong Kong Physiotherapy Journal 29:25-30

Pick M 2001 Presentation 'Beyond the neuron'. JBMT /University of Westminster Conference: Integrative bodywork – towards unifying principles. University of Westminster, London

Pilat A 2011 Myofascial induction. In: Chaitow et al Practical physical medicine approaches to chronic pelvic pain (CPP) and dysfunction. Elsevier, Edinburgh

Pohl H 2010 Changes in the structure of collagen distribution in the skin caused by a manual technique. J Bodyw Mov Ther 14(1):27-34

Purslow P 2010 Muscle fascia and force transmission. J Bodyw Mov Ther 14:411-417

Rabago D et al 2005 A systematic review of prolotherapy for chronic musculoskeletal pain. Clinical Journal of Sport Medicine 15(5):376-380

Rolf I 1977 Rolfing: reestablishing the natural alignment and structural integration of the human body of vitality and well being. Healing Arts Press, Rochester, VT

Roman M et al 2013 Mathematical analysis of the flow of hyaluronic acid around fascia during manual therapy motions. J Am Osteopath Assoc 113:600-610

Sackett DL, Rosenberg WM, Gray JA, Haynes RB, Richardson WS 1996 Evidence based medicine: what it is and what it isn't. BMJ 312(7023):71–2

Sarasa A, Chiquet M 2005 Mechanical signals regulating extracellular matrix gene expression in fibroblasts. Scand J Med Sci Sports 15: 223-230

Schleip R 2003a Fascial plasticity: a new neurobiological explanation. Part I. J Bodyw Mov Ther 7(1):11–19

Schleip R 2003b Fascial plasticity: a new neurobiological explanation. Part II. J Bodyw Mov Ther 7 (2):104–116

Schleip R 2012 Strain hardening of fascia: static stretching of dense fibrous connective tissues can induce a temporary stiffness increase accompanied by enhanced matrix hydration. J Bodyw Mov Ther 16:94-100

Schleip R, Müller DG 2013 Training principles for fascial connective tissues: scientific foundation and suggested practical applications. J Bodyw Mov Ther 17(1): 103-115

Schwind P 2006. Fascia and membrane technique. Churchill Livingstone, Edinburgh

Simmonds N et al 2012 A theoretical framework for the role of fascia in manual therapy. J Bodyw Mov Ther 16 (1):83-93

Solomonow M 2009 Ligaments: a source of musculoskeletal disorders. J Bodyw Mov Ther 13(2):136-154

Smith J 2005 The techniques of structural bodywork. Structural bodywork. Churchill Livingstone, London

Standley P 2007 Biomechanical strain regulation of human fibroblast cytokine expression: an in vitro model for myofascial release? Presentation at Fascia Research Congress, Boston

Standley P, Meltze, K 2008 In vitro modeling of repetitive motion strain and manual medicine treatments: potential roles for pro- and anti-inflammatory cytokines. J Bodyw Mov Ther 12 (3):201-203

Stecco L, Stecco C 2009 Fascial manipulation. Practical Part. Piccini, Padova, p 396

Tozzi P 2012 Selected fascial aspects of osteopathic practice. J Bodywork Mov Ther 16(4):503-519

van der Wal J 2009 The architecture of the connective tissue in the musculoskeletal system. In: Fascia research ii: basic science and implications for conventional and complementary health care. Elsevier GmbH, Munich

Ward RC 2003 Myofascial release concepts. In: Basmajian JV, Nyberg RE (eds) Rational manual therapies. Williams & Wilkins, Baltimore, MD, pp 223-241

Weisman M et al 2014 Surface electromyographic recordings after passive and active motion along the posterior myofascial kinematic chain in healthy male subjects. J Bodyw Mov Ther: in press

Yelland M J et al 2004 Prolotherapy injections, saline injections, and exercises for chronic low-back pain: a randomized trial. Spine 29(1):9-1

SECTION II

SELECTED FASCIAL MODALITIES

The recent series of Fascia Research Congresses (2007 Boston, 2009 Amsterdam and 2012 Vancouver) – and the numerous research studies and scientific papers that they reported and generated – has made apparent a degree of understandable fascial confusion as to the clinical relevance of some research findings. In addition, new and often unvalidated fascia-related therapeutic methods regularly appear, almost always involving slight modifications of methods that have been used for years.

To assist in clarifying what we already know, and what we still need to know, this section examines the methods and evidence for 15 well-established manual approaches that either target or significantly influence fascial function – each written by an acknowledged expert.

The insights in these chapters, set alongside the introductory chapters that offer background summaries of current research knowledge, provide a foundation for informed awareness of fascia's role, its potential problems and how to evaluate these, as well as how different forms of manual therapy may be able to assist the restoration of normal function.

Chapter 6

THE BOWEN TECHNIQUE

Michelle Watson, Julian M Baker

Introduction

The field of manual therapies now contains a growing range of methods and modalities – many claiming to benefit fascia-related health problems. A need for validation of the various approaches is clearly called for (Hansen & Taylor-Piliae 2011) and this chapter discusses the origins, approach, research and mechanisms behind one such modality – a 60-year-old therapy that originated in Australia, the Bowen technique.

Origins

In the 1950s, Thomas Bowen (1916–1982) created a form of manual therapy that is now called 'Bowen', 'Bowtech', 'Bowen therapy', 'Bowenwork', or 'the Bowen technique', which is known for its light touch and described as a series of soft tissue manipulations. Bowen's approach to bodywork was described as intuitive, where observation and touch were his primary tools due to his profound deafness. In 1975, a report commissioned by the Victorian Government confirmed that he was treating approximately 13 000 patients a year, claiming a success rate of greater than 80% in both chronic and acute conditions (Hansen & Taylor-Piliae 2011). Bowen's approach to bodywork was subtle, gentle and non-invasive, compared with many styles of manipulation of that time that involved much greater force and speed. He described himself as an osteopath and attempted to join the register of osteopaths in 1982, but was turned down. A headline in the *Geelong Advertiser* of 31 March 1982 read 'Red tape ties healing man's hands', detailing disappointment at his rejection.

Bowen's work was observed by a number of people over the years, some of whom continue to teach various interpretations of the technique today.

Approach and technique

With over 40 000 Bowen accredited practitioners worldwide, the technique has been categorized as a form of complementary or alternative medicine (CAM). The treatment approach is unique to the individual being treated, may involve multiple regions of the body, and is based upon the belief that the manual moves applied, stimulate or encourage the processes of healing and regeneration.

Each Bowen procedure consists of three stages: the slack in the skin is taken up, variable pressure is applied, and then a rolling-type maneuver is introduced over the selected soft tissues (see Fig 6.2). In between various moves there are pauses in the treatment, to allow time for the gentle stimulus to be responded to by the central nervous system. These breaks are a fundamental signature of the Bowen technique, and usually last 2–5 minutes,

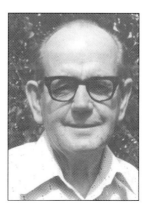

FIGURE 6.1 Thomas Bowen.

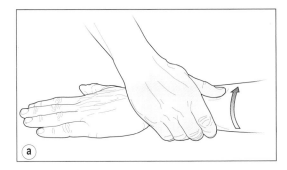

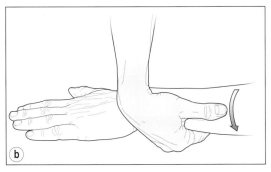

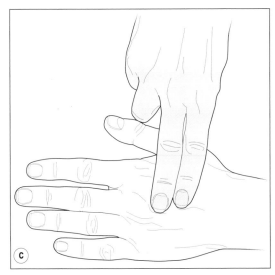

FIGURE 6.2 (a) Skin slack preceding the rolling-type move. (b) End of the rolling-type move. (c) Here the skin slack is drawn in the opposite direction to the intended move. Only at the point of the move will the 'eyeball pressure' be applied. *Figures (a–c) © Julian Baker.*

often between a set of 4–8 moves and depending on the individual patient. The length of these pauses and their frequency are determined by a selection of variables, some of which may include: the rapid changes in tissue tension, erythema, temperature changes in the skin, and reports of any sensory alteration from the patient. It is the Bowen therapist who makes the clinical decision about the pattern of these treatment pauses, and it is an established practice that the therapist will leave the room during these breaks in order to encourage an autonomic nervous system response (Baker 2013).

Whilst there are a couple of specific contraindications to aspects of the procedures, the Bowen technique has been found to be appropriate for people of all ages and in all degrees of health. With regard to the two Bowen procedures that are contraindicated, there has been a long held belief that the procedure that deals with the coccyx should be avoided during pregnancy, although the reasoning behind any risk has not been explained in detail or investigated. More recent interpretations have suggested that treatment of the coccyx region can be used safely after the first trimester. The second contraindication relates to the breast procedures which are discouraged in any woman who has had breast implants. This appears to have occurred after a spate of negligence claims against surgeons following breast implants. Insurers recommended some time ago that the breast procedures be avoided in those patients with implants. Again, no evidence exists with regard to any potential risk to the patient. Although no adverse reactions to treatment have been published, it is not uncommon for recipients of the technique to report: stiffness, soreness, flulike symptoms, temporary increases in the presenting pain and symptoms, and tiredness. These reactions are usually experienced within 24 hours of treatment, but are often short-lived, lasting for an average of 2 days. Such observations are surprising in view of the gentle pressure used and the minimal amount of time that the therapist is in the treatment room (Baker 2013).

The amount of pressure applied, the anatomical location and sequence progression of Bowen procedures, as well as the frequency of treatment sessions, are all determined by three factors: the subjective examination (the history-taking), an observation of the body's posture and symmetry, and the 'feel' of the tissues. A Bowen procedure is described as being very precise, involving mobilization of the soft tissues in a specific way. It involves a rolling-type maneuver, not a flick, designed to disturb the tissue in order to create a centralizing focus for the central nervous system (CNS). The pressure applied to the tissues is described as 'eyeball-type' pressure and is often mistaken to mean the amount of pressure that can be comfortably applied to an eyeball. However, it actually describes a pressure which is sensory without being invasive or painful. It is widely accepted that Bowen procedures should never be considered painful, although access to the deeper tissues is not precluded.

In the early stages of Bowen training, novice practitioners are taught a variety of procedures in order to offer examples of the technique. The advanced Bowen therapist will then follow the principle that the Bowen technique is a system, rather than being simply a series of moves. The procedures would then be applied more intuitively, on a foundation of a comprehensive understanding of human anatomy, physiology, pathology and dysfunction. The Bowen approach is considered to be 'holistic', inasmuch as it addresses body-wide issues, whilst avoiding treatment of a diagnosis, or of a condition or disease, and is not prescriptive. Bowen therapists do not diagnose, or give specific treatments for certain conditions. Neither do they alter or prescribe medications unless qualified to do so, or make claims about treatment outcomes unless there is a foundation of supportive scientific evidence.

Patient acceptance of this light pressure technique is high, both as a stand-alone approach and as part of a more general manual therapy intervention. In 2012/13 a questionnaire was sent from the European College of Bowen Studies (ECBS) to 1030 volunteer individuals who received Bowen treatment from students of the technique. It asked for yes or no answers to the following questions: a) if they found the Bowen technique to be of benefit, b) if they would have the Bowen technique again and c) if they would recommend it to others, to which 93% of respondents answered positively to all three questions.

In 2002 the Bowen technique was accepted in the UK by the Chartered Society of Physiotherapy as a treatment tool that could be used 'within the remit of physiotherapy.' Bowen treatment can therefore be applied as an adjunct to other established physiotherapy assessment and treatment protocols and is currently practiced in UK hospitals as well as in private clinics.

Summary of published literature

The following is a brief summary of the published literature on the Bowen technique during the last 10 years. Systematic reviews are included, as are research designs where measurements of specific outcomes are taken. Due to the large number of published single case studies, it was not possible to consider conclusions from that model of research.

Pain

- Hipmair et al. (2012) investigated the effect of Bowen therapy on 91 patients in the postoperative phase of a total knee replacement. Three single-blinded, randomly allocated groups were involved: group A underwent two Bowen treatments between days 2 and 10; group B received a manual sham therapy (which mimicked the Bowen moves, and consisted of 'soft touches' in proximity to the usual area of a Bowen procedure) and group C, the control group, received no additional treatment. Postoperative pain was assessed using the visual analogue scale (VAS) between days 1 and 10. The results showed no statistically significant difference in average pain score between the three groups over the 10 days, although the Bowen group alone did show a statistically significant decrease in pain in the first 2 days (p = 0.001 and =0.008, respectively).
- Morris et al. (submitted for publication) conducted research into the Bowen technique and low back pain entitled: *A pilot study to investigate the use of The Bowen Technique as a treatment for people who live with chronic, non-*

specific low back pain (CNSLBP). Thirty-seven single-blinded participants were allocated into two groups: an experimental (Bowen) group, and a control ('sham Bowen') group. The sham involved sweeping the back of the hand across the body, with a similar pressure and location to that of the actual Bowen maneuvers. Each participant received three weekly treatments, with completion of a questionnaire 1 week and 4 weeks post-treatment. Twenty measurements were taken including: pain, levels of function, psychosocial/somatic changes and general health. The Bowen group recorded a positive change by the second follow-up in 20 of the categories. By contrast the Sham group showed an improvement in 12 categories at the same time point. The study recommended that with some modifications it was feasible to conduct a larger-scale trial into the effectiveness of the Bowen technique as a treatment for the management of CNSLBP on a biopsychosocial level.

Range of motion

A single blinded randomized controlled trial by Marr et al. (2011) involving 116 asymptomatic volunteers examined the effects of a single Bowen treatment on hamstring flexibility levels over 1 week. The results showed that a single treatment of Bowen produced immediate increases in the flexibility of the hamstring muscles, both within-subjects (p=0.0005) and between-subjects (p=0.008), with improvements lasting for 1 week without further treatment (p=0.0005, mean increase in flexibility of 9.73°).

Employee health and the workplace

In 2005, Dicker examined the effects of a 6-week program using Bowen technique on levels of stress and physical health in 31 Hospital and Community Health Service staff in a group setting. Quantitative and qualitative data indicated that the Bowen technique was successful in reducing pain (78% reported improvements), improving mobility (79%), reducing stress (82%), improving energy and well-being (64%) and sleep (50%).

Functional recovery

- In 2011 Duncan et al. performed a pilot study on 14 chronic stroke sufferers, looking at the potential impact of Bowen as a therapy after stroke. All participants were assessed against the following outcome measures: Barthel index, motor assessment scale (MAS), grip strength, nine hole peg test (9-HPT), timed up and go (TUG), key pinch test, mini-mental state examination (MMSE) and the SF-36. The 14 patients received 13 sessions of Bowen treatment over 3 months. Measurements of gross motor function (MAS) showed statistically significant improvement. Improvements were also noted in relation to physical wellbeing as well as social functioning, and were all statistically significant; however, grip strength reduced.

Systematic review

- Hansen and Taylor-Piliae (2011) conducted a systematic review of the literature relevant to Bowen between 1985 and 2009. Out of 309 citations, 15 articles met the inclusion criteria. The review concluded that Bowen offers a non-invasive, affordable approach to improving health, most notably in pain reduction, frozen shoulder and migraine. However, lack of documented and systematic scientific evidence prevents widespread recommendations.

How can gentle pressure affect change within tissues?

The effects of the Bowen technique are not well understood, remain unproven and have caused controversy amongst scientists and clinicians. Until recently, the mechanisms behind the claims have mostly been attributed to the mechanical properties of the tissues, and little to do with the nervous system (Schleip 2003a). The explosion of scientific research during the past decade, looking into skin, fascia and the effects of manual therapies, has produced a variety of models that may help to explain the observed changes due to Bowen. The most common hypotheses for the treatment effects resulting from Bowen are namely: *proprioception and interoception.*

Proprioception

In 1907, Sherrington was the first to publish work that introduced the terms proprioception, interoception, and exteroception. Since then his pioneering system of classification has kept scientists searching for specialized nerves that transmit information about the constantly changing environment within the body. For the purposes of this chapter proprioception is defined as: 'the ability to sense the position and location, orientation, and movement of the body and its parts' (van der Wal 2012). More simply, it is the ability to function without vision, such as walking in complete darkness without falling over. Definitions of proprioception that suggest a subconscious or psychological awareness of the body are not included in this chapter. Similarly, explanations of exteroception, an awareness of the environment external to the body, are also excluded.

Historically, changes due to Bowen treatment were thought to stimulate the proprioceptive mechanoreceptors in the ligaments, tendons, muscles, and joints; notably the Golgi receptors, muscle spindles, Pacini, paciniform and Ruffini receptors. These pressure, velocity and tension sensitive receptors form part of a feedback loop in response to changes in length and tension relationships within the muscles and associated tissues, and in joint alignment. The effects thought to result from stimulation of these receptors include changes in: muscle tension and tone; movement range; pain; and sympathetic nervous system activity (Schleip 2003a, 2003b). However, research in the 1990s revealed two new facts: that Golgi tendon organs could not be stimulated by passive movement or by passive stretch of myofascial tissue, ligaments or tendons (Jami 1992). This is important to note as Bowen maneuvers are, for the most part, applied to the body passively, without any active contraction of the part. The muscle had to be actively contracting to influence these particular proprioceptors

(Schleip 2003a). Secondly, research by Burke and Gandevia in 1990, discovered that approximately 10% of Golgi receptors are located around the tendon, lying in series with the tendon, hence their inability to detect passive loading. Over 80% of the Golgi receptors were found in other locations: in the muscular part of myotendinous junctions; in the attachments of the aponeuroses; and in the joint capsules and ligaments of peripheral joints (Schleip 2003). The involvement of such deeply located receptors (the Golgi receptors), seems to be improbable, as part of any neurophysiological explanations for the effects of the light touch of Bowen maneuvers, lying as they are, deep to the skin, within the muscles, joints, capsules, tendons, ligaments and deep fascia.

The question therefore remains: how does the 'light' touch of Bowen, and the absence of loading, stretching or motion of the body, stimulate these deeper receptors?

Recent findings go some way to help explain this question. The skin is usually the first tissue to be touched during any manual therapy and is densely innervated by many types of receptors that detect changes in touch, pressure, vibration, temperature and pain. The many roles of the skin include: communication about the internal and external environment of the body; temperature control; balance of water and electrolytes; an immune response to protect from pathogens; and reaction to physical, chemical and thermal factors (Paoletti 2006).

Our understanding of how deeply the skin can communicate, and how widespread its connections range, has advanced significantly in the past decade. The skin is contiguous with the subcutaneous and superficial fascia, also referred to as the hypodermis (Abu-Hijleh et al. 2006). Research into the extracellular matrix (ECM, see discussion in Ch. 1 of this layer of connective tissue) has shown that the ground substance sends out projections towards the surface of the skin, which are cylindrical, acting almost like periscopes, which surround nerves and blood vessels, thus allowing the deep fascia a route of communication with the surface of the body (Paoletti 2006). These cylinders are called Heine cylinders and are 'visible' evidence of an organ of communication from the skin down to the bone (Heine 2006,

Paoletti 2006). The fibers in this layer also contain collagen, elastin and reticulin, allowing connections through to the deep fascia and bone. In addition to adipocytes, the fibroblasts in the superficial layer are responsive to mechanotransduction, giving rise to a wide variety of sensations and communication signals (Langevin, 2006). Such receptors may even account for the commonly reported 'sudden tissue release' phenomenon, described sometimes as a palpable drop in tension beneath a therapist's fingers, usually in less than 2 minutes (Schleip 2003).

Thus when a clinician's hands contact the skin, there is a direct communication route to the deeper structures (Langevin 2006). Furthermore, the organization of the nervous system seems to more markedly involve the sensory nerves, rather than the motor nerves. Schleip (2003) states that in a typical muscle nerve only 20% of its sensory component supplies the muscle spindles, Golgi receptors, pacinian, and Ruffini endings, known as type I and II nerves. Approximately 80% belong to type III and IV sensory nerves, which are now termed interstitial

muscle receptors and are abundant – with the highest concentrations being within the fascia and periosteum (Schleip 2003). More than 80% of these type III and IV nerves are unmyelinated (type 4) and originate in free nerve endings in the skin and superficial fascia. Figure 6.3 (see also Plate 6) shows the superficial positioning of the free nerve endings just beneath the skin and the beginnings of connectivity beneath this layer, whilst also revealing the access to a variety of other receptors just beneath the skin. Figure 6.4 demonstrates the congruent layers of the human body from skin to bone, as seen by the existence of the loose 'areolar' fascia superficial to the deep fascial layers, in a female right mid-thigh.

Interoception

Now called intrafascial mechanoreceptors, these free nerve endings give rise to a sense known as interoception. This can be described as the sense of well-being of the body, and includes a wide range of physiological sensations, such as muscular ef-

FIGURE 6.3 Diagram of receptors within skin and superficial fascia. See also Plate 6. *From Constantin 2006 Inquiry into biology. McGraw-Hill Ryerson, p.429, Fig. 12.27. Reproduced with permission of McGraw-Hill Ryerson Ltd.*

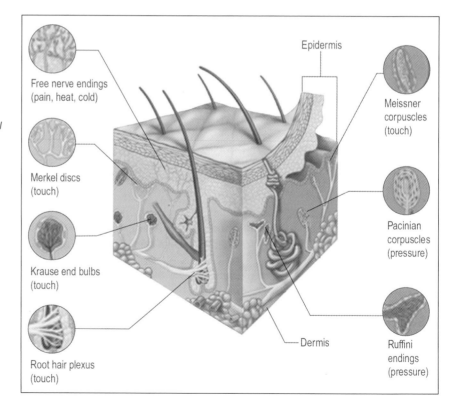

Free nerve endings (pain, heat, cold)

Merkel discs (touch)

Krause end bulbs (touch)

Root hair plexus (touch)

Epidermis

Meissner corpuscles (touch)

Pacinian corpuscles (pressure)

Dermis

Ruffini endings (pressure)

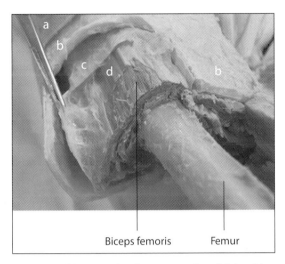

Biceps femoris   Femur

FIGURE 6.4 Dissection showing cross-section of right mid-thigh. © Julian Baker.
Key to lettering on dissection: a = skin; b = superficial fascia/adipose layer; c & d = reflected layers of deep fascia.

fort; tickling; itching; pain; hunger; thirst; warmth; cold; distension of the organs such as the bladder, bowels and esophagus; and sensual or pleasant touch (Richards 2012, Schleip & Jäger 2012). Research has confirmed that some of the free nerve endings are indeed mechanoreceptors, sensing change in mechanical stimuli (light touch, pressure and stretch) and are commonly found in hairy skin. This is in addition to their ability to respond to pain, heat and cold, previously thought to be their primary function (Schleip & Jäger 2012).

How does this relate to Bowen as a therapy? The presence of numerous free nerve endings in the skin and superficial fascia, as receptors of light touch, suggests a possible mechanism for the effects of the Bowen technique and other gentle soft tissue techniques. The existence of an anatomical route of communication from the surface of the skin through to the bone further suggests a mechanism for explaining the deeper changes seen following treatment. It is noteworthy that the pathway of these free nerves ends in the insular cortex in the brain, which is involved in consciousness and is usually linked to emotion and control of the body's homeostasis. The functions of the insular cortex include perception, motor control, self-awareness and cognitive functioning. In contrast,

dysfunction can also change the way afferent information is perceived. For example, Song et al. (2006) conclude that irritable bowel syndrome creates abnormal processing of pain from the bowel to the insular cortex and that this results in loss of inhibition of pain within the brain – sensitization. The effect of a parent stroking or cuddling a child not only provides a sense of well-being, but also neural stimulation that promotes physical growth. Touch also plays a vital role in the process of connective tissue change, which can only be lengthened and remodeled through collagen deposition. Growth factor, although at its peak in childhood, still plays an important role in the laying down of connective tissue in adults (van den Berg 2012). Somatotrophin, a growth hormone secreted by the pituitary gland, has a direct effect on connective tissues, stimulating fibroblasts and the mast cells to produce collagen fibers and build fascia and tendon (Juhan 2003).

This 'well-being' touch, now being linked to interoception in adults, may offer an insight into how a non-invasive, gentle touch, such as that provided by Bowen treatment, could create the reported responses that are not always immediately apparent following treatment. It would appear that, in order to be considered as an interoceptive stimulator, much less pressure is required than that traditionally associated with fascial manipulation (Schleip & Jäger 2012).

How much pressure is therefore required to stimulate the proprioceptors, rather than the interoceptors, is an important question and is currently unknown. The effect of the velocity of the technique is also of interest, but as yet unconfirmed. Lederman (2005) suggests that each form of manual stimulation is coded in the form of a frequency. Mechanoreceptors communicate with the CNS through conversion of mechanical stimulation into electrical signals that are encoded through different frequencies. As a more simple analogy, with our eyes closed we can distinguish between a violin and a cello playing due to a learned signature of sound vibration through the ear. In the same way, it would seem that the body is able to sense differences in touch and movement through analysis of frequencies and patterns. The opportunity now exists for science to explain the effects of different therapeutic techniques and how the body identifies 'good' from 'bad', as far as manual therapy is concerned.

How much pressure is needed during treatment?

This is an important clinical consideration. During the planning of a Bowen treatment, there are many complex factors to consider in the reasoning process, some of which have already been discussed. The subjective examination and knowledge of anatomy, physiology and pathology will, in the first instance, give the clinician a plan of the tissue types and dysfunctions to be targeted. During the process of palpation, each patient will also give the clinician a unique feeling about the state of their tissues, such as: the presence of fibrosis; trigger points; any localized heat or swelling; and the level of resistance to being touched. The reasons for tissue resistance, or thickening, are multi-factorial and can include the effects of current and previous pathologies, the chronicity of the problem, congenital factors affecting tone and stiffness, the presence of scar tissue, the sensory awareness of that individual, and the current pain status. These merely describe the physical factors, which are no less important that the emotional, psychological and environmental factors that may also have an effect on the findings during palpation and assessment.

Ultrasound imaging of chronic tissue injury or inflammation has commonly shown pathological changes to the structure of connective tissues. Where pathology exists, an increase in the thickness of the connective tissues surrounding a muscle is frequently seen in the lumbar spine, compared with those who did not have back pain (Langevin & Kawakami 2012). Experienced manual therapists may be able to feel tissue changes in relation to thickening, relative stiffness, depth, mobility, hydration and heat across the interfaces.

The actual pressure then applied to the tissues by a Bowen therapist will be guided by their own skill in recognizing a 'normal' versus an 'abnormal' feel of tissues, and by their ability to grade the pressure required in any therapeutic intervention. To some extent this is also dependent on the therapists own experience, intuition, balance, stability, and history of injuries. As a result, it is to be expected that variations in pressure will be applied during treatment, not only between different therapists, but also between different treatments and body regions. In the absence of normative data examining how different pressures affect the tissues, it should be accepted that an experienced clinician will use intuition and clinical experience to guide the gradation of force, and would use the least pressure possible to create the desired effect.

The region to be treated will also inform the decision as to how much pressure to apply. Each area will vary in its anatomy dependent on its function(s). Thus, if the main function of the part is for mobility, the fascial arrangement of the part will be different to that where stability is ultimately required. The shoulder is primarily an area of incredible three-dimensional mobility, and the 'feel' of the tissues will reflect that function. The presence of bony prominences may also produce a greater sensitivity to pressure. In contrast, the lumbar spine is, in essence, an area of loading and stability, transmitting the forces to and from the pelvis, trunk and limbs. Therefore the greater depth of tissues beneath the skin, and multiple layers of fibrous connections, may allow for greater manual pressure and depth, again within the realms of comfort.

Finally, during a Bowen maneuver, or repeat maneuver, the tone or tension in the tissues may begin to change, allowing access to much deeper structures, without the need for any increase in pressure or discomfort.

How does Bowen restore function?

When trying to understand how Bowen restores function, there are many neurophysiological and psychological processes to consider. For the purposes of this chapter, the focus will be on the fact that multiple body regions are treated in a single Bowen session.

This is felt to be a key aspect behind the success of the therapy. To better understand this concept, the topic of biomechanical alignment will be considered.

In order to stand up against gravity the human body attempts to optimize each posture by balancing the internal levels of tension against the external forces acting against it, such as gravity and ground reaction forces (see Fig. 6.5). To prevent inflammation, or injury, each movement or activity needs to be balanced, smooth, energy-efficient and successful, with an optimal loading through the tissues, to minimize unwanted friction, shear and strain. For this to succeed, muscles and their connective tissues need to move in an integrated and multidimensional manner, requiring real-time communication with other parts, both adjacent and at some distance.

Figure 6.5 illustrates the optimal standing posture (first pose), where the line of gravity shows the most efficient balance of forces, or, more simply, the least effort needed to stay upright. This image is then followed by five additional examples of postural change, often seen clinically, showing the shift in line of gravity and risk of potential dysfunction.

During a clinical assessment it is common to find asymmetry within our patients and also within ourselves. The debate over whether or not we should try to influence symmetry or not, is beyond the realms of this chapter, as is the topic of whether or not the human body is supposed to be symmetrical, in view of the asymmetrical positioning of its organs. However, postural asymmetry, in addition to the presence of dysfunction and complaints of symptoms, may be an indicator of a history of imbalance of forces and loading through the tissues, and warrants further examination during the assessment.

It will always be a matter of conjecture for any therapist to establish, beyond reasonable doubt, the exact origin or nature of any biomechanical imbalance, so that any successful treatment might aim to reduce speculation and guesswork. A first Bowen treatment may therefore involve several options. The first treatment is generally standardized and will target common areas of stress loading, and often those areas where pathological loading is evident following examination.

In 2011, Marr et al. performed a randomized controlled trial which looked at the effects of Bowen on flexibility. They concluded that a single standardized treatment of the Bowen technique demonstrated immediate increases in the flexibility of the hamstring muscles, both within subjects (p=0.0005) and between-subjects (p=0.008), maintaining improvements for 1 week without further treatment (p=0.0005, mean increase of 9.73°). They hypothesized that the most

FIGURE 6.5 Postural changes with altering line of gravity. *Reproduced with permission from Healus © 2014.*

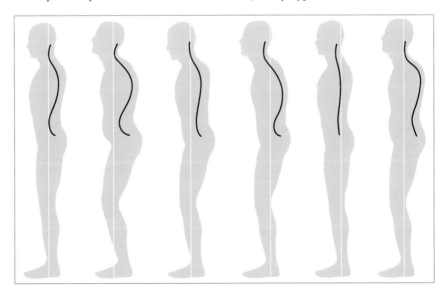

likely explanation was the result of stimulation of anatomically relevant body regions in support of the action of knee extension. The Bowen maneuvers were applied along the posterior layer of the thoracolumbar fascia (as described by DeRosa & Porterfield 2007), and included soft tissue moves over the fascial linkage of the latissimus dorsi to the gluteus maximus. This was followed by stimulation of the hamstring and adductor muscles, where anatomical continuity exists through to the gluteus maximus and into the lumbopelvic slings (DeRosa & Porterfield 2007). In other words, the Bowen treatment that was delivered provided a planned direction of manual stimulation throughout the extensors of the spine, trunk and lower limbs. It may be relevant to note that peripheral information, via the mechanoreceptors, reaching the central nervous system, has been reported to affect both agonist and antagonist muscles (Lederman 2005), possibly serving to activate one and inhibit the other, potentially offering an explanation for reciprocally functional changes.

Summary and recommendations

It is hoped that the research discussed in this chapter, regarding proprioception, interoception and fascial connectivity, may go some way towards offering potentially credible explanations regarding the effects of application of the Bowen technique and other 'light touch' therapies. A clear neural pathway of communication from the surface of the skin, to the bone, has been identified. Studies have also demonstrated the means whereby superficial and gentle manual stimulation may initiate changes in the deeper tissues. How much force to optimally apply, in order to generate a desirable therapeutic response, is currently being investigated. How the processes of proprioception and interoception overlap, and how integral they are in the processing of sensory and motor information in functional recovery, is as yet unknown.

Both chronic and acute presentations have been shown to benefit from Bowen treatment.

However, the technique itself does not yet address functional re-education or rehabilitation needs. A wider skill set, or referral to other practitioners, is currently needed in order for some patients to realize their full recovery potential. It is also acknowledged that additional research is required before general recommendations can be made about Bowen as the stand-alone therapy it aspires to be. In 2014, the first diploma in Bowen studies is due to be launched in the UK, through ECBS, with plans to do the same through the Bowen Association of Australia.

References

Abu-Hijleh MF et al (2006) The membranous layer of superficial fascia: evidence for its widespread distribution in the body. Surg Radiol Anat 28(6): 606–619

Baker J 2013 Bowen unravelled: a journey into the fascial understanding of the Bowen Technique. Lotus Publishing, Chichester

Burke D, Gandevia SC 1990 Peripheral motor system. In: Paxines G (ed) The human nervous system. Academic Press, San Diego, pp 1-133.

DeRosa C, Porterfield JA 2007 Anatomical linkages and muscle slings of the lumbopelvic region. In: Vleeming A, Mooney V, Stoekart R (eds) Movement, stability and lumbopelvic pain, 2nd edn. Churchill Livingstone, Edinburgh, pp 47-62

Dicker A 2005 Using Bowen technique in a health service workplace to improve the physical and mental wellbeing of staff. Aust J Holist Nurs 122, pp 34-42

Duncan B, McHugh P, Houghton F, Wilson C 2011 Improved motor function with Bowen therapy for rehabilitation in chronic stroke: a pilot study. Journal of Primary Health Care 31, pp 53-7. Available online at http://www.rnzcgp.org.nz/assets/documents/Publications/JPHC/March-2011/JPHCCaseSeriesReviewDuncanMarch11.pdf . Accessed 28 July 2013

Hansen C, Taylor-Piliae RE 2011 What is Bowenwork? A systematic review. Journal of Complementary Medicine 17(11):1001-1006. doi: 10.1089/acm.2010.0023

Heine H 2006 Lehrbuch der biologischen Medizin. 3. Aufl.Hippokrates, Stuttgart

Hipmair G et al 2012 Efficacy of Bowen Therapy in postoperative pain management – a single blinded (randomized) controlled trial. Available at http://therapy-training.com/research/bowen-pain-research.html. Accessed 23 February 2014

Jami L 1992 Golgi tendon organs in mammalian skeletal muscle: functional properties and central actions. Phys Rev 73(3):623-666

Juhan D 2003 Job's body, handbook for bodywork, 3rd edn. Station Hill Press, Barrytown, NY, p. 84

Langevin HM 2006 Connective tissue: a body-wide signalling network. Med Hypotheses (66):1074-1077

Langevin HM, Kawakami Y 2012 Imaging ultrasound. In: Schleip R, Findley TW, Chaitow L, Huijing PA (eds) Fascia: the tensional network of the human body. Churchill Livingstone Elsevier, Edinburgh, pp 483-487

Lederman E 2005. The science and practice of manual therapy, 2nd edn. Churchill Livingstone, Edinburgh

Marr M, Baker J, Lambon N, Perry J 2011 The effects of the Bowen technique on hamstring flexibility over time: a randomised controlled trial. J Bodyw Mov Ther 15(3): 281-90 doi:10.1016/j.jbmt.2010.07.008

Morris MF, Ellard DR, Patel S 2014 The Bowen Technique and low back pain: a pilot study to investigate the use of The Bowen Technique as a treatment for people who live with chronic, non-specific LBP. J Bodyw Mov Ther: submitted

Paoletti S 2006 The fasciae. Eastland Press, Seattle

Richards S 2012 Pleasant to the touch. The Scientist [Online]. Available online at: http://www.the-scientist.com/?articles.view/articleNo/32487/title/Pleasant-to-the-Touch/. [Accessed July 2013]

Schleip R 2003a Fascial plasticity – a new neurobiological explanation. Part 1. J Bodyw Mov Ther 7(1):11-19

Schleip R 2003b Fascial plasticity – a new neurobiological explanation. Part 2. J Bodyw Mov Ther 7(2): 104-116

Schleip R, Jäger H 2012 Interoception. A new correlate for intricate connections between fascial receptors, emotion and self recognition. In: Schleip R, Findley TW, Chaitow L, Huijing PA (eds) Fascia: the tensional network of the human body. Churchill Livingstone Elsevier, Edinburgh, p 93

Schleip R, Findley TW, Chaitow L, Huijing PA (eds) 2012 Fascia: the tensional network of the human body. Elsevier Churchill Livingstone, Edinburgh

Sherrington CS 1907 On the proprioceptive system, especially in its reflex aspect. Brain 29(4): 467–485

Song GH et al 2006 Cortical effects of anticipation and endogenous modulation of visceral pain assessed by functional brain MRI in irritable bowel syndrome patients and healthy controls. Pain 126 (1-3):79–90 doi:10.1016/j.pain.2006.06.017

van den Berg F 2012 The physiology of fascia. An introduction. In: Schleip R, Findley TW, Chaitow L, Huijing PA (eds) Fascia: the tensional network of the human body. Elsevier Churchill Livingstone, Edinburgh, pp149-155

van der Wal JC 2012 Proprioception, mechanoreception and anatomy of fascia. In: Schleip R, Findley TW, Chaitow L, Huijing PA (eds) Fascia: the tensional network of the human body. Elsevier Churchill Livingstone, Edinburgh, pp 81-87

Chapter 7

CONNECTIVE TISSUE MANIPULATION AND SKIN ROLLING

Elizabeth A. Holey, John Dixon

Introduction

Connective tissue manipulation/massage (CTM) or bindegewebsmassage is a manual therapy applied with the therapist's hands in contact with the patient's skin. It is more correctly described as a manual reflex therapy as the effects are believed to occur through stimulation of cutaneovisceral reflexes which induce an autonomic reflex response. The ability to harness this response to achieve clinical outcomes directs the clinical decision-making when using the therapy to treat dysfunction. The modality is applied with the longest digit (third finger), or thumb of the therapist's hand, through a lifting stroke, which carefully targets each interface within the skin to create a shear force. Superficial layers may have to be treated before the deep fascial layer, which is where the potent autonomic effects are thought to occur. A pattern of strokes must be learned to enable access to the fascia where it is relatively superficial, attaching to bone and between muscle fibers, for example. The reflex connective tissue (CT) zones utilized are based on those first identified by Henry Head more than 100 years ago (Head 1898). They are particularly interesting as reflex areas as they can be seen, palpated and anatomically understood (Schuh 1992, Holey 1995).

Skin rolling

A skin rolling technique is often used in CTM, at the superficial fascial layer. The same shear force is created at the fascial/skin interface, but, with the patient in a side lying position, the skin layer is lifted up against gravity away from the spine. If the therapist feels tension at the end of the roll and continues to roll the skin, then the autonomic nervous system (ANS) will be stimulated. This is also commonly used as a technique in its own right, either as part of classical (Swedish) massage, within myofascial release techniques and in trigger point therapy. Some proponents grasp the skin within their palm to roll tissue against underlying tension.

Background

CTM originated in Germany in the 1930s. The story of its discovery by Elisabeth Dicke in the 1930s is helpful in understanding the range of problems CTM can help. A physiotherapist, Dicke relieved her lumbar pain by using a pulling and stretching technique on the soft tissues of her back. During this massage, she found that the tissues over her buttock area had become tight and thickened and as they released, the circulation improved to her leg. This had a dramatic consequence in that the amputation she had been waiting for, due to a severe arterial condition, was no longer required. The buttock area coincided with Head's arterial (lower limb) zone. Dicke continued the treatment with the help of a colleague. As they continued the technique in other areas where the tissues were felt to be similarly affected, a stomach disorder improved. Head's stomach zone is over the left side of the ribcage. Dicke recognized the reflex links and subsequently developed CTM as a modality (See Fig. 7.1)

FIGURE 7.1 Head's zones.

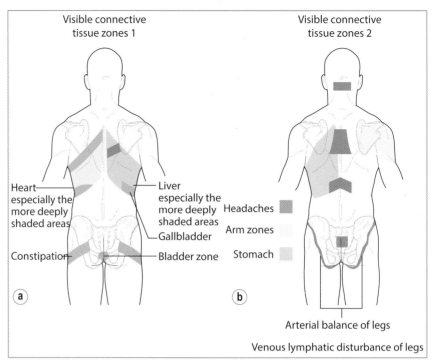

This history summarizes the clinical decision-making that is still relevant today. A seemingly musculoskeletal problem (such as Dicke's back pain) would be assessed in the usual way. The presence of a CT zone and the potentially connected symptoms of circulatory and visceral problems would indicate that an autonomic CTM approach would be effective. The interconnectedness of these problems helps to explain the physiology of CTM. Dicke's main problem was an arterial one. Arteries have a sympathetic nerve supply *(nervi vascularis)*. Dicke's arterial dysfunction influenced the superficial tissues that shared the same spinal segment and they became painful. The nutritional state of the connective tissues was affected, resulting in altered fluid balance, thickenings and indurations that she could feel in her low back/buttock area, which she later identified as the arterial reflex zone. The stomach was similarly affected through its sympathetic nerve supply. Dicke demonstrated a self-perpetuating dysfunction loop connecting:

$$\text{arterial system} \rightarrow \text{ANS}$$
$$\uparrow \qquad\qquad \downarrow$$
$$\text{skin \& fascia} \leftarrow \text{ANS} \leftarrow \text{viscera}$$

resulting in pain. All the dysfunctions in the loop improved with fascial manipulation. The cycle was broken by lowering the level of sympathetic activity, enabling balance restoration and improved function (Holey 2006).

There is some research evidence to support the proposed theoretical mechanisms underpinning CTM, but the evidence base is neither complete nor strong. CTM has been observed to have an effect on physiological measures of autonomic function. Controlled clinical studies are very limited but some evidence shows CTM can improve blood pressure, blood flow, and pain (Goats & Kier 1991, Kaada & Torsteinbo 1989, Brattberg 1999).

Skin rolling can be used in a number of ways. The varying effects depend on the amount of force used and the way in which it is combined with other therapeutic tools. Where it works with the feeling of tissue tension (end-feel), its effect will progress from a relaxing technique to an autonomic reflex effect. Where it stretches beyond the end-feel, gradually increasing the tension felt by the therapist, it will have a mechanical stretching effect. The authors have called these three different applications of skin rolling: grades 1, 2 and 3, respectively, for clarity within the text. There has been little scientific study on the effects of skin rolling as a separate technique to other bodywork approaches. For example, Fitzgerald et al. (2009) conducted a feasibility study, which compared myofascial therapy (including a derivative of CTM) against 'global therapeutic massage' in male and female patients who were suffering from chronic pelvic pain (possibly involving symptoms including interstitial cystitis, painful bladder syndrome), and reported results which warrant further study. In addition to the feasibility results, there were some positive clinical results in both groups, the myofascial group being slightly better, but inferences in relation to effectiveness of skin rolling or CTM are very limited.

Objectives

The problems likely to respond positively will fit into four categories:

1. Visceral problems such as chronic postoperative pain: CTM can be used to reduce sympathetic overactivity and therefore pain (Holey 2000).
2. Hormonal problems such as pre-menstrual syndrome or menopausal symptoms. CTM is used supra-segmentally to enhance autonomic imbalance and reduce symptoms (Holey 2000).
3. Pain manifesting as musculoskeletal pain. This may be local and mechanical, such as chronic low back pain or intractable nerve root pain, but it may be secondary to a visceral 'event' such as surgery and is a result of sympathetic irritation through the spinal segment or zonal changes. Shin splints/anterior compartment syndrome, which shows tight fascia and altered circulation, responds well to CTM. Thickened, adherent (not keloid) or painful scars can respond very well to skin rolling (Fourie 2012). Pain caused by postural imbalance or movement dysfunction, thought to be due to tightening along the fascial train can be helped by grade 3 skin rolling.
4. Autonomic imbalance shown by fatigue (parasympathetic) or irritability, sleeplessness (sympathetic) that is not caused by other

medical problems. Myofascial therapy practitioners will use grade 3 skin rolling in these cases (Andrade 2013).

CTM is most effective where there is autonomic imbalance contributing to symptoms and this is more certain when the symptoms fit into three or four of the categories above.

The aims of treatment are to:
- Reduce pain – through post-synaptic inhibition of pain impulses
- Increase circulation – by enhanced sympathetic stimulation to blood vessels
- Normalize the tissues in zonal areas and in connected dermatomes by reducing tension and swelling, and stretching tissues at the interfaces
- Balancing the sympathetic and parasympathetic components of the ANS.

The therapist must have the ability to distinguish these symptoms from the same ones that, in a different pattern, result from conditions requiring medical attention. This is possible through an in-depth understanding of pathophysiology, patient examination and clinical reasoning.

Skin rolling is a versatile technique that can be included within a variety of therapeutic approaches. Within massage, it is a soothing and relaxing grade 1 stroke. It can be used at grade 2 by myofascial therapists, bodyworkers and trigger point therapists as part of a range of strokes that are aimed at loosening and stretching tightened fascia and thereby potentially influencing the whole of the fascial network. When it pushes into grade 3, it stimulates the ANS.

Assessment

Assessment should follow the approach normally taken by the individual therapist. In patients presenting for physical therapy, osteopathy or chiropractic, for example, the pain and dysfunction presented will often appear to have a musculoskeletal component. CTM 'cues' should be listened for during the **subjective** assessment, which should include questions eliciting the extent of autonomic imbalance. Pain that does not follow a dermatomal distribution or worsens during menstruation or bouts of constipation is an indicator, as is paresthesia – burning, tingling or a sensation of crawling or water running under the skin, which is reproduced when palpating thickened tissues around the sacrum. Other signs of autonomic imbalance include an inability to sleep and relax. The balance between fluid input and output may be inadequate as when a patient drinks copious amounts of coffee but only empties the bladder twice in a whole day and has 'puffy' ankles. The symptoms may have started following a 'visceral event' such as a kidney infection or surgery.

During the objective assessment, in addition to the usual tests, the recognition of skin and subcutaneous tissue changes in CT zones (Holey & Watson 1995) signal autonomic dysfunction and are used to confirm the subjective impression that autonomic imbalance is contributing significantly to the patient's symptoms. They are most easily observed on the back. The patient should sit with the back exposed down to the coccyx, with ankles, knees and hips flexed to 90° and fully supported. The lumbar spine should be slightly extended but not hyperextended, to place the connective tissues under comfortable tension. The tissue changes will become apparent when,

after approximately 30 seconds the tissues have adjusted against gravity. Chronic fascial tension is seen as an in-drawn area, surrounded by tissue fluid. More acute changes tend to show in superficial swellings.

The symptoms described by the patient should be linked with potential causative factors in the history and the relevant active zones to gain an understanding of how the pain, stiffness, autonomic disturbance and CT changes have created and perpetuate each other. This will inform a reasoned treatment plan.

Mechanisms

The theoretical model of physiological mechanisms underpinning CTM

CTM produces both mechanical and reflex effects, but is understood to work by mechanisms that are distinct from traditional massage techniques. Whilst CTM produces an immediate local response of swelling, it seems that the main mechanisms of action are neurophysiological via the ANS, which is stimulated at the fascial interfaces.

It is believed that when problems or imbalances in the CT zones occur, they change the discharge frequency of neurons. Other cells in the spinal cord are chemically alerted and the synapse becomes 'irritated' and its transmission threshold becomes lowered. The ANS responds with a heightened state of activity which spills over throughout the spinal segment. This corresponds to the osteopathic 'facilitated segment' concept. CTM is proposed to normalize any tonic imbalance in parasympathetic and sympathetic activity, usually to increase parasympathetic and decrease sympathetic output (for which there is some evidence, see below).

CTM is understood to elicit a shear force at the connective tissue interfaces between skin and fascia. The precise mechanisms of action have not been clarified; it should be noted that well-controlled studies in the area are few in number, and much of the detailed theory needs further evidence. It is important that skin/fascial interfaces are targeted accurately to achieve the precise effects of CTM as distinguished from other soft tissue modalities. This is because these interfaces contain vascular plexi of blood vessels that are innervated by autonomic nerve endings (Holey 2000). Fascia itself is similarly well innervated (Simmonds et al. 2012). The precise detail of the site(s) of stimulation is lacking, and the theoretical model has changed slightly over the years. But it is believed that the shear force of CTM stimulates cutaneovisceral reflexes via the nerve endings surrounding the horizontal circulatory plexi, which in turn elicits a strong effect on the ANS (see Fig. 7.2). It has been proposed that the primary mechanism is via the sympathetic nervous system at vascular plexi, as most blood vessels have only sympathetic innervation. However, with our increasing knowledge of fascia, and with the awareness that the ANS receives input from various somatosensory afferents, it may be a broader set of receptors that are stimulated, including, for example, fascial or cutaneous mechanoreceptors.

Wherever the precise stimulus occurs, CTM seems to produce effects both general and segmental. The general (or supra-segmental) effect produces a more evenly balanced autonomic system, with feelings of relaxation, improved energy and sleep patterns. This may have some similarities with traditional massage, but the more potent effect of CTM also may be due to the release of endorphins. The segmental effect is believed to be a key factor in clinical treatment. It gives an improved functioning of tissues linked by the same spinal segment of the reflex zone under treatment. This can be seen as enhanced hydration and texture of the skin, increased circulation, better muscle tone and visceral function. Alongside this, pain improves and there is lowered tissue stiffness, which, as Pohl (2010) speculates based on viewing ultrasound scans after manipulating the skin, could be partially due to a wider distribution of tissue fluid in the dermis with relaxation of skin fibroblasts.

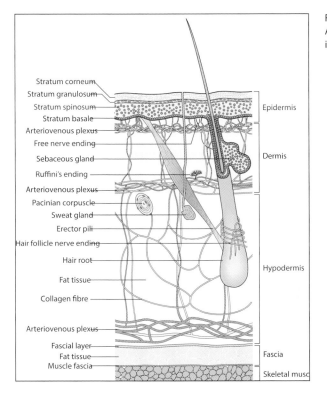

FIGURE 7.2 Layers of the skin and circulatory plexi. Adapted from Holey & Cook 1995, originally published in Schuh 1992.

Stratum corneum
Stratum granulosum
Stratum spinosum
Stratum basale
Arteriovenous plexus
Free nerve ending
Sebaceous gland
Ruffini's ending
Arteriovenous plexus
Pacinian corpuscle
Sweat gland
Erector pili
Hair follicle nerve ending
Hair root
Fat tissue
Collagen fibre
Arteriovenous plexus
Fascial layer
Fat tissue
Muscle fascia

Epidermis
Dermis
Hypodermis
Fascia
Skeletal muscle

Evidence for the proposed mechanisms and effects of CTM

There is not a large volume of high quality scientific evidence for the **proposed mechanisms** of CTM. Some studies have shown measurable physiological responses in autonomic function from CTM.

- Holey et al. (2011) observed an immediate moderate increase in diastolic (but not systolic) blood pressure in healthy women after a single CTM session. No change in heart rate or foot temperature was seen.
- Kisner and Taslitz (1968) also showed that CTM increased sympathetic activity, with the effect seemingly on diastolic blood pressure.
- In contrast, Reed and Held (1988) found no effects in healthy people.
- Horstkotte et al. (1967) investigated the effect of CTM in men with occlusive arterial disease. The group (n=18) receiving CTM showed an immediate reduction in peripheral blood flow followed by an increase after 2 weeks.
- Thirty minutes of CTM in people with various types of pain caused moderate increases in levels of plasma beta-endorphins, but not in the vasodilator vasoactive intestinal polypeptide (Kaada & Torsteinbo 1989).

Regarding the different types of CTM strokes, there is evidence of a physiological difference in the effects of the fascial and the preparatory flashige techniques (see *Protocol* below). Holey et al. (2011) report that fascial technique produces an observable reddening of the skin and an increase in skin temperature, from 15 minutes after treatment, lasting at least an hour (the end of data collection). This was not observed with the flashige technique (see below).

As some of the studies of CTM on the ANS have been carried out on healthy participants, it must be remembered that if CTM is proposed to rebalance the ANS, then little effect may be expected in healthy people and greater responses may occur in clinical groups. Much more research is needed to determine the detailed mechanisms of CTM.

Regarding the **clinical effects** of CTM in patient groups, good scientific evidence is rare. This is because the majority of published CTM clinical studies are limited in either applying CTM alongside another treatment or in being uncontrolled or case studies. Combined studies add little to the evidence base for CTM; inferences cannot be made about the actual CTM effect. Uncontrolled studies have various potential problems such as placebo effects. Currently, the authors know of only three controlled studies of CTM from which inferences can be made about clinically relevant outcome measures in patient groups.

- A high quality study, in which 98 people with type 2 diabetes and peripheral arterial disease were randomized to receive CTM or a placebo control for 15 weeks, was carried out by Castro-Sanchez et al. (2011). They found the CTM group displayed significant improvements in various outcomes such as differential segmental blood pressure, blood flow, temperature and oxygen saturation at the foot, and walking distance scores. The improvements in most measures were still observed after a year.
- A trial of 34 lower limb amputees with Buerger's disease by Ülger et al. (2002) randomized participants to three groups: CTM; interferential therapy; or control (all groups received the control intervention of exercise and prosthetic training). Although no between-group statistical comparisons were carried out, the reduction in pain was significant in all three groups, but of a lower magnitude in the control group.
- In a randomized trial of the effect of 10 weeks of CTM in 48 people with fibromyalgia (Brattberg 1999), it was reported that current pain was significantly better in the CTM group (but average pain did not differ between groups) as was quality of life as measured by the Fibrositis Impact Questionnaire. Hospital Anxiety and Depression Scale scores also showed a trend for a difference between the groups.

Overall, the evidence base for the proposed mechanisms and effects of CTM is small and further research would be welcomed.

Protocol

The contraindications to CTM are: acute inflammation; active infection; malignancy; unstable blood pressure/heart conditions; haemorrhage;

early or late stage pregnancy (some prefer not to treat pregnant women at all); where a resultant heavy menstrual flow would be unacceptable to the patient; and use of anxiolytic drugs.

The fascial stroke is easiest if the patient is sitting, as described above. The preparatory strokes can be applied with the patient side lying. The therapist sits behind.

The therapist should choose from three preparatory strokes (see also p. 125):

- **Skin (haut) technique (Fig. 7.3b)** – a rapid, light brushing with the fingertips to reduce skin tenderness.
- **Flat/shallow (flashige) technique (Fig. 7.3c)** – like the fascial stroke at the fascial interface, to but not beyond the end-feel. It is recommended that this is carried out prior to fascial strokes, but not usually in the same treatment.
- **Subcutaneous (unterhaut) technique (Fig 7.3d)** – a light pushing of the skin layers on the fascia, not quite to the end-feel. This reduces tension in the skin and ensures that subsequent attempts to access the fascial layer is achievable and comfortable to the patient.

The preparatory strokes may be performed for the first two or more sessions, if necessary.

The fascial stroke (Fig.7.3a).

The pad of the middle finger (or the thumb if the patient is side-lying) makes contact with the skin and the distal interphalangeal joint is flexed until the fingertip, but not the nail, is on the skin and the tension in the skin layers is gathered up. Tension is felt at the skin–fascial interface. The therapist then slowly and gently lifts the tissues against gravity into the end-feel but not sufficiently to cause pain. After a pause, the tissue is released. Each stroke is repeated up to six times. The strokes follow the prescribed pattern known to access the fascia in superficial places (Fig. 7.4). The 'basic section' is always treated first, to avoid overstimulating the sympathetic nervous system. This is the section from the coccyx tip to the lower costal margin. With many patients, the symptoms resolve without leaving this area, otherwise progression is in following the affected zones or, in the case

of limb symptoms (such as chronic nerve root pain), the dermatomes.

The principles of treatment are:

1. **The skin must be displaced in relation to the underlying layer.** This creates a shear force at the tissue interface which stimulates mechanoreceptors. It also activates mast cell secretion, including histamine, nitric oxide, vasoactive intestinal polypeptide (a vasodilator) and heparin. The CTM fascial stroke should produce a triple response reaction of reddening and swelling in a line (wheal) as these cells are present in large numbers around blood vessels (Theoharides et al. 2010). Inaccurate or excessive strokes will produce skin irritation and discomfort.

2. **Work caudad to cephalad.** Treatment should start at the apex of the sacrum, to reduce potential unwanted reactions, which, if the principles are not followed, can include dizziness and sweating, fainting, extreme tiredness or irritability and restlessness. These effects are often delayed and uncontrolled, so must be avoided. They are most likely to happen if the skin is over dense sympathetically-supplied areas (such as between the scapulae). To desensitize the skin area, which is reflexively linked to the parasympathetic nervous system, the 'bladder zone' (as the bladder has a parasympathetic nerve supply) should be treated first. This reduces sympathetic activity.

3. **Work superficial to deep.** A shear force is applied to the interface between the deep fascia, the target tissue, and the skin, to create a potent autonomic effect. The treatment will be painful where edema is in superficial fascia and skin, or there is excess skin tension. Pain increases sympathetic activity so will undermine achievement of the intended outcomes. Adverse reactions are avoided by use of preparatory strokes which remove tissue fluid and tension.

4. **Target appropriate tissue interfaces to stimulate the fascia.** As well as using recommended stroke patterns, which correlate to places where the deep fascia lies

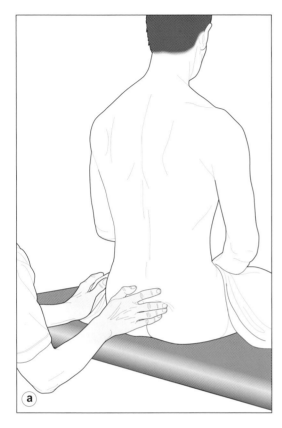

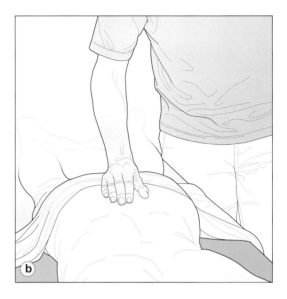

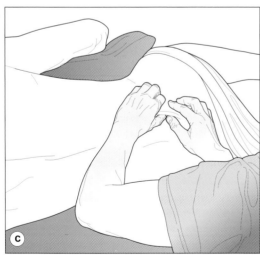

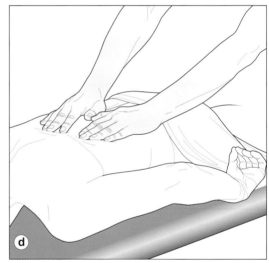

FIGURE 7.3 The four strokes of CTM.

superficially under the skin, the correct tissue interface should be targeted, to reduce the possibility of unwanted reactions and making the treatment as effective as possible. Stimulation of the deep fascia is recognized when a non-painful sharp or 'cutting' sensation is felt by the patient.

As the effects are delayed, progress is not normally seen immediately after treatment, so thorough evaluation at the next session is vital. For this reason, treatments are best spaced over 3 consecutive days until the sensitivity of response is understood by the therapist. Thereafter, twice weekly is acceptable although beneficial results have been seen by the author on once-weekly treatments over 6 weeks. Positive effects should be apparent by the third treatment otherwise the treatment should be stopped. Sessions should stop when improvement reaches a plateau and this will vary between individuals.

Skin rolling (Fig. 7.5).

The therapist places her hands on the skin with the thumbs abducted and the fingers adducted, forming a kite-shaped space between the index fingers and thumbs. Contact is made with the skin and the fingers pulled towards the thumbs, bringing a roll of tissue with them. This tissue can contain skin or muscle. The fingers relax their pressure, allowing the thumbs to gently push the tissue roll forward, avoiding pinching the tissues. By the time the thumb tips have met the index fingers, the roll has virtually disappeared (Holey & Cook 2011). Keeping the thumbs in contact with the skin, the fingers lift and are replaced along the aspect being treated, so the hands 'roll and walk, roll and walk'.

The direction of roll varies with the underlying anatomy, against the tension lines, to maximize the mobility of the skin. Muscle and tendons can also be rolled in this manner. A grade 1 skin roll will roll the layers of skin on each other in a gentle technique. Grade 2 will go deeper into the tissues, and roll the skin loosely on the fascial layer. Grade 3 will roll into the end-feel at the interface between the skin and fascia and care must be taken not to push into pain. The therapist must be aware of potential autonomic effects. To roll muscle, the muscle belly is grasped, beyond the depth of the fascia. This is a deep technique and less mobility will normally be expected.

Progression of treatment is dictated by the symptoms, but the stroke can be applied across adherent scars, moved around an area of tightness or recovering injury or over the whole of the skin in a relaxing massage.

Effects on the fascia

These techniques rely on accurately targeting the interface between the tissue layers and the fascial stroke of CTM and grade 3 skin rolling

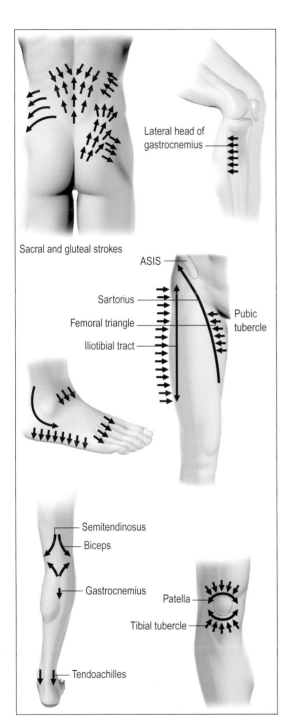

Sacral and gluteal strokes

Lateral head of gastrocnemius

ASIS

Sartorius

Femoral triangle

Iliotibial tract

Pubic tubercle

Semitendinosus

Biceps

Gastrocnemius

Patella

Tibial tubercle

Tendoachilles

FIGURE 7.4 The pattern of CTM strokes, based on work by E. Dicke and H. Tierich-Leube.

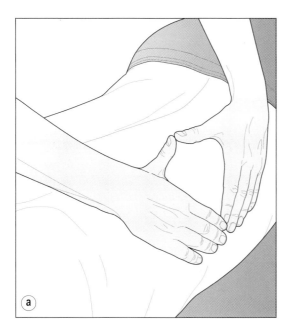

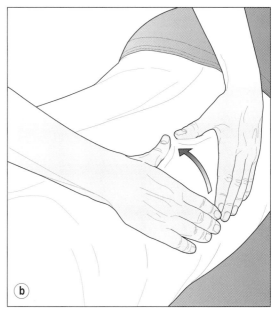

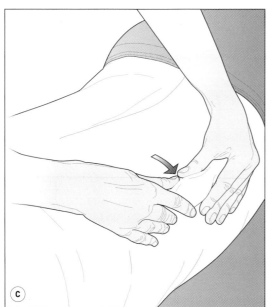

FIGURE 7.5 Skin rolling.

will primarily influence the ANS. The patient describes a feeling of looseness – for example, being able to bend more easily the next day, which could be a result of increasing circulation at the interface. The effects on the fascia it-

self by these techniques are not proven, but the theories include:

- A stretch in one part of the fascial network may influence other parts of the fascial network, along fascial 'trains' which describe pathways of force transmission (Myers 2009).

- The biotensegrity model whereby altering the tension in one part of the fascial network improves force transmission and improves movement (Levin & Martin 2012).

- The mechanostimulatory effects on the fascial myofibroblasts may impact positively on tissue stiffness. The enhanced circulation caused by stimulation at the horizontal circulatory plexus at the fascial-skin interface may have an anti-inflammatory effect on the myofibroblasts, reducing fascial tone (Schleip et al. 2012).

- Shear forces on the blood vessel wall are known to release nitric oxide (NO) and it has been suggested that NO also may relax myofibroblasts (Schleip et al. 2012).

- The cytokine TGF-β1, a myofibroblast stimulator, is increased by sympathetic stimulation. CTM balances the ANS in a parasympathetic direction, so it is possible that as it

Exercise

CT zone recognition

Ask your model/patient to sit as for a CT assessment (see Fig. 7.3a) in a very good light.

Support feet so the hips and knees are at 90°.

Observe: look at the contours of the body surface, thinking about the underlying muscles. Take those into account when you observe any indrawn areas of tissue, subtle swellings (puffiness), skin folds.

Palpate: place the flat of your fingertips on the skin and move the skin on the underlying fascial layer, pushing upwards against gravity until you feel the fascial tension. Note any discrepancies between the right and left sides. Look at the fold of skin above your fingers – is it the same on both sides? Look at the tension gathered up below your fingers – does it stop where you expect the restrictions of bone to be or is it within the skin itself?

Now gather a roll of skin between your fingertips and thumb and gently roll upwards on either side of the spine. Do areas where the roll starts to be lost due to underlying tension match your previous findings? Can you see any parts of the skin having an 'orange peel' appearance?

Now very gently tap any apparent puffy areas. Can you observe tiny ripples of fluid in the skin?

Compare your findings with the Head CT zones map (Fig. 7.1) and see if you can identify any zones.

reduces sympathetic activity, this reduces levels of TGF-β1 (see Ch. 1), which in turn reduces fascial contractility and creates a feeling of looseness in the fascia (Bhowmick et al. 2009).

References

Andrade C-K 2013 Outcome-based massage. Lippincott Williams and Wilkins, Philadelphia

Brattberg G 1999 Connective tissue massage in the treatment of fibromyalgia. Eur J Pain-London 3: 235–244

Bhowmick S, Singh A, Flavell RA et al 2009 The sympathetic nervous system modulates CD4(+)FoxP3(+) regulatory T cells via a TGF-beta-dependant mechanism. J Leukocyte Biol 86:1275–1283

Castro-Sanchez AM, et al 2011 Connective tissue reflex massage for type 2 diabetic patients with peripheral arterial disease: randomized controlled trial. Evid Based Complement Alternat Med (eCAM) 8: 1–12

FitzGerald MP, Anderson RU, Potts J et al 2009 Randomized multicenter feasibility trial of myofascial physical therapy for the treatment of urological chronic pelvic pain syndromes. J Urol 182: 570–580

Fourie W 2012 Surgery and scarring. In: Schleip et al (eds) Fascia: the tensional network of the human body. Churchill Livingstone Elsevier, Edinburgh

Goats GC, Kier KA 1991 Connective tissue massage. Br J Sports Med 25:131–133

Head H 1898 'Die Sensibilitaetsstoerungen der Haut bei Viszeral Erkrankungen.' Berlin. Cited in: Bischoff I, Elminger G 1963 'Connective tissue massage' in Licht S (ed) Massage, manipulation and traction. Waverley Press, Baltimore, pp 57–83

Holey LA 1995 Connective tissue manipulation: towards a scientific rationale. Physiotherapy 81: 730–9

Holey EA 2000 Connective tissue massage: a bridge between complementary and orthodox approaches. J Bodyw Mov Ther 4: 72–80

Holey EA 2006 Connective-tissue manipulations. In: Carriere B, Feldt CM (eds) The pelvic floor. Georg Thieme Verlag, Stuttgart

Holey LA, Watson M 1995 Inter-rater reliability of connective tissue zone recognition Physiotherapy 81: 369–72

Holey E, Cook E 2011 Evidence-based therapeutic massage. A practical guide for therapists, 3rd edn. Churchill Livingstone Elsevier, Edinburgh

Holey LA, Dixon J, Selfe J 2011 An exploratory thermographic investigation of the effects of connective tissue massage on autonomic function. J Manipulative Physiol Ther 34: 457–462

Horstkotte W, Klempien EJ, Scheppokat KD 1967 Skin temperature and blood flow changes in occlusive arterial disease under physiological and pharmacological therapy. Angiology 18: 1–5

Kaada B, Torsteinbo O 1989 Increase of plasma beta-endorphins in connective tissue massage. General Pharmacology 20: 487–489

Kisner CD, Taslitz N 1968 Connective tissue massage: influence of the introductory treatment on autonomic functions. Phys Ther 48:107–119

Levin SM, Martin D-C 2012 Biotensegrity the mechanics of fascia. In: Schleip et al (eds) Fascia: the tensional network of the human body. Churchill Livingstone Elsevier, Edinburgh

Myers T 2009 Anatomy Trains, 2nd edn. Churchill Livingstone Elsevier, Edinburgh

Pohl H 2010 Changes in the structure of collagen distribution in the skin caused by a manual technique. J Bodyw Mov Ther 14: 27–34

Reed BV, Held JM 1988 Effects of sequential connective tissue massage on autonomic nervous system of middle-aged and elderly adults. Phys Ther 68:1231–1234

Schuh I 1992 Bindegewebsmassage. Fischer-Verlag, Stuttgart

Schleip R, Jager H, Klinger W 2012 Fascia is alive. Schleip et al (eds) Fascia: the tensional network of the human body. Churchill Livingstone Elsevier, Edinburgh

Simmonds N, Miller P, Gemmell H 2012 A theoretical framework for the role of fascia in manual therapy J Bodyw Mov Ther 16:(1) 83–93

Theoharides TC et al 2010 Mast cells and inflammation. Biochim Biophys Acta 1822, 2010:21–33

Ülger OG, Yigiter K, Sener G 2002 The effect of physiotherapy approaches on the pain patterns of amputees for Buerger's disease. Pain Clinic 14: 217

USE IT OR LOSE IT: RECOMMENDATIONS FOR FASCIA-ORIENTED TRAINING APPLICATIONS IN SPORTS AND MOVEMENT THERAPY

Robert Schleip, Divo Gitta Müller

Introduction

In sports science as well as in recent sports education, the prevailing emphasis had been on the classical tirade of muscular training, cardiovascular conditioning and neuromuscular coordination (Jenkins 2005). Comparatively little attention had been given to a specifically targeted training of the involved connective tissues. This common practice is in contrast to the role that the muscular connective tissues play in sports associated overuse injuries. Whether in running, soccer, baseball, swimming or dancing, the vast majority of associated repetitive strain injuries occur in the collagenous connective tissues – such as tendons, ligaments or joint capsules – which seem to be less adequately prepared and less well adapted to their loading challenge than their muscular or skeletal counterparts (Renström & Johnson 1985, Hyman & Rodeo 2000, Counsel & Breidahl 2010).

This chapter offers evidence and insights into the role, and the potential for the training, of the muscular connective (i.e. fascial) tissues, involved in sport and movement activities.

Sports science discovers fascia

A range of sometimes confusing words and terms have been used to describe connective tissues in different contexts (Schleip et al. 2013). This chapter follows the terminology suggested by Findley (2012), since it is most suitable for analyzing multijoint force-transmission and the proprioceptive properties of fascial tissues. Here all fibrous collagenous connective tissues, which are part of a body-wide interconnected tensional network, are recognized as fascial tissues. Joint capsules, intramuscular connective tissues, ligaments, and tendons are seen merely as local specifications of this tension-resistant fibrous network. Dense planar connective tissues with a multidirectional fiber arrangement, often referred to as 'proper fascia', are not regarded as separate functional entities but as gradual continuations of adjacently positioned specialized tissues, such as retinaculae, septi or aponeuroses (Schleip et al. 2012.

While electromyography allowed a precise measurement of muscular activity, until recently the assessment of fascial properties was mostly confined to subjective evaluations. However, advances in ultrasound measurement as well as in histology have resulted in a drastic increase of fascia-related studies within the field of sports medicine. The first congress on 'Connective tissues in sports medicine', hosted at Ulm University in 2013, has defined the dynamic impetus of this rapidly growing field. While earlier studies on Australian kangaroos had already shown that their impressive jumps of up to 13 meters are mostly due to the high storage capacity of their tendons (Kram & Dawson 1998), more recent ultrasound examinations in running and jumping humans revealed that the latter also express a similarly impressive elastic 'catapult capacity' in the Achilles tendon and related aponeuroses (Sawicki et al. 2009). At least when assessed in our current Western movement culture, the elastic storage quality in running and hopping tends to be highest between 13 and 16 years of age and then subsequently decreases as we age (Legramandi et al. 2013).

The higher storage capacity of collagenous tissues in young people is associated with a stronger crimp expression within their collagen fibers (Torp et al. 1975). Adequately tailored exercise in older rats has been shown to re-introduce a similar crimp formation as is present in younger ones (Wood et al. 1988). Similarly, it has been shown that the elastic storage capacity in human tendons can be significantly improved by regularly repeated strong mechanical loading of these tissues (Reeves et al. 2006) (Fig.8.1).

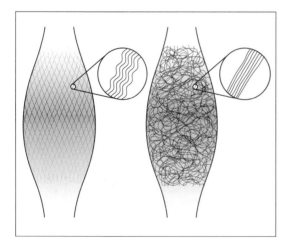

FIGURE 8.1 Collagen fiber architecture is responsive to mechanical loading. Healthy fasciae (left image) express a clear two-directional (lattice) orientation of their collagen fiber network and their fibers show a stronger crimp formation. Lack of exercise, on the other hand, tends to induce a multi-directional fiber architecture and a reduction in crimp formation, leading to a loss of springiness and elastic recoil (right image). *Illustration with friendly permission of FASCIAL-FITNESS.COM.*

Habitual barefoot running seems to involve a higher storage capacity within the lower leg when compared to shod running (Tam et al. 2013). Interestingly this is less the case when running with minimalistic shoes (Bonacci et al. 2013), possibly due to the role of proprioceptive stimulation involvement by barefoot contact with the ground. However, transition to more natural footwear should be performed more gradually than is even recommended by conservative instructions due to the high likelihood of overuse injuries such as bone marrow edema during the change-over time (Ridge et al. 2013). Renewal of fascial tissues is a relatively slow process, taking several months and more (Neuberger & Slack 1953, Babraj et al. 2005).

Plyometric training, also referred to as 'jump training,' is hardly new in the field of sports education. The prevailing theory had been that the involved stretch–shortening cycle in these movements leads to increased motor unit activation via the myotatic stretch reflex (Wilk et al. 1993). In contrast to this muscular-oriented explanation focus, a more recent examination demonstrated that a plyometric training for 14 weeks leads to a significant increase in the passive component of the series elastic component (mainly involving the tendon structures) and an associated decrease in the active part of the muscular contraction (Fouré et al. 2011). Congruently, an increase in tendon cross-sectional diameter could be observed in response to plyometric training (Houghton et al. 2013) signifying that the adaptational response included a morphological tissue adaptation within the tendon.

Due to methodological difficulties the high expression of elastic recoil properties of fascial tissues in humans had been proven – until recently – for lower leg structures only. The impressive study by Roach et al. (2013) has now extended that to the human shoulder girdle: his team demonstrated that the ability of humans to throw projectiles at much higher speed – compared with other primates – involves an increased elastic energy storage in the human shoulder girdle structures, and that this capacity is associated with anatomical changes that evolved 2 million years ago during the evolution of the species *Homo erectus,* which probably provided a significant survival benefit in the hunter and gatherer conditions of our ancestors.

Training of elastic recoil properties

The commonly accepted Wolff's law states that dense connective tissues are able to adapt their morphology to mechanical loading. While this general law had originally been developed with a main focus on skeletal tissues, Davis' law applies this general principle particularly to soft connective tissues. It proposes that these tissues tend to adapt their architecture to the specific mechanical demands imposed on them, provided that these demands are strong enough, and occur in a regular manner (Nutt 1913). More recently this concept has been taken further by the mechanostat theory of Harold Frost, emphasizing that tendons, ligament and fascia adapt their cross-sectional diameter and correspondingly also their stiffness in response to the muscular forces imposed onto them (Frost 1972). However the threshold value of mechanical loading to trigger adaptational effects for tendon is significantly higher for tendons than for muscle. While exercises performed at only 50% of maximum voluntary contraction power are sufficient for triggering an adaptational response in muscle fibers, the involved tendinous connective tissues show very little adaptational response at that impact level; they do require much stronger loads in order to respond. Arampatzis et al. (2007) have shown that for the Achilles tendon and aponeuroses a strain of 4–5% tends to be required for eliciting an adaptational response, while a strain of 2–3% is clearly not sufficient. Note that the high impact loading required for an adaptational response may then be only 35% below the amount of strain at which tendon injuries do occur (Wren et al. 2001)

Once the necessary threshold (of approximately 4–5% strain) has been reached, the adaptational response of the fibroblasts seems to be largely independent of the quantity of strain application involved in an exercise session. It is possible that only five or 10 elastic bounces may be required

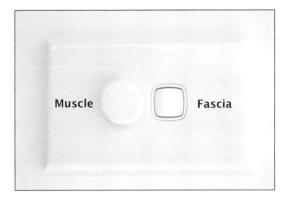

FIGURE 8.2 Simplified analogy for the different responsiveness of myofiber and collagen remodelling. Myofibers respond in a dose-dependent manner to the amount of loading. The stronger these fibers are loaded during training, the more effectively the training effect will be in terms of an increased muscle size and strength. In contrast the training response of collagen renewal works more like a flip switch that turns on a light in an on-off manner. However, the threshold of this flip switch is fairly high and usually demands stronger impacts than are normally applied during daily life situations. *Illustration with friendly permission of FASCIAL-FITNESS.COM (modified from istockphoto.com/0263938).*

for an adaptational response, while adding 100 or more repetitions tends to have very little additional effect (Magnusson et al. 2010) (Fig.8.2).

Based on these considerations suggestions for fascia-oriented movement training have recently been described (Schleip & Müller 2013). These recommendations consist of four basic application forms, which will be discussed in the remainder of this chapter:

- elastic recoil
- fascial stretch
- fascial release
- proprioceptive refinement.

Among these, elastic recoil exercises deserves primary attention.

An example of such exercises is given in Figure 8.3. Note that for an optimal utilization of elastic recoil properties the main movement should be initiated with a preparatory counter movement in the opposite direction.

- Figure 8.3 shows a backward stretch and swing of the arms and tool (Fig 8.3a) prior to the forward swinging motion.

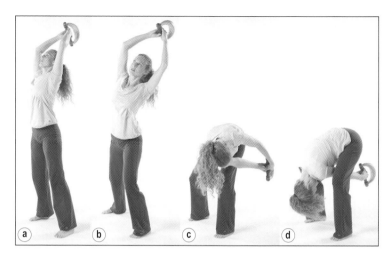

FIGURE 8.3 (a–d) Example of an elastic recoil exercise: the Flying Sword. The movement is initiated by a preparatory counter movement (pre-stretch in the opposite direction). Various angular variations are explored during repetitively swinging applications. *Illustration with friendly permission of FASCIAL-FITNESS.COM.*

- The subsequent forward movement (Fig. 8.3b) is then initiated, involving a proximal body part, such as the pelvis or sternum.
- Finally, this proximal initiation is followed by the more distal body parts in a sequentially delayed manner, similar to the orchestration in a flexible whip (Fig. 8.3b–d).
- More advanced practitioners can be instructed to experiment with two additional steps before commencing:
  - Before the preparatory counter movement a softening and refinement of the somatic perception is initiated. For the duration of one relaxed breath or more the practitioner will go into a state of open attention, checking his body for any unnecessary muscular holding patterns and fostering a sense of curious attention for detecting small details in their perception during the subsequent phases.
  - This is followed by a subtle multidirectional spatial expansion, which is envisioned to involve an extension of the body-wide 'diving suit' being made up of the most superficial layer of dense fasciae covering the whole body. For the thorax this may involve a minute increase in width, depth and length (of only few millimetres each) while it may also be accompanied by an almost invisible extension of the limbs. While this second step is often referred to as 'iron shirt' in martial arts practices, it can also be

seen as an increase in tensegrity-like omnidirectional pre-tension in the body wide fascial network (Levin & Martin 2012).

Interestingly, such expansional movements tend to trigger potentially important psychological, behavioral and endocrine-related alterations; studies by Carney et al. (2010) demonstrated an increase in testosterone levels as well as a decrease in cortisol – in as little as 1 minute after a voluntary postural change, as described. These changes have been shown to result in increased feelings of power and tolerance for risk.

Table 8.1 Steps in an ideal orchestration of fascial elegance

Step	Emphasis
Pre 1	Open attention
Pre 2	Tensegral expansion
1	Preparatory counter movement
2	Proximal initiation
3	Distal delay

Listening to the acoustic feedback in many elastic recoil movements can be a helpful guide. The less sound is created by the practitioner – e.g. in jumping barefoot on the ground – the better. In analogy to the legendary Ninja warriors, who supposedly moved without making any sounds, this feature is referred to as 'Ninja quality' in fascial training.

Timing and rhythm are crucial in elastic recoil movement. This was impressively shown in the investigation of Heglund et al. (1995) with women from West Africa, who can carry large loads on their heads without any additional energy expenditure due to their pendulum-like storage and release of kinetic energy during gait. When testing these women in a laboratory environment it was revealed that their impressive energy consumption was dependent on walking at their preferred speed. When asked to walk at different speeds than they had intuitively chosen, the women expressed the same load-dependent increase in energy expenditure as was found in untrained Western control subjects.

In elastically swinging recoil motions the ideal speed and rhythm are dependent on the inherent resonant frequency, which itself is a product of the material stiffness as well as the pendulum length. This suggests that a particular musical dance rhythm may allow some dancers to swing, hop and bounce with minimal energy expenditure, while another rhythm may be better suited for other dancers. In addition, a voluntary adjustment of pendulum length and of fascial stiffness (via muscular contraction) may also allow a partial adjustment of the dancer's resonant frequencies towards the given external rhythm.

This suggests that elastic recoil movements can result in higher loads being safely imposed on fascial tissues. However, this should not be performed without a proper warm-up (as with the other training elements described below) as well as with a heightened somatic mindfulness. Following the findings of Magnusson et al. (2010) such loading is recommended, once or twice per week only, in order to lead towards an optimal collagen renewal.

Stretching recommendations for fascial health

Figure 8.4 a shows an example of a fascia-oriented stretch application. Following the excellent review of pandiculating movements in animals by Bertolucci (2011), the practitioner is asked to explore expansional stretch variations that involve several joints and are felt in large membranous fascial areas. Rather than precisely repeated muscular elongations, angular variations should be explored. While 'melting' stretches, in which the elongated muscles are intentionally relaxed, are utilized to reach intramuscular connective tissues as well as extramuscular connections between different muscle bellies, dynamic (more active) stretches can be added in which the elongated muscle fibers are simultaneously activated in order to reach the more serially arranged tendinous structures (Schleip & Müller 2013).

The benefits of such stretching depend on the application context. While static stretches tend to decrease vertical jump height immediately afterwards, dynamic stretching can have a positive effect on this performance (Hough et al. 2009). Dynamic stretching, as examined here, can include mini-bounces in the long-stretched position, i.e. at the end-range position at which the targeted myofascial tissues are maximally stretched. These mini-bounces should be performed in a soft and mindful manner, utilizing

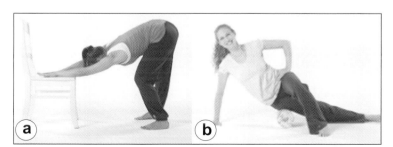

FIGURE 8.4 Examples of fascial stretch and fascial release. The so-called 'cat stretch' simulates the pandiculations observed in cats and other feline predators. (a) Use of a foam roller on the other side exemplifies the fascial release applications, in which fascial tissues– here the iliotibial tract – can be subjected to sponge-like squeezing in a 'slowmotion' manner. (b) *Illustrations with friendly permission of FASCIAL-FITNESS.COM.*

sinusoidal speed changes only rather than any abrupt and jerky accelerations or decelerations. Note that during the deceleration phase of such bounces the muscle fibers will be briefly activated in an eccentric manner, while hardly any muscle activation will then be necessary during the subsequent accelerating phase of each mini-bounce. For best results such gentle mini-bounces should be alternated with phases of melting stretches, performed for at least several breaths and possibly longer.

Melting stretches practiced throughout the year can provide health related range of motion benefits (Behm & Chaouachi 2011). A recent study on rats by Corey et al. (2012) demonstrated that static stretching may also have an anti-inflammatory effect when slowly applied to previously inflamed connective tissues.

Fascial release: use of foam rollers

Figure 8.4b demonstrates a typical fascial self-treatment using a foam roller. Such treatments have shown to improve range of motion (MacDonald et al. 2013). Additionally, in the treated fascial tissues a decreased arterial stiffness and improved endothelial function have been observed; both of which are most likely enhanced by the documented increased expression of the gaseous transmitter substance nitric oxide (Okamoto et al. 2013).

For a treatment of too flaccid fascial tissues, a more vigorous application using repeated rapid motions can be explored in order to increase local collagen production (Pohl 2010; see Ch. 7 on connective tissue manipulation). However, when working on chronic scar tissues, hypertoned fascial tissues and pathological adhesions, the implementation of super-slow rolling movements are recommended, which induce a low fluid shear-strain motion on the fibroblasts of the treated tissues (see Ch. 18 on the treatment of scarring). Such gentle fibroblast stimulation may subsequently trigger release of the enzyme MMP-1, a potent agent for desynthesizing collagen fibers (Zheng et al. 2012).

A crucial and indispensible ingredient: proprioceptive refinement

The body-wide fascial network has been described as a sensory organ (Schleip et al. 2012). Various authors have confirmed the presence of proprioceptive as well as nociceptive nerve endings in fascial tissues (van der Wal 2009, Stecco et al. 2008, Tesarz et al. 2011). Providing mechanical stimulation may stimulate polymodal receptors, belonging to so-called wide-dynamic-range neurons, which tend to provide an analgesic effect on the level of the spinal cord (Wang et al. 2012). Mindful attention to the local tissue stimulation can be a key factor in the therapeutic utilization of this mechanism (Moseley et al. 2008).

Bouncing movements can lead to increased likelihood of injury particularly when performed with an outwardly oriented high performance attitude. Clinical experience has shown that the probability of subsequent strain injuries is highest when showing these movements to middle-aged men with a high achievement orientation, accompanied by a lack of refined somatic perception. Proprioceptive refinement should be fostered in such individuals – and in all fascia-oriented movements.

To avoid the dampening function of the reticular formation – a portion of the central nervous system that inhibits the delay of sensory signals, which it considers 'as expected'– non-habitual fascial stimulations should be explored, using body positions and joint angulations that are rarely utilized during normal sedentary behaviour. In a comparative study of Alexander (2004) an intriguing correlation between joint usage and degenerative joint diseases was observed: the less a joint is utilized in the anatomically available range of motion, the more this joint is prone towards osteoarthritis, possibly due to lack of usage of an available range of joint motion. A chimpanzee-like creative usage of our available joint range

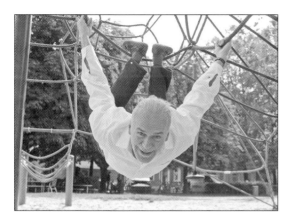

FIGURE 8.5 Stimulating ape-like loading of the anatomically available range of joint motion. Towards completion of the long hours of deskwork associated with the writing of this chapter, one of the authors explored a nearby children's playground for stimulating fascial stretches combined with some monkey-like swinging motions. ©*FASCIALNET.COM*.

of motion could possibly induce a similar healthy tissue physiology as is expressed in our arboreal relatives (Fig. 8.5).

Fascial fitness training: an important addition to general health care

Renewal of collagen tissues happens much slower than that of muscle fibers (Babraj et al. 2005). Application of the above described applications will therefore not be visible in a matter of weeks; it usually takes 3–9 months to see the tissue remodelling effects from the outside as well as 'feel' them in palpation. However, in contrast to muscular training the gained effects will not be lost as quickly (e.g. when having to stop training because of health or work-related reasons) and are therefore of a more long-lasting sustainable quality. Fascial training does not compete with neuromuscular or cardiovascular training, both of which can have very important health effects that are not possible with fascial training only.

In contrast, fascial training is suggested as a sporadic or regular addition to comprehensive movement training. It promises to lead towards remodelling of the body-wide fascial network in such a way that it works with increased effectiveness and refinement in terms of its kinetic storage capacity as well as a sensory organ for proprioception. Further research is necessary to validate whether it does indeed fulfil its basic promise of an increased protection against repetitive strain injuries in muscular connective tissues.

References

Alexander CJ 2004 Idiopathic osteoarthritis: time to change paradigms? Skeletal Radiol 33(6):321-324

Arampatzis A, Karamanidis K, Albracht K 2007 Adaptational responses of the human Achilles tendon by modulation of the applied cyclic strain magnitude. J Exp Biol 210(Pt 15): 2743-2753

Babraj JA et al 2005 Collagen synthesis in human musculoskeletal tissues and skin. J Physiol Endocrinol Metab 289(5): E864-869

Behm DG, Chaouachi A 2011 A review of the acute effects of static and dynamic stretching on performance. Eur J Appl Physiol 111(11):2633-2351

Bertolucci LF 2011 Pandiculation: nature's way of maintaining the functional integrity of the myofascial system? J Bodyw Mov Ther 15: 268-280

Bonacci J et al 2013 Running in a minimalist and lightweight shoe is not the same as running barefoot: a biomechanical study. Br J Sports Med 47(6): 387-392

Carney DR, Cuddy AJ, Yap A 2010 Power posing: brief nonverbal displays affect neuroendocrine levels and risk tolerance. J Psychol Sci 21(10):1363-8

Corey SM, Vizzard MA, Bouffard NA, Badger GJ, Langevin HM 2012 Stretching of the back improves gait, mechanical sensitivity and connective tissue inflammation in a rodent model. PLoS One 7, e29831

Counsel P, Breidahl W 2010 Muscle injuries of the lower leg. Seminars in Musculoskeletal Radiology 14, 162-175

Findley TW 2012 Fascia science and clinical applications: a clinician/researcher's perspectives. J Bodyw Mov Ther 16 (1): 64-66

Fouré A, Nordez A, McNair P, Cornu C 2011 Effects of plyometric training on both active and passive parts of the plantar flexors series elastic component stiffness of muscle-tendon complex. Eur J Appl Physiol 111(3):539-548

Frost MF 1972 The physiology of cartilaginous, fibrous, and bony tissue. C C Thomas, Springfield, IL

Heglund NC, Willems PA, Penta M, Cavagna GA 1995 Energy-saving gait mechanics with head-supported loads. Nature 375(6526):52-54

Hough PA, Ross EZ, Howatson G 2009 Effects of dynamic and static stretching on vertical jump performance and electromyographic activity. J Strength Cond Res 23(2):507-512

Houghton LA, Dawson BT, Rubenson J 2013 Effects of plyometric training on achilles tendon properties and shuttle running during a simulated cricket batting innings. J Strength Cond Res 27(4):1036-1046

Hyman J, Rodeo SA 2000 Injury and repair of tendons and ligaments. Physical Medicine and Rehabilitation Clinics of North America 11, 267e288

Jenkins S 2005 Sports science handbook. In: The essential guide to kinesiology. Sport & Exercise Science, vol. 1. Multi-science Publishing, Brentwood

Kram R, Dawson TJ 1998 Energetics and bio mechanics of locomotion by red kangaroos (Macropus rufus). Comparat Biochem Physiol B120, 41-49

Legramandi MA, Schepens B, Cavagna GA 2013 Running humans attain optimal elastic bounce in their teens. Sci Rep 3:1310

Levin P, Martin DC 2012 Biotensegrity: the mechanics of fascia. In: Schleip R, Findley T, Chaitow L, Huijing P (eds) Fascia: the tensional network of the human body. The science and clinical applications in manual and movement therapies. Churchill Livingstone Elsevier, Edinburgh, pp 137-146

Magnusson SP, Langberg H, Kjaer M 2010 The pathogenesis of tendinopathy: balancing the response to loading. Nature Reviews Rheumatology 6:262-268

MacDonald GZ et al 2013 An acute bout of self-myofascial release increases range of motion without a subsequent decrease in muscle activation or force. J Strength Cond Res 27(3):812-821

Moseley GL, Zalucki NM, Wiech K 2008 Tactile discrimination, but not tactile stimulation alone, reduces chronic limb pain. Pain 137:600-608

Neuberger A, Slack H 1953 The metabolism of collagen from liver, bones, skin and tendon in normal rats. Biochem J 53:47-52

Nutt JT 1913 Diseases and deformities of the foot. EB Treat, New York

Okamoto T, Masuhara M, Ikuta K 2013 Acute effects of self-myofascial release using a foam roller on arterial function. J Strength Cond Res: Epub ahead of print

Pohl H 2010 Changes in the structure of collagen distribution in the skin caused by a manual technique. J Bodyw Mov Ther 14(1):27-34

Reeves ND, Narici MV, Maganaris CN 2006 Myotendinous plasticity to aging and resistance exercise in humans. Exp Physiol 91:483-498

Renström P, Johnson RJ 1985 Overuse injuries in sports. A review. Sports Med 2: 316-333

Ridge ST et al 2013 Foot bone marrow edema after a 10-wk transition to minimalist running shoes. Med Sci Sports Exerc 45(7):1363-1368

Roach NT, Venkadesan M, Rainbow MJ, Lieberman DE 2013 Elastic energy storage in the shoulder and the evolution of high-speed throwing in Homo. Nature 498(7455): 483-486

Sawicki GS, Lewis CL, Ferris DP 2009 It pays to have a spring in your step. Exercise and Sport Sciences Reviews 37:130-138

Schleip R, Jäger H, Klingler W 2012 What is 'fascia'? A review of different nomenclatures. J Bodyw Mov Ther 16(4):496-502

Schleip R, Müller DG 2013 Training principles for fascial connective tissues: scientific foundation and suggested practical applications. J Bodyw Mov Ther 17(1):103-115

Stecco C et al 2008 Histological study of the deep fasciae of the limbs. J Bodyw Mov Ther 12(3): 225-230

Tam N, Astephen Wilson JL, Noakes TD, Tucker R 2013 Barefoot running: an evaluation of current hypothesis, future research and clinical applications. Br J Sports Med (Epub ahead of print) doi: 10.1136/bjsports-2013-092404.

Tesarz J, Hoheise, U, Wiedenhofer B, Mense S 2011 Sensory innervation of the thoracolumbar fascia in rats and humans. Neuroscience 194:302-308

Torp S, Arridge RGC, Armeniades CD et al 1975 Structure-property relationships in tendon as a function of age. Colston Papers No. 26. Butterworth, London, pp 197-221

van der Wal J 2009 The architecture of the connective tissue in the musculoskeletal system -an often overlooked functional parameter as to proprioception in the locomotor apparatus. Int J Ther Massage Bodywork 2(4):9-23

Wang W et al. 2012 Acute pressure on the sciatic nerve results in rapid inhibition of the wide dynamic range neuronal response. BMC Neurosci 13:147

Wilk KE, et al 1993 Stretch-shortening drills for the upper extremities: theory and clinical application. J Orthop Sports Phys Ther 17(5):225-239

Wood TO, Cooke PH, Goodship AE 1988 The effect of exercise and anabolic steroids on the mechanical properties and crimp morphology of the rat tendon. Am J Sports Med 16: 153-158

Wren TA, Yerby SA, Beaupré GS, Carter DR 2001 Mechanical properties of the human achilles tendon. Clin Biomech 16(3):245-251

Zheng L et al 2012 Fluid shear stress regulates metalloproteinase-1 and 2 in human periodontal ligament cells: involvement of extracellular signal-regulated kinase (ERK) and P38 signaling pathways. J Biomech 45(14): 2368-2375\

Chapter 9

THE FASCIAL MANIPULATION® METHOD APPLIED TO LOW BACK PAIN

Antonio Stecco, Stefano Casadei, Alessandro Pedrelli, Julie Ann Day, Carla Stecco

Introduction

Myofascial tissue is gaining increasing attention in the field of medicine and manual therapy. Its anatomy, physiology and biomechanical behavior have been object of numerous research papers that are influencing the development of treatment modalities for musculoskeletal dysfunctions.

Studies concerning myofasciae have primarily focused on the anatomy and pathology of specific areas, such as the abdominal fascia, the Achilles tendon enthesis organ, plantar fascia or the iliotibial tract. While these studies are important, they do not provide a vision of the human fascial system as an interrelated, tensional network of connective tissue.

Fascia is the connecting element that unites all parts of the musculoskeletal system. It is continuous with ligaments, joint capsules and the outer layer of the periosteum. Whilst these structures vary in their denomination and composition, in terms of percentage of collagen or elastic fibers, together they form the so-called soft tissues.

While more and more authors are now associating the causes of many pathological conditions to a lack of balance within the tridimensional myofascial system, specific indications for treatment are not always provided.

Low back pain is one problem that clinicians address on a daily basis. The Fascial Manipulation® approach to low back pain will be discussed in this chapter.

The Fascial Manipulation method

Luigi Stecco, physiotherapist and author of the Fascial Manipulation method (Stecco 2004), has focused on the relationship between muscles, deep fascia and its components (epimysium, perimysium and endomysium – see Ch. 1) to develop a new approach to musculoskeletal dysfunctions that takes into account movement limitation, weakness, and distribution of pain. Based on the idea of fascia as the uniting element between the various body segments, this method also considers fascia as having a potential role as a coordinating component for motor units of unidirectional muscle chains.

The thoracolumbar fascia region is one area of fascia that has been closely examined and its implications in low back pain have been considered (Langevin et al. 2009). The thoracolumbar fascia is a large, diamond-shaped sheet that forms part of the deep fascia. It consists of three layers of cross-hatched collagen fibers (Benetazzo et al. 2011) that cover the back muscles in the lower thoracic and lumbar area before slipping through these muscles to attach to the sacral bone (see Fig. 1.5). These layers insert onto the transverse and spinous processes of the lumbar vertebrae. They also attach themselves to the iliac crest near the dimples of the low back and fuse with the posterior surface of the sacrum. Furthermore, the thoracolumbar fascia links with most of the body. It connects with:

- the deep structures of the spine by extending down to the spinal muscles, spinal ligaments, vertebral column and spinal canal
- the upper limbs, head and neck by virtue of its links with the trapezius and latissimus dorsi
- the lower limbs by melding with the gluteus maximus
- the midline of the abdomen by means of its posterior and middle layers that fuse laterally to form the lateral raphe, a weave of connective tissue that joins with the transversus abdominis and internal oblique muscles. These muscles wrap around to the front of the body, surrounding the rectus abdominis and merging at the linea alba.

Thoracolumbar fascia is clearly a part of an extensive network of interrelated structures that merit consideration as a whole. Unbalanced tension between any of these related structures could lead to the development of low back pain

Fascial Manipulation aims at interpreting the passage of compensation from one segment to another and the evolution from an initial, segmental disturbance to a more generalized dysfunction. 'Manus sapiens potens est' (Fig. 9.1), the logo coined for this method, means 'A knowledgeable hand is powerful', suggesting that only by understanding the origin of a problem can manual therapies resolve them rapidly and efficiently. Numerous

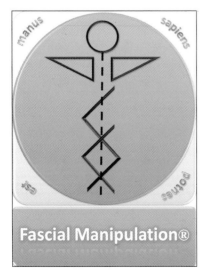

FIGURE 9.1 Fascial Manipulation® logo.

histological, biomechanical, and functional studies have been undertaken to verify some of the hypotheses proposed by Stecco, focusing on the anatomy of the superficial (Lancerotto et al. 2011) and deep fascia (Stecco et al. 2009), innervation (Stecco et al. 2007), and the possible mechanisms of action of the manual technique itself.

Stecco's biomechanical model

Stecco and Stecco (2009) divide the body into 14 functional segments: the head (subdivided into three: eye, ear, jaw); neck; thorax; lumbar; pelvis; scapula; humerus; elbow; wrist; fingers; hip; knee; ankle and foot.

Each functional segment is composed of portions of muscles (mono- and biarticular fibers), that tense or move their fascia (deep and epimysial) and the associated joint components (tendons, ligaments, capsule). Thus, several components form each segment:

- active components (muscular fibers)
- passive components (the joint and its components)
- and a force transmitting element (fascia).

Latin terms are used to distinguish these 14 segments from simple joints (Fig. 9.2).

The myofascial unit

Six myofascial units (MFUs) govern each functional segment, controlling its movements on the three spatial planes (sagittal, – also known as median; frontal – also known as coronal; and horizontal) (Day et al. 2012).

A MFU is a functional unit formed by:

- motor units innervating mono- and biarticular muscle fibers
- the joint moved in only one direction when these fibers contract
- the fascia that connects these fibers to the articular and periarticular components (menisci, ligaments, tendons, capsule)
- the nerve components involved in this contraction.

Thus, different vectors act on each segment. Between the two principal vectors of every MFU (monoarticular fibers and biarticular fibers), there are many smaller vectors formed by sin-

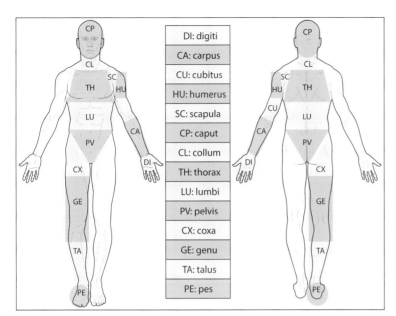

| DI: digiti |
| CA: carpus |
| CU: cubitus |
| HU: humerus |
| SC: scapula |
| CP: caput |
| CL: collum |
| TH: thorax |
| LU: lumbi |
| PV: pelvis |
| CX: coxa |
| GE: genu |
| TA: talus |
| PE: pes |

FIGURE 9.2 Fourteen body segments with associated Latin names and abbreviations.

gle muscle fibers situated some distance apart. If we analyze all of these fibers, we can see how the monoarticular fibers are deeper and more voluminous than the biarticular ones. Partially free to slide in their fascial sheaths, the deep monoarticular muscle fibers transfer their tension to the superficial fascial layers via the continuity of the endomysium, perimysium and epimysium. The monoarticular fibers can exert strength and stability during movement while the biarticular fibers transmit tension between adjoining segments. While regional specializations in fascial structures do exist (Stecco et al. 2009a) the same 'architecture' can be found in every MFU.

Due to this multiplication of vectors, each MFU has a fine control over a specific movement. The continuity of endomysium with perimysium and epimysium permits harmonious synchronization of all these tensional forces.

Each MFU has two functionally different areas. The first is on the deep fascia covering the muscle belly and can be considered as the active component of the MFU. Known as the center of coordination (CC), according to the Fascial Manipulation model, the forces involved in muscle fiber contraction converge in this small area. The second area is a passive component. It is situated around the joint that is moved by MFU muscle

fiber contraction. Called the center of perception (CP), this is where the patient feels the movement resulting from MFU activity (in a physiological situation) or pain (in a pathological situation).

Center of coordination

The term center of coordination (CC) infers that the fascia is potentially involved in feedback concerning movement of body segments due to its connections to muscle spindles, Golgi tendon organs and other mechanoreceptors. The CC is a small area of deep fascia where muscular forces of a MFU, generated by the contraction of mono and biarticular fibers, converge.

This myofascial tension or force converges at a CC because:

- part of the epimysial fascia is free to slide over the underlying muscle fibers
- part of the fascia is anchored to the bone, so stretch can converge in one point
- part of the fascia is inserted onto the bone, partially separating the tensioning of one MFU from the successive one.

CCs are usually situated within the deep fascia overlying a muscle belly and are not close to the joint. Nociceptors embedded in these areas are not normally stretched or irritated by movement therefore these areas are rarely spontaneously symptomatic.

Center of perception

The center of perception (CP) is where traction produced by MFU muscle-fiber activity is perceived. The CP of each MFU is located in a circumscribed area over the joint capsule, tendons and ligaments. This is the area commonly indicated by the patient as being symptomatic.

According to Stecco et al. (2013), impeded sliding between collagen fiber layers within the fascia of a malfunctioning MFU could produce atypical afferent information from mechanoreceptors embedded within the fascial component of the MFU. Consequent anomalies in motor unit recruitment could result in unaligned joint movement. Over time, joint conflict, friction, inflammation of periarticular soft tissues, pain or joint instability can develop, with symptoms arising in the corresponding CP.

New terminology for movement

To simplify the interpretation of myofascial dysfunctions, Stecco describes movement in terms of directions on the three spatial planes. In classical terminology, the hip joint flexes when the femur moves forward but at the knee, the same direction of movement is called extension. In Fascial Manipulation terminology, all forward movements on a sagittal (medial) plane are called antemotion and all backward movements retromotion. Adduction and abduction are substituted by latero- (from the center to the periphery) and mediomotion (from the periphery to the center), and intra- and extra-rotation are used every time a joint moves on the horizontal plane. Thus, movements on the sagittal plane are governed by the MFUs of ante- and retromotion, movements on the frontal (coronal) plane by the MFUs of latero- and mediomotion and movements on the horizontal plane by the MFUs of intra- and extrarotation (see Table 9.1).

Due to its rich innervation, directional afferents originating from the fascial part of each MFU could contribute to proprioceptive information (Stecco et al. 2010). Consequently, the deep fascia component is considered as being potentially active in movement coordination and peripheral motor control.

Fascial mediation of agonist-antagonist interaction

Agonists are group of muscles that contract to provide the force required to produce a particular movement. Antagonists are the muscles that oppose the action of the agonists. In Stecco's model, agonist and antagonist MFU interaction is important for myofascial force transmission and the coordination of movement, as also demonstrated by other studies (Huijing & Baan 2003). As the agonist MFU is activated during movement (albeit forwards, backwards or sideways), the antagonist MFU adapts according to the angle of inclination of the body part (reciprocal inhibition).

In almost every MFU, many monoarticular fibers insert onto the intermuscular septum that separates two antagonist MFUs. The intermuscular septa, together with the epimysial sheaths, could play a direct role in the regulation of the muscular fibers of the two MFUs.

For example, the MFU for elbow extension has its own antagonist myofascial unit that coordinates elbow flexion (Fig. 9.3). When the elbow extends, the monoarticular fibers contract and the intermuscular septum (where they insert) is stretched. The monoarticular fibers of the antagonist MFU (elbow flexion) insert on the other side of this same septum meaning that during extension, its monoarticular components are stretched a little too, causing embedded stretch receptors to fire. Therefore, fascia can be considered as an active component in agonist-antagonist activity.

Table 9.1 Terminology used in Fascial Manipulation® to describe movement on the three spatial planes

Sagittal plane	Frontal plane	Horizontal plane
Antemotion (AN)	Mediomotion (ME)	Intrarotation (IR)
Retromotion (RE)	Lateromotion (LA)	Extrarotation (ER)

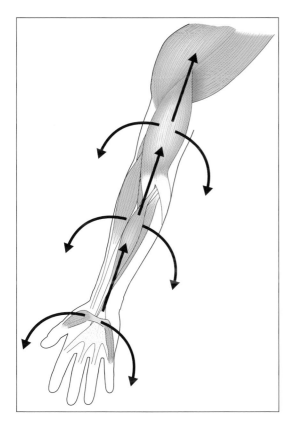

FIGURE 9.3 Fascial connections among synergic muscles in the anterior region of the upper limb.

The myofascial sequences

Stabilization by monoarticular vectors and synchronization between adjacent segments by biarticular muscular fibers allows for precision and stability of each segment during movement. The biarticular muscle fibers composing each MFU connect unidirectional MFUs responsible for movement in only one direction to form myofascial sequences (MFS). Part of the biarticular fibers from each MFU also insert onto the deep fascia of adjacent segments forming myotendinous expansions that link one segment to the next (Stecco et al. 2008, Stecco et al. 2009b) and providing the anatomical substratum of the MFS.

For example, the anatomical continuity of the MFS on the sagittal plane in the lower limb can be traced from antemotion talus (dorsiflexion of the foot), which is carried out by tibialis anterior, extensor digitorum longus and extensor hallucis longus muscles. These muscles originate from the condyles of the tibia and the fibula, from the intermuscular septa and the overlying fascia. The tendinous expansion of the quadriceps tensions the anterior fascia of the leg proximally, whereas the previously listed muscles traction it distally. The fascia lata connects with the anterior fascia of the leg, and is tensioned distally by its insertions into the intermuscular septa of the vastus medialis and lateralis. Moreover, it is continuous with the ileopsoas fascia, which inserts onto the vastus medialis that tensions it distally, together with the sartorius. Ileopsoas fascia continues above over the fascia of the iliacus and psoas minor muscles. The iliacus fascia is involved in antemotion of the pelvis (antiversion of the pelvis) together with the inferior rectus abdominis, which is surrounded by the lateral raphe. This weave of connective tissue joins the abdominal muscles and the middle and posterior layers of the thoracolumbar fascia.

In the antagonist sequence, retromotion of the foot is activated just prior to the push-off, or toe-off, phase of the gait cycle. In this phase, the foot is slightly supinated, bringing the lateral compartment, comprising the abductor digiti minimi, in contact with the ground. Abductor digiti minimi originates from the plantar aponeurosis, which is the continuation of the Achilles tendon of triceps surae (Fig. 9.4 and Plate 7).

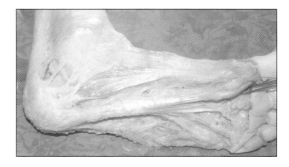

FIGURE 9.4 Dissection of the plantar aponeurosis. While a longitudinal continuity along the main axis of the foot is evident, the plantar aponeurosis also continues with the medial and lateral fasciae of the foot (fascia of the abductor hallucis and abductor digiti minimi muscles, respectively). See also Plate 7.

The contraction of the triceps surae stretches the popliteal fascia and the fibers of the gastrocnemius inserted into it. A few fibers of the biceps femoris, as well as some fibers of the semitendinosus and semimembranosus, tension the popliteal fascia and the fascia of the leg proximally. These latter muscles participate both in retromotion genu (knee flexion) and retromotion coxa (hip extension); therefore, they not only tension the popliteal fascia but also the sacrotuberous ligament. This myofascial concatenation is tensioned during the push-off phase of each step. The sacrotuberous ligament continues proximally with the thoracolumbar fascia. The erector spinae muscles originate from the thoracolumbar fascia and during *retromotion lumbi* (extension of the spine) they become tensors of the retromotion sequence of the lower limb.

Similar anatomical continuity is found in each MFS. Sequences on the same spatial plane (sagittal, frontal, or horizontal) are reciprocal antagonists; therefore, altered areas along the fascia of one MFS can potentially compromise the entire spatial plane related to that MFS.

> ### Key Point
>
> In English, **densification** is a neologism coined by Stecco to describe the palpable sensation of lack of sliding between interfascial and intrafascial layers.

Clinical reasoning

In cases of low back pain, clinicians apply Stecco's biomechanical model to interpret the spread of tensional compensations from one segment to another. A tensile alteration in any given MFU causes a counter tension in another MFU along the same sequence, as a means of preserving the fascia's basal tension. Such tensile adjustments are a remedy that often creates acute pain because the free nerve endings in this segment of fascia are subjected to excessive, abnormal traction. The body then compensates this tension as a means of re-establishing equilibrium. Compensatory tension can be symmetrical (in the antagonist sequence) but, with reference to the MFU where the compensation originated, it could be localized in a proximal or distal segment. In the trunk, each MFU of antemotion and retromotion can act with the contralateral side of the body. For example, it is possible to find that a hypertonic left sided component of the antemotion MFU in the lumbar region is compensated by a right sided component of retromotion.

In summary, if the basal tension of the fascia is altered by the formation of a **'densification'** compensations can develop either in the symmetrically antagonist MFU or along the ipsilateral sequence, or in the contralateral sequence.

Low back pain is always approached through an accurate examination of each individual case in order to identify the densified CCs that are involved in compensations. While both descending and ascending compensations are common, some examples of ascending compensations that originate in the foot and spread upwards on the three planes are described below:

- On the sagittal plane, a restriction within a toe extensor tendon (e.g. hammer toe) can provoke contraction of the triceps surae causing the knee to hyperextend in compensation for the increase in the angle of the ankle joint. The hyperextended knee (*genu recurvatum*) causes anteversion of the pelvis with consequent shortening of the iliopsoas muscle. An exaggerated lumbar lordosis results, leading to a dorsal kyphosis and, in an attempt to neutralize the other curves, an exaggerated cervical lordosis may form.
- In the frontal plane, lowered arches (flat feet) often produce a medial deviation of the knee (*genu valgus*). Hip abduction (frontal plane) ensues, with a lowered iliac crest due to a restriction of the tensor fascia lata. This variation in pelvic alignment initially inclines the vertebral column to the same side and, in time, produces compensation in the opposite side.

- On the horizontal plane, misalignment can begin with a unilateral hallux valgus. This alteration can be bilateral but to simplify the analysis only one limb is considered here. Intrarotation of the forefoot (*hallux valgus*) is compensated by eversion of the talus due to contraction of the peronei muscles (*talus valgus*). The knee and the hip intrarotate, bringing the pelvis forward on the same side and causing contralateral compensation in the trunk.

Therefore, it can be seen that the biomechanics of the lumbar spine are strictly connected to the correct functioning of the ankle and knee because of the fascial continuity between these three anatomical segments.

For example, it is common to find the origin of low back pain in a now 'silent' knee or ankle that suffered a strain or tendinitis years ago (see Case Example). That is because the fascial system is a complex network that runs the entire length of the body and connects all of its parts. It responds to mechanical traction induced by muscular activity in different regions and plays a relevant role in epimuscular force transmission in every spatial plane and trajectory of movement.

Analysis might reveal that:

- Various painful areas are distributed along a sequence; for example, if pain is localized in the medial part of the thigh, knee and ankle then one could hypothesize a dysfunction of the mediomotion sequence of the lower limb.
- Various painful areas are distributed on one plane: if pain is localized in the right side of the lumbar region plus lateral right thigh and medial lower leg, then one could hypothesize a dysfunction on the frontal plane.

Clinicians aim to elaborate a valid hypothesis that explains the compensatory pathways chosen by the body to counterbalance one or more fascial densifications. This hypot hesis is fundamental in developing a correct therapeutic plan and for validation during on-going assessments.

Assessment

> ### Key Point
>
> **Silent CCs** are asymptomatic areas of deep fascia that can be deduced from the patient's symptoms and located by using knowledge of the continuity of the sequences on the three planes.
>
> Application of the Fascial Manipulation® method involves compilation of a specific assessment chart that assists the selection of CCs to treat, and provides concise documentation of treatment sessions. Patient's personal data and history, an abbreviated description of the presenting symptoms, including pain location, characteristics, and chronicity, and identifiable painful movements are all noted.
>
> Patients are encouraged to report any concomitant pain because even minor painful areas are useful in indicating the disturbed sequence or plane.
>
> The following questions are taken into consideration:
> - In which plane have the various compensations developed?
> - What could have been the initial trauma that determined these compensations?
> - Are they ascending or descending compensations?
> - Are there any hidden compensatory strategies **(silent CCs)?**

Multisegmental problems are approached through the analysis of chronological events involved in each individual case. Asymptomatic previous disturbances are frequently the cause of presenting pain because fascia often repairs a trauma with an excess of fibers and densification, neutralizing the lack of elasticity due to established densifications by extending tension along the same sequence. Neither the body nor pharmacotherapy removes these excess fibers because they are normal collagen fibers and are not recognized as being inappropriate.

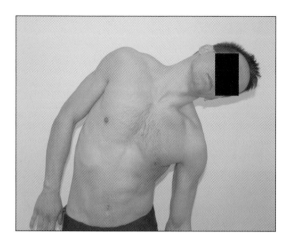

FIGURE 9.5 Example of movement assessment of the LA-LU myofascial units (MFU): the right side stretches during an eccentric contraction; the therapist notes the amplitude and whether lateral flexion is harmonious or whether other compensations appear. The patient may report pain or tension.

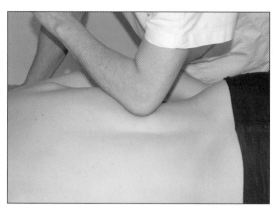

FIGURE 9.6 Example of palpatory (sensitivity) test of RE-LU center of coordination (CC) located in the erector spinae's deep fascia, lateral to L1.

Once the clinician has formulated a hypothesis, movement and palpation assessments are then performed.

Movement assessment

Clinicians evaluate the mobility of two or more joint segments on all three planes by using codified movement tests (Fig. 9.5) to determine the more compromised plane of movement. The most painful or limited movement in the majority of segments suggests which MFS or plane may be implicated in the dysfunction.

As mentioned above, pain in the pelvis or the lumbar region may be merely the latest counter compensation, the cause being a now silent knee segment or a previous ankle problem.

Palpation assessment

Once altered movements are noted, palpatory tests guide therapists in selecting the combination of densified CCs to be treated (Fig. 9.6). All six CCs of the implicated segments are palpated and compared. CCs that are painful, densified and from which a referred pain expands towards the CP are the most likely candidates for treatment.

Treatment

Treatment consists of a deep friction over the CCs. Therapists use the olecranon of their elbow, their knuckle, or fingertips over densified CCs, creating localized hyperaemia through friction.

Treatment is directed toward the fascia because of its particular characteristics:

- Elasticity: fascia is an elastic tissue with established limits, which permits involvement in motor coordination and perception of motion. Different studies do suggest that fascia is richly innervated. Nerves passing through the deep fascia are surrounded by loose connective tissue. Therefore, they are subjected to traction when the fascia lengthens. However, when these nerves terminate in neuroreceptors (e.g. free nerve endings) they insert directly into the collagen fibers. The abundance of free and encapsulated nerve endings could activate specific patterns of proprioceptors, potentially providing directional and spatial afferent information.

- Plasticity: external stress, such as repeated mechanical stimuli, thermal stress and chemical or metabolic dysfunctions, can alter fascia. External mechanical stimuli stimulate protein turnover and fibroblast activity within fascia, altering the mechanical properties of its extracellular matrix. These characteristics and the reported abundant innervation of deep fascia indicate that it could have the capacity to perceive mechanosensitive signals.

- Malleability: 'densification' is not a permanent and irreparable pathological condition. Fascial tissue is easily accessible and it possesses a strong capacity for repairing and regenerating itself. Just as stressful stimuli can modify fascial consistency, manipulation of specific areas can restore its physiological condition.

In general, if a traumatic stimulus causes local inflammation, rest and physiological movement induce reorganization of collagen fibers along the lines of traction and a normal healing process of the damaged area ensues. Repeated inflammation (overuse, repetitive strains) increases the number of collagen fibers resulting in a chaotic redistribution of these fibers at the CCs (see Table 9.2). Trauma, disuse with consequent diminished circulation, repetitive motion and poor posture can cause the ground substance of the connective tissue to dehydrate, contract and harden resulting in lack of sliding between collagen bundle layers.

Densification of a CC may cause hypertonicity within a MFU, which can be responsible for incorrect joint movement. If the soft tissues surrounding a joint (CP) do not stretch according to physiological lines, then receptors embedded in these tissues signal the dysfunction as pain.

Under physiological conditions, CCs are not hypersensitive nor do they produce referred pain when stimulated. Normally, the elasticity of the fascia allows it to adapt to compression without straining embedded nerve endings. Densified CCs increase overall tension, lowering the pain threshold of the free nerve endings, and minimal compression can then be sufficient to set off local as well as referred pain. This process can also involve the CP of the implicated MFU, the CP of the antagonist MFU, or the entire MFS, which can explain the irradiation of pain along this structure. These stresses can apparently resolve spontaneously through compensations and a densified CC often becomes silent (similar to latent trigger points) and pain is no longer felt at the CP. This seemingly balanced condition is unstable and, whenever the body is no longer capable of maintaining these compensations, chronic fascial densifications become active, and pain presents again.

The alteration of a CC can cause joint pain (in the CP) as well as a joint blockage. In the latter case, if it is a recent lesion then it is possible to intervene directly with joint mobilizations. Freeing the articulation reduces the painful afferent and eliminates MFU hypertonicity. However, if the chronicity of the problem has created a true 'densification' of the CC, manipulation applied directly to the CC is required (Pedrelli et al. 2009).

Hyaluronic acid, located in considerable amounts in the ground substance of the loose connective tissue layer between the deep fascia and the surface of muscle (Stecco et al. 2011), normally acts as a lubricant but, under pathological conditions, it aggregates, increasing ground substance viscoelasticity, resulting in densification (Stecco et al. 2013). Manipulation is required to act on a densified CC for a sufficient amount of time for the friction against the fascia to produce heat (Borgini et al. 2010). This heat is needed to modify the consistency of the ground substance and to initiate the inflammatory process required for healing.

Table 9.2 Physiological and pathological reactions of fascia to stress

Repeated mechanical stimuli	Chronic dysfunction
Inflammation	Repeated inflammation
Repair	Collagen fiber hyperplasia
Reorganization of collagen fibers	Collagen fiber dysplasia
Healing	Ground substance densification

If a tensional balance in the fascia is restored, physiological movements can align new collagen fibers along the normal lines of force. It is therefore important not to focus treatment at the sites of pain, which is often merely the consequence of the dysfunction. The aim is always to trace back to initial disturbances.

Treatment begins once the assessment has defined the CCs to be treated. Treatment of the sequences is characterized by the fact that the selected CCs must be part of a plan for restoring global postural equilibrium.

It is imperative to:

- Choose a proximal CC and a distal one to release fascial tension.

- Choose one or more CCs of the antagonist sequence.

After having manipulated two points then it is useful to re-assess movement. If symptoms have improved then it can be taken as an indication to continue with that sequence or plane, otherwise it is best to re-elaborate the therapeutic program. Treatment can vary in its intensity or depth for the following reasons:

- Superficial friction is used whenever the disturbance of the deep fascia has extended itself to the subcutaneous loose connective tissue.

- Static compression or stretch is used when there is a localized swelling.

Case Example

Fascial Manipulation applied to low back pain

LR is a 50-year-old male who has been suffering from low back pain for 1 year. Symptoms were resistant to treatment of any kind.

He had never suffered from backache prior to this and a CAT scan has excluded a prolapsed disc. Pain, localized along the right posterior side of the **lumbar region** and pelvis, had begun 1 year ago after a tennis match and since then it has never completely disappeared but it has varied in intensity. Symptoms are accentuated with running and bending forward.

Two segments (LU, PV) are indicated as the site of pain distributed in the posterior part (RE) of both segments. This could indicate the sequence of retromotion but this would mean considering only the present situation without considering other potential causes. Certainly, by treating the CC of RE-LU and RE-PV it is likely that the patient will have some relief but at the first attempt at running it may well recur. When asked *'Have you ever had pain in the past in any part of your body? Did you ever suffer from fractures or ankle sprains? Did something happen to your knees in the past?'* the patient recalls having a right first metatarsal fracture when aged 40 (10 years ago) and he remembers rupturing his right Achilles tendon 1 year later (9 years ago).

From this data it was possible to hypothesize that the spasm in the retromotion sequence (RE-

TA, RE-LU, RE-PV) may have been determined by a compensation created by the antagonist antemotion sequence (AN-PE) that had not caused any problems for 10 years. It required an intense physical stress, such as a long tennis match, to decompensate the tensile equilibrium.

Movement assessment revealed pain along the posterior leg during the test for antemotion talus (ankle) and pes (foot). Palpation assessment revealed densification of five CCs (RE-LU, AN-PV, RE-TA, AN-TA and AN-PE).

The AN-PE and RE-TA CCs were treated first. Post-treatment movement assessment demonstrated that the pain in the lumbar region had decreased from 8 to 3 on the VAS scale. The other three CCs were treated in order to complete the tensile balance.

The patient was pain-free after the first treatment, therefore the following advice was given: *'When the treated points are no longer tender you can recommence running. The first run should be brief and you should stop if any pain reappears. Try again after 2 days and if the pain is felt again then ask for a second appointment.'*

The athlete called after 10 days to say that he had some pain during the first run but during the following run, no disturbance had been felt.

- Deep friction is used when granulation tissue or densification of the fascial tissue is present. Here the intention is to infiltrate through the loose subcutaneous connective tissue to reach the deep fascia.

As treatment is usually at a distance from the site of pain or the inflamed area, this technique can be applied during the acute phase of a dysfunction.

Conclusion

The Fascial Manipulation method indicates a new manner for comprehending the possible connections between different sites of pain, introducing interesting perspectives for clinicians involved in the manual treatment of musculoskeletal dysfunctions such as low back pain.

Acknowledgment

The authors are grateful to Luigi Stecco for his unfailing support.

References

Benetazzo L et al 2011 3D reconstruction of the crural and thoracolumbar fasciae. Surg Radiol Anat 33(10):855–62

Borgini E, Antonio S, Julie Ann D, Stecco C 2010 How much time is required to modify a fascial fibrosis? J Bodyw Mov Ther 14:318–25

Day JA, Copetti L, Rucli G 2012 From clinical experience to a model for the human fascial system. J Bodyw Mov Ther 16 (3):372–80

Huijing PA, Baan GC 2003 Myofascial force transmission: muscle relative position and length determine agonist and synergist muscle force. J Appl Physiol. 94:1092–107.

Lancerotto L et al 2011 Layers of the abdominal wall: anatomical investigation of subcutaneous tissue and superficial fascia. Surg Radiol Anat 33(10):835–42

Langevin HM et al 2009 Ultrasound evidence of altered lumbar connective tissue structure in human subjects with chronic low back pain. BMC Musculoskelet Disord 10:151

Pedrelli A, Stecco C, Day JA 2009 Treating patellar tendinopathy with Fascial Manipulation. J Bodyw Mov Ther 13: 73–80

Stecco A et al 2009a Pectoral and femoral fasciae: common aspects and regional specializations. Surg Radiol Anat 31: 35–42

Stecco A et al 2009b Anatomical study of myofascial continuity in the anterior region of the upper limb. J Bodyw Mov Ther 13:53–62

Stecco A, Gesi M, Stecco C, Stern R 2013 Fascial component of the myofascial pain syndrome. Curr Pain Headache Rep 17(8):352

Stecco A et al 2014 Ultrasonography in myofascial neck pain: randomized clinical trial for diagnosis and follow-up. Surg Radiol Anat Apr; 36(3):243-53

Stecco C et al 2007 Anatomy of the deep fascia of the upper limb. Second part: study of innervation. Morphologie 91:38–43

Stecco C et al 2008 The expansions of the pectoral girdle muscles onto the brachial fascia: morphological aspects and spatial disposition. Cells Tissues Organs 188:320–9

Stecco C et al 2009 Mechanics of crural fascia: from anatomy to constitutive modelling. Surg Radiol Anat 31:523–9

Stecco C et al 2010 The ankle retinacula: morphological evidence of the proprioceptive role of the fascial system. Cells Tissues Organs 192:200–10

Stecco C et al 2011 Hyaluronan within fascia in the etiology of myofascial pain. Surg Radiol Anat. 33(10):891–6

Stecco L 2004 Fascial manipulation for musculoskeletal pain. Piccin, Padova

Stecco L, Stecco C 2009 Fascial Manipulation, practical part. Piccin, Padova

Chapter 10

FASCIAL UNWINDING

Paolo Tozzi

Introduction

Fascial unwinding (FU) comprises a dynamic functional indirect technique usually applied to the myofascial–articular complex, aimed at releasing fascial restrictions and restoration of tissue mobility and function. The therapist initially induces motion in the body, usually by lifting and holding the worked area, so as to reduce the influence of gravity and to overcome reactive postural tone (Minasny 2009). The operator engages the restricted tissues/joint by unfolding the pattern of dysfunctional vectors associated with the inherent fascial motion. The effective movement will be felt as a spontaneous expression from dysfunctional tissue tension: shearing, torsional or rotational component may develop in a complex three-dimensional pattern that needs to be supported, amplified and unwound, until release is perceived.

Background

Although the vital role of fascia has been intuitively known since the origins of osteopathy – *'By its action we live and by its failure we die'* (Still 1902) – the term *unwinding* applied to fascial treatment seems to have been more recently introduced by V.M. Frymann DO (1998). FU originated from, and has been most widely described, in the osteopathic field (Ward 2003), mainly in relation to the release of physical features associated with fascial restrictions, or the unwinding of the so-called craniosacral mechanism (Frymann 1998). More recently, a somatoemotional component has been included in which it is suggested that FU might be used to release

trauma-induced energy, stored in the myofascial system (Upledger 1987). It has been described as: *'a manual technique involving constant feedback to the osteopathic practitioner who is passively moving a portion of the patient's body in response to the sensation of movement'* (ECOP 2006). In this sense, FU has been considered as a form of indirect myofascial release: *'the dysfunctional tissues are guided along the path of least resistance until free movement is achieved'* (Minasny 2009). The unwinding process may also occur spontaneously during the application of other techniques. Muscles, ligaments, and fascia have been ascribed as the agencies for such motion (Frymann 1998).

FU has been demonstrated to be an effective integrative technique for:

- neck pain (Tozzi et al. 2011)
- low back pain (Tozzi et al. 2012)
- adult scoliosis (Blum 2002)
- tension-type headaches (Anderson & Seniscal 2006).

Objectives

As it is safe and gentle in its application, FU has been used by osteopaths, craniosacral therapists and generally by myofascial body-workers to correct somatic dysfunctions, to release pain, muscoloskeletal tension and fascial restriction (Ward 2003), especially following injury (Frymann 1998) or surgery.

FU can be performed in ways that involve the whole body (possibly requiring the simultaneous cooperation of two operators in such cases) or on any single articulation or group of articulations, particularly involving the neck, arms or legs, as these are mobile regions where strain and trauma commonly manifest.

FU is generally indicated for any myofascial condition, including those related to sport injury, such as tennis elbow, plantar fasciitis, shin splints, muscular and tendinous injury rehabilitation (Weintraub 2003), or to any repetitively strained or overused joint and related myofascial structures.

Assessment

In evaluating fascial restrictions, it is important to view the body as a whole, considering the continuity and connectivity of fascia through its kinetic chains (Myers 2009) (Fig. 10.1; see also Fig. 1.5). A disruption at any point in any of these chains can have an effect elsewhere. Abnormal points of tension within this system, following a recent or longstanding injury, surgery, or any sort of repetitive strain, creates adaptive compensatory patterns, following the path of least resistance. This can lead to altered structural alignment, impaired movement patterns, joint restrictions, pain, poor energy levels and decreased vitality. A body-wide postural assessment should be accurately performed, together with hands-on assessment of the tone and texture of the myofascial tissue, joint range of motion, muscle testing and subjective complaints of pain and/or loss of function.

Protocol

FU is a dynamic technique that requires a state of relaxation from the patient, as well as high sensitivity and fine palpation skills from the practitioner. The operator supports the patient and palpates for fascial tensions and allows any spontaneous movement to manifest (Fig.10.2).

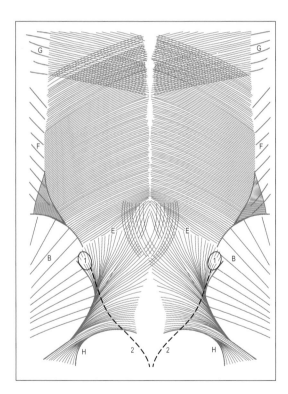

FIGURE 10.1 The deep layer of the thoracolumbar fascia (TLF) and its attachments. The deep layer of the TLF is a good example of tensional continuity of the myofascial system. This fascia attaches to: (B) gluteus medius; (E) erector spinae muscle; (F) the internal oblique; (G) serratus posterior inferior; (H) the sacrotuberous ligament; (1) PSIS; (2) sacrum. *Adapted from Vleeming et al. (1995).*

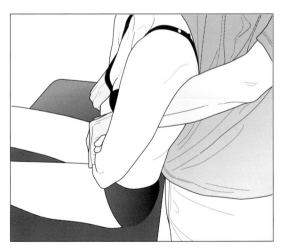

FIGURE 10.2 FU hold for thoracolumbar fascia. The patient sits on the couch with their arms crossed, while the operator stands behind. The therapist places their hands underneath and through the patient's arms, contacting the patient's lumbopelvic region with the lateral part of their hip region. By using the patient trunk as leverage and the lumbopelvic region as fulcrum, lumbar tissues tensions are unwound up to the point where a release is felt.

The patient gives constant feedback to the examiner as the practitioner supports the structures, amplifying the range and intensity of movement, guided by inherent fascial tensions, until a spontaneous release is perceived. The unwinding process can be carried out on the whole body, or any part of the body, especially limbs and neck. The neck or extremities can be treated regionally or used as levers to manipulate the trunk. However, not everyone is responsive to FU; for example, if the patient is unable to relax, therefore alternative strategies should be used. In some cases unwinding may happen spontaneously while the therapist is applying other techniques, for example, neck unwinding may occur spontaneously during the performance of myofascial release technique (Weintraub 2003) or suboccipital decompression.

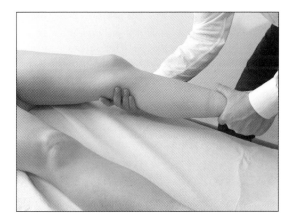

FIGURE 10.3   FU hold for the lower limb. The patient lies supine. The therapist supports the leg under the knee and ankle joints. To promote the unwinding process, the therapist applies a mild compression towards the hip joint.

FU application:

1. **Evaluation:** after a thorough assessment of the myofascial system, the operator identifies the dysfunctional body region to be worked on, including its dysfunctional vectors – that is the preferential directions of tissue motion, perceived by the practitioner as movements towards 'ease'. These usually mirror directions of injury or trauma, suffered by involved tissues. A shearing, torsional or rotational component generally arises in a complex three-dimensional pattern. The operator approaches the involved area with a gentle touch.

2. **Induction:** the therapist initially induces motion in the body, usually by lifting and holding the area in a relaxed position, so to reduce the influence of gravity and overcome reactive proprioceptive postural tone (Minasny 2009). Alternatively, a distraction or compression force on related joints can be added to prompt the process. For example, in leg unwinding, with the patient supine, the operator lifts and supports the leg under the knee and ankle, while a mild compression towards the hip joint can be added to promote the unwinding process (Fig. 10.3).

3. **Unwinding:** the practitioner should sense movements arising from the inherent motion of dysfunctional tissues, that should not be directed or forced but just supported and followed. Such patterns of motion are mostly unpredictable: usually following a spiral path, sometimes very subtle, sometimes extremely vigorous, either rhythmic or random, but always at its own individual rate. The intention is to hold tissues in a balanced and relaxed state, remaining sensitive to fascial signals that spontaneously express the inherent tensional patterns. **Note:** The unwinding process should not be allowed to occur as a 'fulcrumless' circular repetitive motion, since that would be unlikely to produce any therapeutic effect. Instead, a precise fulcrum should be identified, around which tissues may express their dysfunctional pattern: this should be a point of major restriction that is being addressed.

4. **Still point (not always present):** the unwinding process may occasionally cease, resulting in a still point where no motion occurs and tissues are 'silent'. The patient's cooperation may be requested at this stage; for example, involving forced respiration, to promote tissue changes and release.

5. **Release:** a collapse of myofascial tension may be felt together with warmth and a 'melting' sense in the tissues that are being worked on. A release may take seconds to be obtained when working on recent and mild

restrictions, whereas longstanding or severe injuries may require more than one session. *'The principle of this profound technique is to place the patient in the position that they were in at the moment of injury, and permit fascia to go through whatever motions are necessary to eliminate all the forces imposed by the impact'* (Frymann, 1998). In some cases, an emotional release may occur, or be induced, during the unwinding process.

6. **Reassessment:** tissue should be re-examined after release has been achieved, and a sense of balanced tension within and around the myofascial tissue should be verified. Any combined therapeutic exercise and traditional manual modalities may then be found to be more effective in achieving enhanced function.

FU has been indicated for myofascial conditions following injury or surgery.

It has also been demonstrated to be a beneficial integrative technique:

- To reduce pain and improve sliding fascial mobility in patients with non-specific neck pain (Tozzi et al. 2011)
- To reduce pain and improve visceral mobility in people with low back pain (Tozzi et al. 2012)
- In the treatment of adult scoliosis (Blum 2002), spondylolisthesis (Ward 2003) and of tension-type headaches (Anderson & Seniscal 2006).

No injuries have been reported in the literature as attributed to indirect or fascial techniques (Vick et al. 1996). However, a myalgic flare may occur within the first 12 hours after treatment, usually lasting only a few hours, and similar to the muscle pain after a vigorous workout (Ward 2003).

Self-unwinding

It is possible to learn how to gently self-unwind fascia during a guided meditation session, by connecting with the myofascial system and its tensional patterns. This experience may show how the body often spontaneously unwinds and suggests the ways it wants to release tension and return to its natural state. Since unwinding the fascia may also release memories of past emotional trauma, an emotional as well as a physical release may be experienced.

Mechanisms

Although fascia has been demonstrated to contract in a smooth-muscle-like manner (Schleip et al. 2005), its ability to unwind has not yet been investigated. In the literature, FU is usually explained as an expression of the body's ability to self-correct from functional disturbances (Frymann 1998). However, the mechanism behind it is still unknown, although Minasny's theory (2009) offers an interesting view:

- When applying FU, the operator initiates the unwinding process through a gentle touch and an induction along directions of ease. This may produce a stimulation of pressure-sensitive mechanoreceptors in the fascial tissue followed by a parasympathetic response (Schleip 2003).
- The latter may induce a state of relaxation in the patient, possibly associated with rapid eye movement or deep breathing (Bertolucci 2008). A change in local vasodilatation and tissue viscosity together with a lowered tonus of intrafascial smooth muscle cells may also take place under parasympathethic influence (Schleip 2003).
- In response to the proprioceptive input from the induction process, the central nervous system (CNS) changes muscle tone and allows muscle action and movements along paths of least resistance.
- At this point of relaxed central activity, ideomotor reflexes occur (Dorko 2003): unconscious reflexes that imply involuntary muscle movement, mostly ascribed to an external force and possibly caused by prior expectations or suggestions. The ideomotor action is generated through voluntary motor control, but is altered and experienced as an involuntary reaction. This is why the patient usually assumes that the therapist is guiding the movement during FU, although when made aware of it can consciously stop it. This indicates a dissociation between voluntary action and conscious experience.

- This unconscious movement or stretching sensation stimulates a response in the tissue, providing a feedback to the CNS, which, in turn, will generate the movements again, as outlined in the theory of ideomotor action (Elsner & Hommel 2001).
- The process is repeated until a release is achieved.

Since tissue release seems to be unrelated to viscoelastic deformation of fascia (Chaudhry et al. 2008), which would, in fact, require much stronger forces or longer durations, neurological reflexive changes in tissue tonus have been proposed to explain the effects of fascial work (Schleip 2003). Minasny (2009) concludes that FU occurs when a physical induction by a therapist prompts ideomotor action experienced as involuntary by the patient. However, other mechanisms may come into play: for instance, cell-based mechanisms seem to exhibit a crucial role in manual fascial work. Some of these are summarized in Table 10.1. See Chapter 1 for detail of mechanotransduction.

Moreover, it has been suggested that most of the changes following fascial work may be the result of a transformation of the ground substance from its densified state (gel) to more fluid (sol) state (Greenman 2003). Such thixotropic changes seem to increase the production of hyaluronic acid, together with the flow within the fascial tissue, thanks to the interplay of calcium ion concentration and unbound water oscillations (Lee 2008). Such interfascial flow may play a role in improving drainage of inflammatory mediators and metabolic wastes; on decreasing chemical irritation of the autonomic nervous system endings, and nociceptive stimuli to somatic endings (Lund et al. 2002); on resetting aberrant somatovisceral and/or viscerosomatic reflexes.

Others have considered piezoelectric properties as an alternative explanation of the change in fascial plasticity. The fascia presents crystalline collagen strands that display a polarity within their molecular structure, and can then generate piezoelectricity: applying an electric stimulus causes mechanical motion (vibration) and applying physical force (tension, compression, or shear) generates electricity (Lee 2008). Therefore, fascia may combine the property of a sol-liquid conductor and of a crystal generator system, which can generate and conduct direct currents, including the ability to store memories and traumas (Oschman 2009) by using energy transmissions as information (Pischinger 1991).

In addition, some therapeutic changes following FU may be related to the anandamide effect on the endocannabinoid system: an endorphin-like system constituted of cell membrane receptors, endogenous ligands and ligand-metabolizing enzymes. This system affects fibroblast remodelling, and may play a role in fascial reorganization, in diminishing nociception and reducing inflammation in myofascial tissues (McPartland et al. 2005). Cannabinoids are also linked to cardiovascular changes, smooth muscle relaxation and perhaps to mood changes through their role on the CNS (Ralevic et al. 2002).

Table 10.1 Cellular mechanisms possibly related to fascial work

Fibroblast response	Strain direction, frequency and duration of a therapeutic load may influence fibroblast functions known to mediate pain, inflammation and range of motion (Standley & Meltzer 2008)
Effector cell response	Mechanical loading stimulates protein synthesis at the cellular level, promoting tissue repair and remodelling (Khan & Scott 2009)
Mechano-coupling	Physical load (often shear or compression) produces a transduction into various chemical signals – within and among cells – leading to a modulation of cell metabolism and response, producing changes in intracellular biochemistry and gene expression (Wipff & Hinz 2008)
Cell–cell communication	Stimulus in one location leads to a perturbation of distant cells, although these have not received any direct mechanical stimulus
Collagen response	Collagen architecture responds to mechanical loading and a therapeuthic load may stimulate connective tissue repair and remodelling (Kjaer et al. 2009)

Some studies have also demonstrated modulation of hypersympathotonia with an improvement in a variety of visceral and psychosomatic features as demonstrated by hemodynamic functions (Rivers et al. 2008), heart rate variability (Henley et al. 2008), and anxiety levels (Fernandez-Perez et al. 2008) following osteopathic fascial work.

Parasympathetic tone may also have an influence as its up-regulation, following manual therapy, has been reported to influence blood shear rate and blood flow turbulence (Quere` et al. 2009).

References

Anderson RE, Seniscal C 2006 A comparison of selected osteopathic treatment and relaxation for tension-type headaches. Headache 46(8):1273–80

Bertolucci LF 2008 Muscle repositioning: a new verifiable approach to neuro-myofascial release? J Bodyw Mov Ther 12:213–224

Blum CL 2002 Chiropractic and pilates therapy for the treatment of adult scoliosis. J Manipulative Physiol Ther 25(4):E

Chaudhry H et al 2008 Three-dimensional mathematical model for deformation of human fasciae in manual therapy. J Am Osteopath Assoc 108 (8):379e390

Dorko BL 2003 The analgesia of movement: ideomotor activity and manual care. J Osteopath Med 6:93–95

Educational Council on Osteopathic Principles (ECOP) 2006 Glossary of Osteopathic Terminology Usage Guide. Chevy Chase, Maryland: AACOM

Elsner B, Hommel B 2001 Effect anticipation and action control. J Exp Psychol Hum Percept Perform 27:229–240

Fernandez-Perez AM et al 2008 Effects of myofascial induction techniques on physiologic and psychologic parameters: a randomized controlled trial. J Altern Complement Med 14:807–811

Frymann V 1998 The collected papers of Viola M Frymann, DO. Legacy of osteopathy to children. American Academy of Osteopathy, Indianapolis

Greenman PE 2003 Principles of manual medicine, 2nd edn. Williams and Wilkins, Baltimore, Ch 1 & 2

Henley CE et al 2008 Osteopathic manipulative treatment and its relationship to autonomic nervous system activity as demonstrated by heart rate variability: a repeated measures study. Osteopathic Med Prim Care 2, 7

Khan KM, Scott A 2009 Mechanotherapy. Br J Sports Medicine 43:247–251

Kjaer M et al 2009 From mechanical loading to collagen synthesis. Scand J Med Sci Sports 19(4):500–510

Lee RP 2008 The living matrix: a model for the primary respiratory mechanism. Explore (NY) 4(6):374–8

Lund I et al 2002 Repeated massage-like stimulation induces long-term effects on nociception: contribution of oxytocinergic mechanisms. Eur JNeurosci 16, 330e338

McPartland JM et al 2005 Cannabimimetic effects of osteopathic manipulative treatment. J Am Osteopath Assoc 105(6):283e291

Minasny B 2009 Understanding the process of fascial unwinding. Int J Ther Massage Bodywork 2(3):10–7

Myers T 2009 Anatomy Trains, 2nd edn. Churchill Livingstone, Edinburgh

Oschman JL 2009 Charge transfer in the living matrix. J Bodyw Mov Ther(3):215–28

Pischinger AA 1991 Matrix and matrix regulation: basis for a holistic theory of medicine. In: Heine H (ed) English edn. Haug International, Brussels p 53

Quere´, N et al 2009 Fasciatherapy combined with pulsology touch induces changes in blood turbulence potentially beneficial for vascular endothelium. J Bodyw Mov Ther 13(3):239e245

Ralevic V et al 2002 Cannabinoid modulation of sensory neurotransmission via cannabinoid and vanilloid receptors: roles in regulation of cardiovascular function. Life Sciences 71:2577e2594

Rivers WE et al 2008 Short-term hematologic and hemodynamic effects of osteopathic lymphatic techniques: a pilot crossover trial. JAOA 108, 646e651

Schleip R 2003 Fascial plasticity: a new neurobiological explanation. Part 2. J Bodyw Mov Ther 7:104–116

Schleip R et al 2005 Active fascial contractility: fascia may be able to contract in a smooth muscle-like manner and thereby influence musculoskeletal dynamics. Med Hypotheses 65:273–277

Standley P, Meltzer K 2008 Effects of repetitive motion strain (RMS) and counter-strain (CS), on fibroblast morphology and actin stress fiber architecture. J Bodyw Mov Ther 12(3):201–203

Still AT 1902 The philosophy and mechanical principles of osteopathy. Hudson-EimberIt, Kansas City, pp 60–65

Tozzi P et al 2011 Fascial release effects on patients with non-specific cervical or lumbar pain. J Bodyw Mov Ther15(4):405–16

Tozzi P et al 2012 Low back pain and kidney mobility: local osteopathic fascial manipulation decreases pain perception and improves renal mobility. J Bodyw Mov Ther16(3):381–91

Upledger JE 1987 Craniosacral therapy II: beyond the dura. Eastland Press, Seattle

Vick DA et al 1996 The safety of manipulative treatment: review of the literature from 1925 to 1993. J Am Osteopath Assoc 96:113–115

Vleeming A et al 1995 The posterior layer of the thoracolumbar fascia: its function in load transfer from spine to legs. Spine 20:753–758

Ward RC 2003 Foundations for osteopathic medicine, 2nd edn. Philadelphia, Lippincott Williams & Wilkins, pp 931–65

Weintraub W 2003 Tendon and ligament healing: a new approach to sports and overuse injury. Paradigm Publications, Herndon, VA, pp 66–67

Wipff PJ, Hinz B 2008 Integrins and the activation of latent transforming growth factor beta1 – an intimate relationship. Eur J Cell Biol 87(8–9):601–15

Chapter 11

BALANCED LIGAMENTOUS TENSION TECHNIQUE

Paolo Tozzi

Introduction

Balanced ligamentous tension (BLT), also known as ligamentous articular strain (LAS), is a non-invasive, safe and fairly common osteopathic technique (Sleszynski & Glonek 2005). According to BLT principles, all joints in the body are balanced ligamentous articular mechanisms that may be altered after injury, infection or mechanical stress. Therefore, BLT was originally conceived as an indirect technique to address articular strains. This initially required a disengagement of tissues from their guarding position, then an exaggeration of the dysfunctional pattern into the direction of ease, up to the point when a ligamentous tensional compromise is reached – where a tensional ligamentous balance is achieved, and a release is felt. Although specifically proposed for articular disturbances, the same principles have been applied to membranous, body fluid flow, fascial and visceral dysfunctions. It has also been shown to be effective in various clinical conditions, by affecting fascial, muscular, and neural structures, together with lymphatic and blood flow.

Background

Reportedly developed by A.T. Still, founder of osteopathy, BLT was greatly expanded by R. and H. Lippincott DO, R. Becker DO, and A. Wales DO (Crow 2010). However, the major contribution to its development came from W.G. Sutherland DO, the 'father of cranial osteopathy'. *In Contributions*

of thought, Sutherland (1998) describes the BLT approach as an application of the principles of cranial treatment to the rest of the body and extremities. The key concept is that every joint in normal condition should be within a balanced state of tension of its capsular and ligamentous elements, responsible for proprioception as well as for muscle response during joint motion and position. *'In normal movements, as the joint changes position the relationships between the ligaments also change, but the total tension within the articular mechanism does not'* (Carreiro 2009). However, when an injury or any articular disturbance occurs, such physiological and tensional balance may be compromised, producing proximal and distal effects. Consequently, the joint or tissue, when taken beyond its physiological barrier remains dysfunctional, failing to return into its normal position, therefore showing a shifting of its normal balance point. BLT aims to restore the tensional and functional equilibrium, by seeking and mantaining a balanced tensional point within tissues involved, from which the inherent body potency may find its way to correction.

Objectives

Mainly used by osteopaths, BLT is usually perceived as a pleasant and relaxing technique by the patient. It has been indicated for:
- Joint injury, articular and myofascial dysfunction (Speece & Crow 2001)
- Chronic pelvic pain in women (Tettambel 2005)

- Coccydynia (Fraix & Seffinger 2010)
- Foot drop symptoms (Kuchera 2010a)
- Lymphatic congestion and local edema (Kuchera 2010b, Nicholas & Nicholas 2011)
- Headache, osteoporosis and acute asthma (DiGiovanna et al. 2005)
- Infants and children (Carreiro 2009)
- Chronic low back pain – it is one of the 14 most commonly used techniques for this condition (Licciardone et al. 2008).

Clinical aims are:

- To correct articular strain
- To release capsular and ligamentous tension
- To normalize joint dysfunction, including acute articular ones
- To balance autonomic activity
- To promote synovial fluid circulation
- Vascular congestion relief
- Nerve entrapment release

Assessment

The choice to apply BLT may be taken when clinical assessment finds any sign of articular strain: loss of function; pain; restriction of joint mobility or of myofascial tissue motility; impairment of fluid dynamics (arterial, venous, lymphatic and synovial); deficiencies in fine and gross motor controls; altered sensation; joint laxity; muscle stiffness or spasm. Such changes may be caused by compensatory patterns, inflammation, infection, macro-trauma or repetitive micro-traumatic events following work, sport- or hobby-related positions and activities. Articular strains may also alter the normal proprioceptive role of the capsular–ligamentous complex leading to an impaired reflex muscular activation (Solomonow 2009). This may consequently alter joint position and body posture, at both a local and global level, predisposing to reoccurring of injuries and to the establishment of chronic dysfunctional patterns.

Protocol

BLT is primarily an indirect technique, safe and non-invasive in its application, associated with light touch and patient cooperation. The operator should avoid causing discomfort or guarding by remaining within the tissue's permitted motion and elastic limits. Throughout the technique, the operator should remain in a perceptive state, looking for diagnostic clues as the patient responds to treatment. When treating a body region, visualization of anatomical features may reinforce the procedure and its therapeutic effect: *'Keep your minds full of pictures of the normal body all the time, while treating the afflicted'* (Still 1899). Although generally simplified to three main steps (Disengage-Exaggerate-Balance), BLT procedure may be extended into seven phases, as summarized in Table 11.1 when applied to the ankle (See also Fig. 11.1).

1. **Functional diagnosis:** should be based upon an accurate assessment of the involved structures, aiming to locate restriction of motion, positional asymmetry, tissue texture change and tenderness (Greenman 2003). An unbalanced ligamentous tension in a given joint results in a tendency for easier movement to occur towards the 'shortened' ligamentous complex, as well as a reduced range of motion when the joint is tested in the opposite directions. It has been noted that *'ligaments do not need to be disrupted for the balance to be distorted'* (Crow 2010). At the end of the evaluation, the operator should have identified which dysfunctional joint vectors to address during the technique.

2. **Disengagement:** either traction or compression may be used at this stage (although the latter is more commonly applied) to initially disengage the joint involved and allow motion to occur with least resistance. *'This is similar to pushing in the clutch on a car to shift gears'* (Speece & Crow, 2001). This force helps the practitioner to feel the inherent tissue motion while seeking for a neutral point.

3. **Exaggeration:** the joint is taken into the direction of injury, exaggerating the position of relative freedom, allowing the expression of strained tissues only up to the point where all forces (such as torsion, shear) balance each other out to a neutral point. In other words,

Table 11.1 Example of BLT application to the ankle joint

1. Functional diagnosis	After having evaluated the ankle joint, the operator may find dysfunctional vectors of plantar flexion, adduction and inversion
2. Disengagement	With the patient lying supine, the operator may hold the ankle as shown in Figure 11.1 and then apply traction or compression, constantly visualizing the anatomy of the area being worked, while sensing the motion expressed from surrounding tissues
3. Exaggeration	The operator exaggerates the dysfunctional pattern of the ankle involved, by applying plantar flexion, adduction and inversion, within tissue permitted motion, up to where a neutral point is found in all directions
4. Balance	The practitioner locates a balance point within the range of ankle plantar flexion, adduction and inversion, where tensional forces are equally balanced in all directions
5. Holding	The operator holds the balance point, while visualizing the anatomy of the ankle. A deep breath may be asked for, to promote a release. The practitioner should bear in mind that a too firm hold may prevent the change from taking place
6. Releasing	The operator may feel a collapse of the tensional pattern within and around the treated ankle, together with other signs of release. A tissue inherent force may bring the ankle back to neutral position and this should be allowed by the practitioner. If a release is not achieved, the exact balanced point may have not been adequately identified . If this is the case, the procedure should be repeated from phase 4 onwards
7. Reassessment	The operator brings the ankle back to neutral and reassesses the joint in all directions. A sense of balanced tissue tension within and around the ankle joint should be found

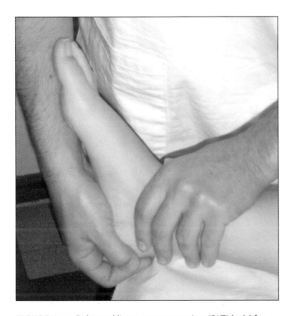

FIGURE 11.1 Balanced ligamentous tension (BLT) hold for the ankle joint. The patient lies supine. The operator holds the heel with the caudal hand and the malleoli with the cephalic hand, while the plantar surface rests on the forearm.

the operator engages ligaments, membranes and fascia towards a position of ease and of least resistance, or simply matching tissues tone, but always remaining within the field of permitted motion. The practitioner should never exaggerate the strain beyond the balance point (Moeckel & Mitha 2008).

4. **Balance:** once all connective tissue tensions are equally balanced, and all the vectors of joint motion are in a state of balance, there should be a sense of poise in a neutral field. *'The articulation is carried in the direction of the lesion position as far as is necessary to cause tension of the weakened elements of the ligamentous structure to be equal to or slightly in excess of the tension of those that are not strained. This is the point of balanced tension.'* (Lippincott 1949). This is the state in which there is minimum resistance to the self-correcting tendency of tissues. It is suggested that balance can be identified not only in ligamentous structures, but also in membranes (balanced membranous tension), fascia (balanced fascial tension) and

fluids (balanced fluid tension). Balanced tension involves a neutral point between freedom of movement and restriction of mobility (Magoun 1976).

5. **Holding:** the balance point is held allowing *'physiologic function within to manifest its own unerring potency'* (Becker 1990). During this phase, tensional and neurological information is elaborated (refining stage) up to when a still point results, before corrective changes. Since ligaments are not under voluntary control, Sutherland (1998) recommended using the inherent forces of the body to promote tissue release: patient cooperation (e.g. respiration, posture, active movement, muscle contraction, eye–tongue movement, patient positioning) may be then requested as an 'enhancing maneuver' to the technique. Such patient assistance may be spontaneous, such as an involuntary muscular movement or a deep breath, but in some way it is useful to overcome *'the resistance of the defense mechanism of the body to the release of the lesion'* (Lippincott 1949).

6. **Releasing:** a release is felt and the joint is brought back into its normal position by the balanced ligamentous tension itself. A sense of melting, softening and fluid reorganization within tissues may be perceived together with warmth, expansion and a restoration of the joint midline.

7. **Reassessment:** the joint is brought back to a neutral position and then reassessed.

During a treatment, the point of BLT tension may also be located to support the application of high velocity thrust to the joint involved, as suggested in the following analogy attributed to A.T. Still: *'If you had a horse tied to a post and you wanted to untie him, you wouldn't first frighten him so that he would pull back on the rope to hold it tight during the untying operation, would you?'* (Fryette 1954).

BLT has been demonstrated as an effective integrative technique to the osteopathic treatment of:

*   Post-infective middle ear effusion (Steele et al. 2010), colonic inertia (Cohen-Lewe

2013), chronic neck and low back pain with a history of standard treatment failure (Gronemeyer et al. 2006)

*   Gastrointestinal disturbances in premature infants, contributing to a reduction in the length of stay in intensive care units (Pizzolorusso et al. 2011), as well as in the management of hospitalized premature infants with nipple feeding dysfunction (Lund et al. 2011)
*   Hospitalized patients with chronic cardiovascular disease (Kaufman 2010) and in the management of subjects at high risk of cardiovascular events (Cerritelli et al. 2011); promoting beneficial hemodynamic effects on the recovery of patients with coronary artery bypass graft (O-Yurvati et al. 2005)
*   Hospitalized patients in general, producing a reduction of anxiety and pain (Pomykala et al. 2008).

BLT has also been shown to be a useful integrative technique with osteopathic treatment for migraine headache, at a lower cost than that provided by allopathic intervention (Schabert & Crow 2009). Finally, BLT is an effective technique in animal practice, having been shown to produce significant changes in dogs with knock knee (Accorsi et al. 2012a) as well as immediate anti-inflammatory effects when applied in dogs with polyarthritis (Accorsi et al. 2012b).

BLT has been indicated for reducing foot drop symptoms when applied to the fibular head and interosseous membrane (Kuchera 2010a); for tenosynovitis and plantar fasciitis (Modi & Shah 2006); for chronic pelvic pain in women (Tettambel 2005) and for coccydynia (Fraix & Seffinger 2010); for headache, osteoporosis and acute asthma (DiGiovanna et al. 2005), and for various conditions affecting infants and childrens – including those with sensory integration disorders (Moeckel & Mitha 2008) – such as brachial plexus injuries and Erb's palsy, suckling dysfunctions, migraine and sinusitis (Carreiro 2009).

BLT is relatively contraindicated in cases of bone fracture, joint dislocation and gross instability, infection, malignancy, severe osteoporosis and open wounds (Nicholas & Nicholas 2011).

Mechanisms

Latest research suggests that muscles, capsules, ligaments and related fascial structures may work together as a unit in maintaining joint function and stability. With regards to anatomical features, ligaments have been shown to be arranged in series, rather than in parallel, with muscle fibers (Van der Wal 2009). They also have been shown to be in anatomical and functional continuity with fascial structures and joint capsules (Willard 1997). It is therefore plausible that when muscle contraction occurs, ligaments and fascia are automatically engaged, working as a connective tissue complex, assisting in joint stabilization, regardless of articular position or phase of muscle contraction (Libbey 2012). Furthermore, from a physiological point of view, afferent mechanoreceptors in ligaments seem to be capable of eliciting a ligamentomuscular reflex that may exert inhibitory effects on muscles related to the joint (Solomonow 2009). This may in turn alter the load on ligaments themselves. This reflex may play a role during BLT application, having an effect on the state of tension of the entire fascio-musculo-ligamento-capsulo-articular complex. In this sense, Sutherland's words (1998) are truly sppropriate: *'The ligaments, not the muscles are the natural agencies for this purpose of correcting the relations and positions of joints.'*

Initially, when BLT is applied, the strained joint receives a disengagement force: this may reduce or remove the 'crimping' of collagen fibers (undulations present when not under tensile loading) around the joint, creating a temporary lengthening of collagenous structures (Threlkeld 1992). Following this, an exaggeration of the dysfunctional pattern is pursued, unloading tissues, possibly decreasing neural inputs, as well as mechanical stress. According to Van Buskirk (1990), positioning a joint into ease may produce an unloading of muscle spindles while possibly loading Golgi tendon organs. This may result in modulation of muscle tone and of related fascial tension. In addition, the activation of mechanoreceptors in ligaments may affect both local blood supply and tissue viscosity, causing either local or systemic effects (Schleip 2012). Moreover, the position of ease may quieten nociceptive input from the dysfunctional area to potentially facilitated spinal levels. Reduction of peripheral biochemical substances (cytokines etc.) that are known to be linked to nociception may dampen local edema and lower sympathetic drive, which may have previously encouraged local vasoconstriction and diminished lymphatic flow in involved joints and tissues.

Subsequently, during BLT application, a position of balanced tension is achieved. At this stage the neurological proprioceptive feedback from involved tissues may be kept at a low level while their involuntary motion quietens and generally passes through a still point. A complex interplay between different body rhythms and fluid dynamics may occur at this point, up to when a release is felt. Sutherland referred to a tide propagating throughout the entire body, including fluids that create an interstitial flow. This concept has recently been supported by research (Chikly & Quaghebeur 2013). In cases of dysfunction the interstitial fluid fluctuation would be impaired, possibly resulting in tissue hypoxia and a build-up of pain-inducing waste products, such as prostaglandins and nitrogenous waste. Restoration of balanced tension (for example, via BLT) may be achieved, re-establishing fluid motion and more normal function.

During the BLT 'balance and hold' phase, the practitioner may request respiratory cooperation. Such contributions may play a role in myofascial relaxation and improvement in joint mobility since respiration seems to have an effect on myofascial tension (Cummings & Howell 1990), even on non-respiratory muscles (Kisselkova & Georgiev 1979) suggesting that they receive input from respiratory centres.

Cellular and fluid exchanges take place within and through the matrix. According to the tensegrity model, the whole body is a three-dimensional viscoelastic matrix, balanced by an integrated system of compressional and tensional forces in dynamic equilibrium. In this perspective, bones are non-touching rods that play the role of compression struts, embedded in a continuous connecting system (the tension system), that is the myofascioligamentous continuum in the body.

Such systems exhibit a balanced tension concurrent with a dynamic ability to adapt to any force introduced anywhere in the system. Thanks to its hierarchical organization, any applied load can influence any part of the entire system, from the cellular to the entire body, and vice versa, by means of the non-linear distribution of forces.

Research has shown that changes in tissue structure may alter the arrangement of the cytoskeleton, which in turn can influence gene expression and cellular metabolism (Chen & Ingber 1999). For instance, fibroblast strain may set in motion a cascade of events that attenuate pro-inflammatory substances, while at the same time stimulating anti-inflammatory signalling pathways (Tsuzaki et al. 2003), thus influencing pain perception. A brief, moderate amplitude (20–30% strain) involving stretching of connective tissue, decreases both TGF-ß1 and collagen synthesis, preventing soft tissue adhesions (Bouffard et al. 2008). Therefore, beneficial light and balanced strain, such as that applied during a BLT session, may be sensed at the cellular level, normalizing tissue structure and function. In this sense, BLT is perhaps one of the best examples of how the concept of tensegrity can be applied in treatment. In addition, it is not only strain magnitude that appears to play a role in tissue response, but also strain duration and direction, since they both seem to differentially regulate cell growth, ion conductances and gene expression, responding accordingly with differential stretch-activated calcium channel signalling (Kamkin et al. 2003).

References

Accorsi A et al 2012a Osteopathic manipulative treatment for knock knee: a case finding. Conference Proceedings. First International Congress of Osteopathy in Animal Practice, 28–29 September. Rome, Italy, p 11

Accorsi A et al 2012b Case-report: impact of OMT on biochemical mediators of inflammation. Conference Proceedings. First International Congress of Osteopathy in Animal Practice, 28–29 September. Rome, Italy, p 10

Becker RE 1990 Foreword. In: Sutherland WG (ed) Teachings in the science of osteopathy. Sutherland Cranial Teaching Foundation, Fort Worth, TX

Bouffard NA et al 2008 Tissue stretch decreases soluble TGF ß1 and Type-1 pro-collagen in mouse subcutaneous connective tissue: evidence from ex vivo and in vivo models. J Cell Physiol 214: 389–395

Carreiro JE 2009 Pediatric manual medicine: an osteopathic approach. Churchill Livingstone Elsevier, Edinburgh

Cerritelli F et al 2011 Osteopathic manipulation as a complementary treatment for the prevention of cardiac complications: 12-months follow-up of intima media and blood pressure on a cohort affected by hypertension. J Bodyw Mov Ther 15(1):68–74

Chen CS, Ingber DE 1999 Tensegrity and mechanoregulation: from skeleton to cytoskeleton. J Osteoarthritis Res Soc Int 7:81e94

Chikly B, Quaghebeur J 2013 Reassessing cerebrospinal fluid (CSF) hydrodynamics: a literature review presenting a novel hypothesis for CSF physiology. J Bodyw Mov Ther 17(3):344–54; epub: 12 Apr

Cohen-Lewe A 2013 Osteopathic manipulative treatment for colonic inertia. J Am Osteopath Assoc 113(3):216–20

Crow WMT 2010 Balanced ligamentous tension and ligamentous articular strain. In: Chila AG (ed) Foundations of osteopathic medicine. Philadelphia, Lippincott Williams & Wilkins, Ch 52

Cummings J, Howell J 1990 The role of respiration in the tension production of myofascial tissues. JAOA 90 (9):842

DiGiovanna DL et al 2005 An osteopathic approach to diagnosis and treatment, 3rd edn., Lippincott Williams & Wilkins, Philadelphia

Fraix MP, Seffinger MA 2010 Acute low back pain. In: Chila AG (ed) Foundations of osteopathic medicine. Lippincott Williams & Wilkins, Philadelphia, Ch 69

Fryette HH 1954 Principles of osteopathic technique. Academy of Applied Osteopathy Carmel, CA, p 62

Greenman PE 2003 Principles of manual medicine, 2nd edn. Williams and Wilkins, Baltimore, Chs 1 & 2

Gronemeyer J et al 2006 Retrospective outcome analysis of osteopathic manipulation in a treatment failure setting. In: 50th Annual AOA Research Conference-Abstracts. J Am Osteopath Assoc 106:471–510

Kamkin A et al 2003 Activation and inactivation of a non-selective cation conductance by local mechanical deformation of acutely isolated cardiac fibroblasts. Cardiovasc Res 57 (3): 793e803

Kaufman B 2010 Adult with chronic cardiovascular disease. In: Chila AG (ed) Foundations of osteopathic medicine. Lippincott Williams & Wilkins, Philadelphia, Ch 55

Kisselkova G, Georgiev V 1979 Effects of training on post-exercise limb muscle EMG synchronous to respiration.J Appl Physiol Respir Environ Exerc Physiol 46:1093–1095

Kuchera ML 2010a Lower extremities. In: Chila, AG (ed) Foundations of osteopathic medicine. Philadelphia, Lippincott Williams & Wilkins, Ch 42

Kuchera ML 2010b Lymphatics approach. In: Chila AG (ed) Foundations of osteopathic medicine. Philadelphia, Lippincott Williams & Wilkins, Ch 51

Libbey R 2012 Ligamentous articular strain technique – a manual treatment approach for ligamentous articular injuries and the whole body. Journal of Prolotherapy 4:e886–e890

Licciardone JC et al 2008 Osteopathic health outcomes in chronic low back pain: the osteopathic trial. Osteopath Med Prim Care Apr 25;2:5

Lippincott, HA 1949 The osteopathic technique of Wm G. Sutherland DO. Yearbook of the Academy of Applied Osteopathy. AAO, Indianapolis, p 1–41

Lund GC et al 2011 Osteopathic manipulative treatment for the treatment of hospitalized premature infants with nipple feeding dysfunction. J Am Osteopath Assoc 111(1):44–8

Magoun HI 1976 Osteopathy in the cranial field, 3rd edn. Journal Printing Company, Kirksville, MO, Ch 5

Modi RG, Shah NA 2006 Comlex review: clinical anatomy and osteopathic manipulative medicine. Blackwell, Malden, MA, Ch 9, 10

Moeckel E, Mitha N 2008 Textbook of pediatric osteopathy. Churchill Livingstone, Edinburgh, Ch 8

Nicholas A, Nicholas E 2011 Atlas of osteopathic techniques, 2nd edn. Lippincott Williams & Wilkins, Philadelphia, Chs 14 & 16

O-Yurvati AH et al 2005 Hemodynamic effects of osteopathic manipulative treatment immediately after coronary artery bypass graft surgery. J Am Osteopath Assoc Oct 105(10):475–81

Pizzolorusso G et al 2011 Effect of osteopathic manipulative treatment on gastrointestinal function and length of stay of preterm infants: an exploratory study. Chiropr Man Therap 19(1):15

Pomykala M et al 2008 Patient perception of osteopathic manipulative treatment in a hospitalized setting: a survey-based study. J Am Osteopath Assoc 108(11):665–8

Schabert E, Crow WT 2009 Impact of osteopathic manipulative treatment on cost of care for patients with migraine headache: a retrospective review of patient records. J Am Osteopath Assoc 109(8):403–7

Schleip R 2012 Fascia as a sensory organ. A target of myofascial manipulation. In: Dalton E. Dynamic body – exploring form, expanding function. Freedom from Pain Institute, Oklahoma City

Sleszynski SL, Glonek T 2005 Outpatient osteopathic SOAP note form: preliminary results in osteopathic outcomes-based research. J Am Osteopath Assoc 105(4):181–205

Solomonow M 2009 Ligaments: a source of musculoskeletal disorders. J Bodyw Mov Ther 13(2):136–54

Speece C, Crow T 2001 Ligamentous articular strain: osteopathic techniques for the body. Eastland Press, Seattle

Steele KM et al 2010 Brief report of a clinical trial on the duration of middle ear effusion in young children using a standardized osteopathic manipulative medicine protocol. J Am Osteopath Assoc 110(5):278–284

Still AT 1899 Philosophy of osteopathy. Journal Printing Company, Kirksville, MO, Ch 1

Sutherland WG 1998 Contributions of thought. In: Sutherland AS, Wales AL (eds) The Sutherland cranial teaching foundation. Ruda Press, Portland

Tettambel MA 2005 An osteopathic approach to treating women with chronic pelvic pain. J Am Osteopath Assoc 105(9 Suppl 4):S20–2

Threlkeld J 1992 The effects of manual therapy on connective tissue. Phys Ther 72:893–902

Tsuzaki M et al 2003 ATP modulates load-inducible IL-1beta, COX 2, and MMP-3 gene expression in human tendon cells. J Cell Biochem 89 (3):556e562

Van Buskirk RL 1990 Nociceptive reflexes and the somatic dysfunction: a model. JAOA 90(9): 792–805

van der Wal J 2009 The architecture of the connective tissue in the musculoskeletal system –an often overlooked functional parameter as to proprioception in the locomotor apparatus. Int J Ther Massage Bodywork 2(4):9–23

Willard FH 1997 The muscular, ligamentous and neural structure of the low back and its relation to back pain. In: Vleeming, A et al (eds) Movement, stability and low back pain: the essential role of the pelvis. Churchill Livingstone, Edinburgh

Chapter 12

INSTRUMENT-ASSISTED SOFT TISSUE MOBILIZATION

Warren I. Hammer

Introduction

An underlying feature of all the methods of fascial therapies discussed in this text involves the creation of tissue deformation. Every cell in the body requires deformation, such as movement, tension and compression, in order to function.

As discussed in previous chapters (see mechanotransduction in Ch. 1), innumerable effects occur from applied tissue deformation. Deformation of tissue is necessary for life, for both tissue generation and reparation processes. Our everyday movements and exercise are an essential source of such deformation. Manual methods might even be considered as an applied, localized, precise form of passive exercise.

A major effect of mechanical load deals with changes at the cellular level, which include changes in cell morphology, cytoskeletal organization, cell survival, cell differentiation and gene expression to produce RNA or necessary proteins (Pirola et al. 1994, Sarasa & Chiquet 2005). The realization that forms of mechanical load are responsible for fibroblastic proliferation (especially collagen type I; Rozario & DeSimone 2010), creation of the extracellular matrix (ECM), release of growth factors (cytokines) and a myriad of chemical reactions by transduction is still in its early stages. Tissue deformation is the major stimulus for mechanoreceptive triggering and proprioception (van der Wal 2012). In addition, tissue deformation is involved in the possible restoration of muscle force transmission (Turrina et al. 2012) because fascia performs along with muscles as a force transmitter.

The question arises: just what exactly are we attempting to change in fascial tissue? Many clinicians speak of freeing fibrotic scar tissue, but while the scar may be stretched it cannot be restored to a functional state. Fibrosis is a normal process that occurs after injury at the end stage of the inflammatory cascade. But severe injury and actual tearing of fibers can result in abnormal fibrous bands of scar tissue in between muscle fibers. Stecco et al. (2013) differentiate fibrosis from what they call fascial densification. They suggest that fibrosis is a macroscopic rearrangement of the composition and conformation of fascial tissue within the dense connective tissue that is easily recognized on MRI, CAT scans and ultrasound. Most clinical results obtained by manual methods may well be the result of restoring the function of the loose connective tissue, containing adipose cells, glycosaminoglycans (GAGs) and hyaluronic acid (HA). A densification in the loose connective tissue, rather than a fibrosis, occurs due to the increased viscosity of tissue. This increased viscosity is caused by the larger HA fragments and HA molecule entanglement. Normalizing of the HA molecule by deep compression, friction, heat and increased alkalinity are factors found to change the 'gel' into a more fluid medium, thus allowing restoration of the normal sliding function of the fascia (see Ch. 1). Stecco and colleagues (2013) hypothesize that the myofascial pain syndrome with its stiffness and pain is caused primarily by a densification of the loose connective tissue.

The use of instruments other than the hands probably dates back thousands of years; for example, in Gua Sha, in which practitioners use instruments such as soup spoons, coins, or slices of water buffalo horn. By 'scraping' the skin (without harming the epidermis), the traditional belief was that pathogenic blood stagnation was being modified, while more normal circulation and metabolic processes were being encouraged. By modifying micro-adhesions in the fascia, via use of scraping tools, the lymphatic system was encouraged to transport and eliminate stagnant fluids. In Greek and Roman baths, curved metal tools known as strigils were used to scrape dirt and sweat from the body, possibly with similar objectives (Kotera-Feyer 1993).

Currently, instrument-assisted soft tissue mobilization (IASTM) involves the use of hand-held instruments that become extensions of the hand, and in many cases reduplicate or improve the clinical results achieved by the hand. Instruments can be made of materials such as stone, stainless steel, wood, plastic, and ceramic. Possibly counterintuitively, IASTM actually enhances palpatory skills for detecting major and minor fibrotic and/or densified tissue. Instruments also permit deeper sustained penetration of tissues when necessary. Loghmani & Warden (2009) demonstrates that using IASTM expedites rehabilitation/recovery. For the practitioner, a very important benefit derived from using IASTM is the reduction of manual stress on his/her hands and joints. Repetitive injury to manual therapists' hands and upper extremities over time has been reported as a major reason for loss of work (Snodgrass et al. 2003). This chapter outlines the safe use of IASTM.

Instrumented Assisted Soft Tissue Mobilization

Possibly the most widley used IASTM method is Graston Technique® (GT), which was formally introduced in 1994. GT employs six proprietary stainless steel instruments (Fig. 12.1) with contoured beveled edges designed to adapt to the various tissue/shapes/curves of the body. Stainless steel has a higher resonating quality than other materials, which allows it to be a better sensor of tissue restriction. Becoming proficient in the use of GT requires professional training.

Most will agree that nothing can replace the hand as a sensory diagnostic tool, but IASTM can be an important modality for clinicians who depend on hands-on therapy. The use of instrumentation has been increasing over the years. According to a recent conversation with GT's president (Arnolt, personal communication 2013):

GT has trained nearly 16 000 clinicians to date, mostly in the USA. The instruments support treatment in more than 1600 outpatient facilities. They are used in more than 70 industrial, armed forces and entertainment sites and are used to treat athletes in some 250 amateur and professional sports organizations. And most importantly, GT is supported in 57 academic institutions. It is the foremost instrument-assisted system being taught in advanced degree programs for physical therapists, athletic trainers and chiropractors today.

IASTM instruments allow practitioners to easily feel and identify myofascial restrictions. Depending upon the fascial technique used, the instruments can be used to apply local pressure or friction to a thickened restricted area. Broad strokes are used for larger areas such as the quadriceps or hamstrings. IASTM can be applied to either superficial or deep layers of fascia. Due to the concentration of pressure and friction tolerable with IASTM, treatment time may be reduced. Ideally, before the use of instruments or hands, a functional examination should be performed including passive, contractile and active motion tests to determine the possible source of the pain. Post-treatment testing is particularly important to determine whether the procedure was successful. As is discussed later, treatment with perturbation, i.e. the patient performing a painful motion to indicate where they feel the pain, is a useful way of revealing and treating the abnormal tissues.

Research

There are numerous case studies and some histological studies that affirm the value of IASTM.

- Early studies emphasized the proliferation of fibroblasts following IASTM. While it is recognized that mechanical load influences many healing effects, fibroblasts play a significant role. *'The repair and maintenance of connective tissues is performed predominately by a mesenchymal cell known as a fibroblast'* (Eastwood et al. 1998). (See Ch. 1 for more on fibroblasts.)

- Fibroblasts affect the synthesis of ECM proteins (Thie et al. 1989).
- Mechanical strain encourages altered gene expression in fibroblasts, encouraging collagen synthesis, for example following trauma (Cui et al. 2004).
- Gehlsen et al. (1999) describe how increased pressure produced a greater proliferation of fibroblasts. They conclude that heavy pressure promotes the healing process to a greater degree than light or moderate pressure.
- Davidson et al. (1997) showed how the use of IASTM promotes healing in rat tendons via fibroblast recruitment and their production of rough endoplasmic reticulum.
- Loghmani & Warden (2009) bilaterally surgically transected the medial collateral ligaments (MCL) of both knees of 20 rats. GT instruments were used on one knee while the opposite knee served as a control. Seven days postoperatively, GT was used for 1 minute to the left MCL 3 times/week for 3 weeks. The treated ligament side was found to be 31% stronger (p<0.01) and 34% stiffer (p<0.001) than the untreated side. The healing time was accelerated, indicating that the use of IASTM could also be responsible for earlier rehabilitation. A general view of the effect of IASTM is that it re-initiates the inflammatory process and stimulates a healing cascade by introducing a controlled amount of micro-trauma to the tissue. This results in a proliferative invasion of blood nutrients and fibroblasts, creating collagen deposition and eventual maturation of the tissue.
- Perle et al. (2003) conducted a prospective multi-center case series of 1004 patients treated by GT and demonstrate that, for the conditions treated (see Applications below), there was a significant decrease in pain (p<0.001) and numbness (p<0.002), and increase in function (p<0.001). Most patients achieved a high percentage of their treatment goals.

Applications

IASTM can be used in most areas where hands are used to apply manual loading. It can be used almost anywhere on the body where there are superficial and deep fascia and retinaculum. Examples include:

- Tendinopathy: osis/itis (epicondylopathy; Sevier et al. 1995), plantar fasciosis
- Neural entrapment areas, i.e. carpal tunnel etc. (Anandkumar 2012)
- Arthritic joint capsules and ligaments (Loghmani & Warden 2009)
- Traumatic or surgical scars, lymphedema
- Thickened fascia that has been shown to be associated with recurrent and chronic low back pain (Langevin et al. 2009)
- Cervical pain, de Quervains's syndrome, epicondylitis, fibromyalgia, IT band syndrome, joint sprain, lower back pain, muscle strain, painful scar, plantar fasciitis, post fracture pain, tendinitis (Perle et al. 2003).

Protocol

Some practitioners have found that their ability to palpate superficial and deep fascia is greatly enhanced when instruments are used and that the time of application is greatly reduced. A superficial or deep application can be applied, depending on the force and the weight of the particular instrument used. It is noteworthy that the depth and force of the instrument may create different results. Yang et al. (2005) hypothesized that repetitive, small magnitude stretching was anti-inflammatory, whereas large magnitude stretching was pro-inflammatory. Standley (2007) demonstrated that manual light myofascial treatment was anti-inflammatory (this was an in vitro study). Treatment of the superficial fascia with light strokes may be important for improving circulation and lymphatic drainage.

IASTM (GT) protocol (Table 12.1) usually relies on an initial tissue warm-up with moist heat or ultrasound, although the friction of the instrument may create sufficient heat by itself. It has been found that the lack of sliding between layers of fascia might be due to molecular entanglement of HA molecules resulting in increased

Table 12.1 IASTM (GT) protocol

Procedure	Rationale
Tissue warm-up At least 3–5 min of either: • Local tissue exercise • Moist heat • Ultrasound or • 10–15 min of cardiovascular exercise	Increase blood flow and tissue warming
Use of GT 2 treatments per week in the same area 30 sec–1 min for localized lesion dysfunction 3–5 min for local region (i.e. shoulder) 8–10 min for treatment of all areas combined	Break-up of soft tissue restriction; creation of new extracellular matrix
Stretching Immediately after IASTM 1–3 30-sec stretches Mattes Active Isolated Stretching* (2 sets of 12)	Lengthen shortened structures; realign fibers
Strengthening High-repetition, low-load 1–2 sets of 15; isotonic rubber tubing, eccentric contraction Cryotherapy (if necessary)	Strengthen weak or lengthened structures Minimize post-treatment inflammation, soreness, and bruising

*Mattes 2000.

viscosity and that increased temperature is necessary to restore normal HA fluidity (Piehl-Aulin 1991) along with compression and friction to restore normal fascial gliding. Clinical experience suggests that the GT instrument should be used with the beveled edge down. Several types of strokes may be employed: strumming, J-stroke, sweeping, framing, swivel brushing, fanning or scooping. Today, practitioners are using a variety of instruments but, as with most procedures, with time and experience it becomes an art, as more effective ways of using the tools are identified. Bruising can occur, but recent experience demonstrates that in most cases satisfactory results can be obtained with only establishing a redness response. If a local inflammation occurs, which is often necessary to stimulate a healing response and the laying down of new connective tissue, it is important to not treat the same area for at least 4–7 days.

There are a variety of applications that can be used with instrumentation (Fig. 12.1). For example, in tennis elbow (lateral epicondylopathy) broad instruments 'GT-4' and 'GT-5' could be used to scan the areas both proximal and distal to the elbow to feel where the most obvious fascial restrictions are located.

Smaller instruments, such as GT-3 and GT-6, can be used for treating the fascial entheses around the lateral epicondyle itself (Figs 12.2–12.4). An example of an IASTM procedure for treating lateral epicondylopathy is to first perform functional testing, such as resisted wrist extension and passive wrist flexion for identification of pain and areas of complaint. Next, scan the arm and forearm on both the dorsal and volar surfaces to identify dysfunctional painful areas, which indicate where fascial restrictions may be present.

As in the treatment of most areas, in this case the elbow, the instruments should be used towards any direction where a barrier may have been identified.

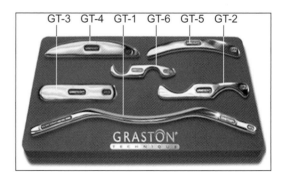

FIGURE 12.1 Graston Technique® Instruments.

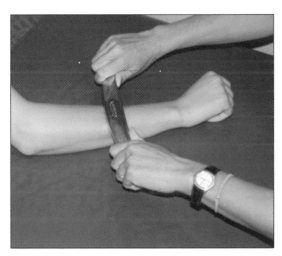

FIGURE 12.2 Scanning for densifications along the dorsal forearm extensor areas using GT-4.

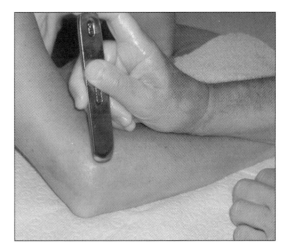

FIGURE 12.4 Treating around the entheses of the lateral epicondyle using GT-3.

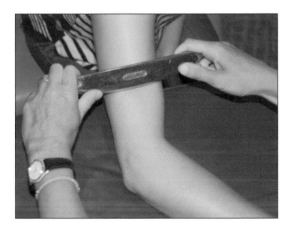

FIGURE 12.3 Scanning for densifications along the arm using GT-4.

They should also be used all over the arms and forearms including the antagonist locations. This is easier than using the fingers to palpate all of the surrounding areas.

Figure 12.4 shows the use of GT-3 (GT-6 is also possible) at the entheses locations around the lateral epicondyle. Information derived from pre- and post-treatment should be compared, based on functional testing; for example, was there improvement after treatment (less pain) on functional testing? What area does post-testing still aggravate?

The original painful site may change location and a new area could be treated and then retested for improvement. On retesting after the first session, it is often found that the patient experiences diminished or no pain. On the second session, re-testing may show decreased pain on functional testing and the clinician can then treat similar areas or new areas that demonstrate palpatory restrictions. If, on the second visit, the patient is worse or does not show any change, it is recommended that the proximal and distal kinetic chain is checked by scanning the neck, shoulder and hand. Patients typically ask how many treatments will be necessary. Although this is impossible to predict, treatment should be terminated when 10 consecutive positive functional tests produce no symptomatology before the treatment is performed. If indicated, the patient can be given stretching exercises to do at home. In the case of lateral epicondylopathy, eccentric exercise has been shown to be very beneficial in the promotion of collagen synthesis and healing (Croisier et al. 2007).

Relative and absolute contraindications (yellow and red flags, respectively) are listed in (Box 12.1):

- It is suggested that only superficial, light strokes are employed initially, especially for patients on anticoagulants.

Box 12.1

Red flags: absolute contraindications (Carey-Loghmani et al. 2010)

Open wound-unhealed suture site/sutures
Thrombophlebitis
Uncontrolled hypertension
Kidney dysfunction
Patient intolerance/non-compliance

Hypersensitivity
Hematoma
Osteomyelitis
Myositis ossificans

Yellow flags: relative contraindications

Anti-coagulant medication
Cancer
Varicose veins
Burn scars

Acute inflammatory conditions i.e., synovitis
Inflammatory condition secondary to infection
Acute rheumatoid arthritis

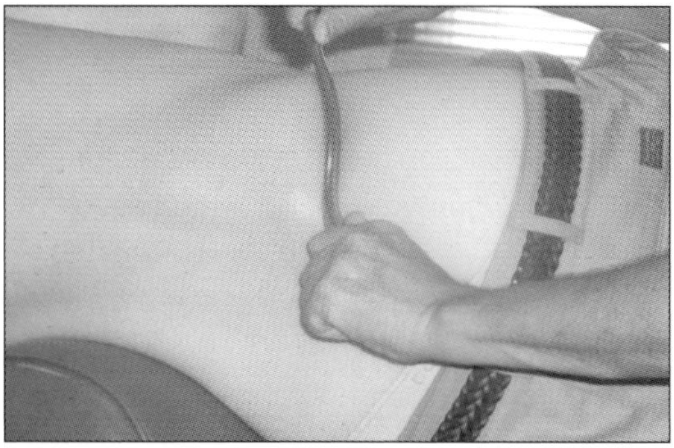

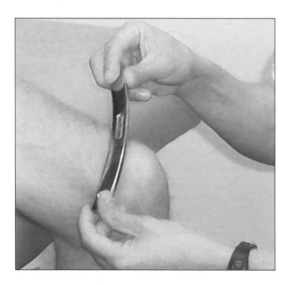

FIGURE 12.5 Use of GT-1 on the quadratus lumborum area.

FIGURE 12.6 GT-5 for quadriceps/retinaculum area.

- Cancer is not an absolute contraindication as palliative treatment may be warranted depending on the type and location of the cancer being treated. Note: increasing blood flow can promote metastases, depending on the phase and type of cancer. It pays to seek medical clearance before proceeding if there is any doubt whatsoever.

Examples of the use of IASTM are shown in Figures 12.5 and 12.6:

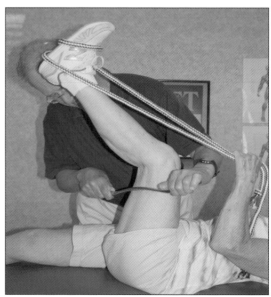

FIGURE 12.7 Treatment of the distal hamstring during active isolated stretch. For the distal hamstring, with the hip flexed 90° the leg is elevated to its maximum and then stretched for a second.

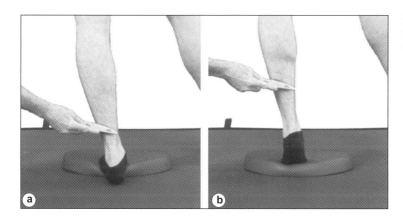

FIGURE 12.8 Increasing proprioception while treating on a balance board with ankle motion.

- Figure 12.5 shows a larger instrument (GT-1) being used on the lateral lumbar area
- Figure 12.6 shows GT-5 for quadriceps/retinaculum area, which is often valuable for treatment of diminished knee flexion post-surgery.

The use of IASTM with movement is becoming more widespread. Approximately 9 years ago, Greg Doerr DC and Tom Hyde DC began to experiment with treating soft tissue/fascial disorders through the use of instruments and incorporated treatment during movement to provoke pain, loss of range of motion and feeling of tightness. Treatments where increased weight (dumbbells etc.) or therabands are used to provoke pain often help to localize areas of restriction. Treatment while the patient stands on a balance board helps to stimulate proprioception. There is some research that points to the value of treatment with motion; for example, proprioceptive acuity improves as movement becomes more dynamic and more active and there is an increase in proprioceptive recruitment with active movements due to increased cortical activity (Chapman et al. 1987, Paalasmaa et al. 1991).

- Figure 12.7 demonstrates treatment of the distal hamstring during active isolated stretch (Mattes 2000)
- Figure 12.8 shows treatment of lower gastrocnemius/soleus area using a balance board during ankle plantar flexion.

In conclusion, IASTM is proving to be an effective method for the treatment of soft tissue dysfunction. It is becoming more widely used in the United States and elsewhere as an increasing number of manual therapy practitioners discover its clinical usefulness.

References

Anandkumar S 2012 Physical therapy management of entrapment of the superficial peroneal nerve in the lower leg: A case report. Physiotherapy Theory Pract

Carey-Loghmani MT, Schrader JW, Hammer WI 2010 Graston Technique: M1 Instruction Manual, 3rd edn. TherapyCare Resources, Indianapolis

Chapman CE et al 1987 Sensory perception during movement in man. Exp Brain Res 68(3):516–24

Croisier JL et al 2007 An isokinetic eccentric programme for the management of chronic lateral epicondylar tendinopathy. Br J Sports Med 41(4):269–75, Epub 2007 Jan 15

Cui W, Bryant MR, Sweet PM, McDonnell PJ 2004 Changes in gene expression in response to mechanical strain in human scleral fibroblasts. Exp Eye Res 78: 275–284

Davidson CJ et al 1997 Rat tendon morphologic and functional changes resulting from soft tissue mobilization. Medicine and Science in Sports and Exercise 29:313–319

Eastwood M, McGrouther DA, Brown RA 1998 Fibroblast responses to mechanical forces. Proc Inst Mech Eng Vol 212 Part H

Gehlsen GM, Ganion LR, Helfst R 1999 Fibroblast response to variation in soft tissue mobilization pressure. Medicine and Science in Sports and Exercise 31 (4), 531–535

Kotera-Feyer E 1993 Die Strigilis. Lang, Frankfurt am Main, pp 63–148

Langevin HM, Churchill DL, Cipolla MJ 2001 Mechanical signaling through connective tissue: a mechanism for the therapeutic effect of acupuncture. FASEB J 15:2275–2282

Langevin HM et al 2009 Ultrasound evidence of altered lumbar connective tissue structure in human subjects with chronic low back pain. BMC Musculoskeletal Disorders 10:151

Loghmani MT, Warden SJ 2009 Instrument-assisted cross fiber massage accelerates knee ligament healing. J Orthop Sports Phys Ther 39:506–514

Mattes AL 2000 Active isolated stretching: The Mattes Method. Aaron L Mattes, PO Box 17217 Sarasota, FL 34276–0217, USA

Paalasmaa P, Kemppainen P, Pertovaara A 1991 Modulation of skin sensitivity by dynamic and isometric exercise in man. Applied Physiology 62: 279–283

Perle SM, Perry DG, Carey MT 2003 Effects of Graston Technique on soft tissue conditions: a prospective case series. In: WFC's seventh Biennial Congress, Orlando, FL, World Federation of Chiropractic, pp 344–345

Piehl-Aulin K 1991 Hyaluronan in human skeletal muscle of lower extremity: concentration, distribution, and effect of exercise. J Appl Physiol 71(6):2493–8

Pirola CJ et al 1994 Mechanical stimuli induce vascular parathyroid hormone-related protein gene expression in vivo and in vitro. Endocrinol 134 2230–2236

Rozario T, DeSimone DW 2010 The extracellular matrix in development and morphogenesis: a dynamic view. Dev Biol 341(1):126–40

Sarasa A, Chiquet M 2005 Mechanical signals regulating extracellular matrix gene expression in fibroblasts. Scand J Med Sci Sports 15, 223–230.

Sevier TL et al 1995 Traditional physical therapy vs Graston Augmented Soft Tissue Mobilization in treatment of lateral epicondylitis. Journal of the American College of Sports Medicine 27:(5)

Snodgrass SJ et al 2003 Factors related to thumb pain in physiotherapists. Aust J Physiother 49:243–250

Standley P 2007 Biomechanical strain regulation of human fibroblast cytokine expression: an in vitro model for myofascial release. Presentation at Fascia Research Congress, Boston. DVD from <www.fasciaresearch.com>

Stecco A, Gesi M, Stecco C, Stern R 2013 Fascial components fo the myofascial pain syndrome. Curr Pain Headache Rep 17:352

Thie M, Schlumberger W, Rautenberg J, Robenek H 1989 Mechanical confinement inhibits collagen synthesis in gel-cultured fibroblasts. Eur J Cell Biol 48,294–301

Turrina A, Martinez-Gonzalez, Stecco C 2012 The muscular force transmission system: role of the intramuscular connective tissue. J Bodyw Mov Ther 17:95–102

van der Wal JC 2012 Proprioception. In: Schleip R, Findley T, Chaitow L, Huijing P et al (eds) Fascia: the tensional network of the human body. Elsevier, Edinburgh

Yang G, Im HJ, Wang JH 2005 Repetitive mechanical stretching modulates IL-1beta induced COX-2, MMP-1 expression, and PGE2 production in human patellar tendon fibroblasts. Gene 363:166–172

Chapter 13

MUSCLE ENERGY TECHNIQUES

Leon Chaitow

Introduction

Muscle energy techniques (MET) originated in osteopathic medicine in the 1950s and include a group of methods that involve either isometric contractions, or isotonic eccentric contractions, in treatment and rehabilitation of musculoskeletal dysfunction.

The most basic and most widely used form of MET involves the careful positioning of an area of the body, just short of a restriction barrier (see notes on barriers in Ch. 5), followed by the use of a brief isometric contraction, in which the degree of moderate force employed by the patient, as well as the direction(s) and duration of that effort, are prescribed by the therapist.

After cessation of the isometric contraction (or sometimes during the contraction), the tissues being treated – soft tissue or joint – are eased to a new position. The contraction effort produces changes – discussed below – that allow tissues to be moved or stretched more comfortably than before the isometric contraction.

The repositioning after the contraction commonly involves a degree of stretching, particularly in chronic settings, or might simply take advantage of a reduction in resistance to movement, that allows painless positioning at a new end-of-range barrier, without stretching.

The 'non-stretch' option is more usually chosen in acute clinical settings or in the treatment of joints (Chaitow 2013).

Definitions

Muscle Energy Technique is defined as *'a form of osteopathic manipulative diagnosis and treatment in which the patient's muscles are actively used on request, from a precisely controlled position, in a specific direction, and against a distinctly executed counterforce'* (ECOP 2009).

An isometric contraction is one in which no visible movement occurs, but in which internal elements of the muscle – actin and myosin – *(see Physiology of contraction in* Ch. 5) interact to produce a shortening of the sarcomere, thereby stretching the *series elastic fascial component* of the sarcomere. See Figure 5.1 in Chapter 5.

Isotonic eccentric contraction: a contraction in which a degree of lengthening occurs – with the muscle-length increasing despite the continuing contraction. In MET methodology eccentric stretching can be slowly or rapidly performed, with quite different outcomes – as explained below.

The processes involved in an eccentric stretch include both lengthening of the *series elastic fascial component,* and also lengthening of the *parallel elastic fascial component.*

The **series elastic components** of sarcomeres store energy when stretched, and contribute to elasticity. They comprise non-contractile – fascia/connective tissue – components of muscle that lie in series with muscle fibers. Tendons are examples of the *series elastic component,* as are the cross-bridges between *actin* and *myosin,* the sliding elements of muscle that allow shortening to occur (see Chapter 5, Fig. 5.1; Huxley & Niedergerke 1954).

The **parallel elastic component** of sarcomeres provides resistive tension when a muscle is passively stretched. These are also non-contractile and consist of the muscle membranes (fascia), which lie parallel to the muscle fibers (see Fig. 5.1).

The origins of MET – quotes from the pioneers

MET was developed in osteopathic medicine in the USA, in the late 1940s, with strong influence from several key figures – some of whom are quoted below:

- **Fred Mitchell Jr DO:** *'Treating joint motion restriction as if the cause were tight muscle(s), is one approach that makes possible restoration of normal joint motion... Regardless of the cause of restriction, MET treatment based on a "short muscle" paradigm is usually completely effective in eliminating blockage, and restoring normal range of motion, even when the blockage is due to non-muscular factors'* (Mitchell & Mitchell 1999).

- **Fred Mitchell Sr DO:** *'Muscle energy technique, with its many ramifications, is a most useful tool in preparation of soft tissues... before articular* [joint] *correction is attempted'* (Mitchell 1958).

- **Edward Stiles DO:** *'He* (Fred Mitchell Sr) *was focused on using muscles to* [treat] *restricted joint function. His main focus was not relaxing muscles but re-establishing joint mechanics'* (Stiles 2012, personal communication).

- **R.E. Kappler DO:** *'The term barrier may be misleading if it is interpreted as a wall or rigid obstacle to be overcome with a push. As a joint reaches the barrier, restraints in the form of tight muscles and fascia, serve to inhibit further motion.* **We are pulling against restraints,** *rather than pushing against some anatomic structure.'* (Kappler 2003).

- **Fred Mitchell Jr DO:** *'The therapist's force is always the counterforce. A common mistake is to ask the patient to "resist my effort". This ignores the factor of intentionality that ensures that core muscles are re-educated and rehabilitated. What works best is to tell the patient the exact direction of the action, the amount of force, and when to stop'* (Fred Mitchell Jr interview, in Franke 2009).

- **Thomas Jefferson Ruddy DO:** Ruddy suggested the use of multiple mini-isometric contractions, [usually] towards the barrier, at a rate slightly faster than the pulse-rate. The patient is asked to introduce a series of these mini-contractions against [practitioner] resistance. For example ... *'contract-relax,' 'contract-relax,' 'contract-relax'* – 10 times. After this, as the patient relaxes, the joint is eased to its new barrier. The process is repeated once more. These contractions should be performed without 'wobble' or 'bounce' (Ruddy 1962).

- **Karel Lewit MD:** *'Strong or moderate force contractions – as initially used in MET – recruited too many of the "wrong" motor units, and results were less that were hoped for. It was Karel Lewit who drastically reduced the force generated by muscle contractions'* (Mitchell Jr 2009).

- **John Goodridge DO:** *'Muscle energy technique is not a wrestling match... A small amount of force should be used at first, with increase as necessary. This is much more productive than beginning with too much force... Localization of force is more important than intensity of force'* (Goodridge 1981).

- **Fred Mitchell Jr:** *'Isolytic* [eccentric isotonic] *contractions with vibratory counterforce, involves light to moderate force, sustained for no more than 15 seconds'* (Fred Mitchell Jr interview, in Franke 2009).

- **Gary Fryer PhD, DO:** *'The features that are required to ensure successful use of MET include: a precise positioning to the barrier; an active and appropriately formulated (strength, timing) muscle contraction, by the patient, against a defined resistance of the therapist, in a precise direction; the number of repetitions, and finally an accurate assessment of the therapeutic outcome'* (Chaitow 2013).

These quotes offer a sense of the evolution of MET, from fairly crude origins (where heavy degrees of patient effort were requested), to the use of subtle, low-force, specifically directed contractions of different types.

The ultimate focus remains the same, however – to normalize and rehabilitate the soft-tissue component of the body when dysfunctional, so allowing more normal, ideally pain-free, function – most particularly involving previously restricted joints. For a summary of the detail of MET application see: *MET protocol summary,* later in this chapter.

Basic MET variations

The elements that make up **standard isometric MET** (see definitions above) always include:

- Identification of a resistance barrier, whether this is the end-of-range of a muscle or a joint. The MET barrier represents the *very first sign of resistance to movement in any particular direction* (see Ch. 5).
- The use of an isometric – or sometimes isotonic eccentric – contraction, starting with the tissues just short of the resistance barrier, with the contraction directed towards or away from that barrier, or in another direction altogether.
- In some instances the isometric contractions are achieved as a series of very brief, rhythmic, 'pulsing' efforts, rather than as sustained 5–7-second contractions.
- Following an isometric contraction – sustained single contraction or a series of pulsed efforts – the now less restricted tissues are taken to a new barrier – or past the new barrier, into stretch. A major effect of the isometric contractions has been described as producing a *'reduced resistance to stretch'* – or *'increased tolerance to stretch'.* As discussed later in the section on *Fascial (and other) mechanisms of MET* (Magnusson et al. 1996).
- MET *isometric* contractions should always involve the patient's effort – against the therapist's resistance. The same benefit will not be achieved if the patient is asked to resist the practitioner's effort.
- Where *eccentric* stretching is used in MET, the patient partially resists the practitioner's effort to stretch muscle, or to move a joint – so that a slow lengthening occurs of the contracting muscle(s).

Instruction examples

1. An example of a typical instruction when using an isometric contraction in treatment of levator scapula (Fig 13.1) might be:

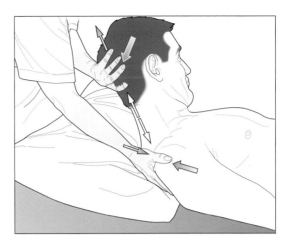

FIGURE 13.1 Hand positions and directions of resisted isometric contraction, and stretch application, in MET treatment of the right side levator scapula.

Start gently and slowly to push your head backwards against my hand, and your shoulder blade upwards against the other hand – using no more than 30% of your available strength, until I ask you to slowly stop pushing.

2. An example of a typical instruction when using an isotonic eccentric contraction of the hamstrings, with the patient lying supine and the leg held so that the hamstrings are just short of their easy resistance barrier (see Fig. 13.2), might be:

Try to bend your knee against my resistance. Starting slowly, build up your effort, using no more than a third of your available strength, and maintain the effort for 5 to 7 seconds, while I gently stretch the muscles, and then slowly relax

After releasing the contraction effort the leg would be straightened to a position where a small degree of stretch of the hamstrings (in this example) was achieved, and held there for between 5 and 30 seconds (depending on how chronic the problem is).

3. Where the practitioner is able to firmly control the area being treated, such as a small joint that is easier to stabilize (compared with long-leverage, as in the hamstring example), rhythmic, brief, pulsed isometric contractions are more useful than sustained ones. After the

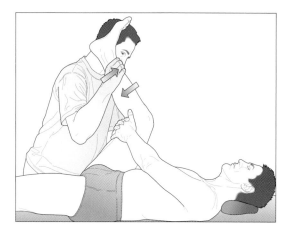

FIGURE 13.2 Hand positions and directions of a slow eccentric stretch application in treatment of the shortened hamstring muscles.

contraction(s), the patient should participate in the movement as tissues are taken to a new position, or into stretch.

4.   An example of a typical instruction when using an isotonic eccentric contraction involving the rectus femoris muscles – with the patient lying prone – might be: *'Try to resist my effort as I try to bend your knee'* (Fig. 13.3). The patient needs to be taught to use just sufficient force to avoid this becoming stressful for either party. In this example it should allow a relatively slow, painless lengthening of the contracting rectus femoris. The abbreviation/acronym for this method is SEIS (slow eccentric isotonic stretch). A more rapid version of this isotonic eccentric stretch is

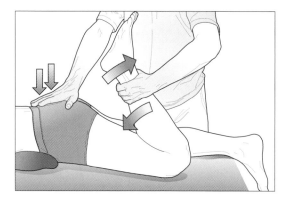

FIGURE 13.3 Hand positions and directions of isotonic eccentric stretch application in MET treatment of rectus femoris.

known as an isolytic contraction. The rationale and clinical usefulness of this is described later in the chapter – see discussion of the work of Parmar et al. (2011), under *Clinical objectives of MET and evidence,* below.

Clinical objectives of MET and evidence

Pain relief, improved mobility, rehabilitation and reducing fibrosis

Some research has suggested that isometric contractions, as used in MET, even without subsequent stretching, may have powerful analgesic effects (Hoeger et al. 2011). Possible mechanisms for this are described later in the chapter under the heading: *Fascial and other mechanisms of MET.*

Lewit and Simons (1984) used MET-type isometric contractions in treatment of 244 patients with myofascial pain, in whom trigger points (TrP) had been identified within affected muscles, which displayed tension and discomfort on stretching. The problematic muscle was passively stretched to a point just short of pain and then the patient performed a gentle isometric contraction for 10 seconds, followed by relaxation and further stretching, three to five times. Treatment resulted in immediate pain relief in 94% of patients, with lasting relief recorded in 63%.

Knebl (2002) compared the use of the Spencer technique – an osteopathic sequence for passive mobilization of the shoulder – with the same protocol using MET in 29 elderly patients with chronic shoulder restrictions and pain. Eight treatment sessions lasting 30 minutes each were performed twice a week at weeks 2, 4 and 6, and once at weeks 10 and 14, over a 14-week period. Both forms of treatments (mobilization with, and mobilization without MET) were found to produce improvements, but a greater increase was found in active and passive flexion in the group receiving MET. When participants were reassessed after the end of the treatment period, there was a trend for the range of motion (ROM) in the MET group to continue to increase, but also a trend for it decrease in those treated with passive mobilization only.

Hunt and Legal (2010) conducted a randomized, single-blinded, controlled study, involving 80 subjects with piriformis spasm and pain, together with the presence of myofascial trigger points in that muscle. Twenty-eight subjects were treated using MET, with the objective of relaxing piriformis; a further 27 subjects were treated with a high velocity low amplitude (HVLA) thrust technique that applied rapid stretch to piriformis; the remainder (25 controls) were treated by a placebo measure. Outcomes involved assessment of pressure pain threshold (using algometry); hip internal rotation range (goniometry); and pain levels, using a visual analog scale. Both the MET and HVLA thrust methods produced an equally significant increase in piriformis extensibility, together with pain relief, compared with the placebo group.

Moore et al. (2011) studied the effects of MET in treatment of shoulder ROM of amateur (college) baseball players. A single application of MET was used on the glenohumeral joint (GHJ) horizontal abductors (19 subjects) and the GHJ external rotators (22 subjects), to improve ROM. The results showed that a single application of a MET procedure, on collegiate baseball players, for the GHJ horizontal abductors provided immediate improvements in both GHJ horizontal adduction and internal rotation ROM.

Parmar et al. (2011) report on the use of slowly applied isotonic eccentric stretching (SEIS) compared with passive manual stretching (PMS) in knee rehabilitation following hip surgery. These orthopedic surgeons noted that while there was no difference in the significantly increased ROM that was eventually achieved (when comparing MET with PMS), those receiving MET showed significantly more rapid pain reduction. They describe the technique used as follows: *'With the patient in a side lying position, the hip was maintained in neutral with adequate stabilization of the pelvis. The knee was then taken to a range where the first resistance barrier was reached. The patient was* then instructed to use 20 to 25% of the knee extensor force to resist the therapist applied flexion force. The knee was then moved to a new [end of] range, till a second resistance barrier was reached and held in that position for 15 seconds and then returned back to full extension. This technique was applied for 5 to 7 repetitions once daily.'

Two key elements to note in this example are:

- The easy end of range – *'first sign of resistance'* – was used. As has been emphasized, this is a MET characteristic, unlike some other approaches where end of range is described as *'first sign of discomfort.'*
- The patient's attempt to extend the knee from that position – using 20 to 25% of available strength (not full strength) – was overcome by the practitioner, making this an isotonic eccentric stretch.

The rationale for use of SEIS and isolytic contractions (ILC) post-surgically is described as follows: *'In immediate post-surgery groups we used SEIS in order to prevent excessive pain and to also allow gradual gentle lengthening, thereby assisting in the remodeling of the injured, as well as the surrounding, soft tissue.*

In chronic phase, we used ILC which is more vigorous, in order to assist in breaking the fibrotic adhesions by controlled microtrauma, thus allowing improvement in elasticity and circulation during remodeling.'

MET and hyaluronic acid (HA). As described in Chapter 1, the sliding function of fascia requires the ample production of lubricants such as HA. This is stimulated by frictional, vibratory mechanisms – something easily incorporated into the application of isolytic or SEIS type stretches (Kuchera & Kuchera 1992).

Wilson et al. (2003) suggest a form of MET for achieving rehabilitation focused on the intrinsic muscles of the spine (such as the rotatores, intertransversarii) – as this can offer marked benefits in terms of spinal stabilization and proprioceptive reeducation. *'A dysfunction of these muscles can lead to incorrect afferent input to the central nervous system, resulting in a distorted view of the spatial relationships of the motion segments. This can lead to an ineffective use and/or disuse of the* *primary dynamic stabilisers of the spine.'* Description of the MET protocol recommended by Wilson et al. (2003) is too lengthy for this chapter. It can be found in full in Chapter 9 of Chaitow (2013). What is required of the patient is explained as follows:

> *It is important for the patient to provide a very small contraction. The focus is to strengthen the small intersegmental muscles. These will quickly become overpowered by the larger prime mover muscles if too great a contraction is elicited. The clinician should bear in mind that the core musculature will activate before the periphery, therefore the muscle contraction should be measured in 'ounces' (grams) instead of 'pounds' (kilos). The following are some examples of useful instructions to give to the patient:*

- *'Meet my force as I pull your leg towards the ceiling, but do not overpower me.'*
- *'Push into my hand as if you were pushing on an egg you did not want to break* (Wilson et al. 2003).'

Note: Pulsed MET would offer an ideal model for this protocol.

Lederman (2011), among others, believes that the best means of resolving dysfunction, such as low back pain, should involve rehabilitation strategies, motor re-education and behaviorally-focused methodologies – rather than manual modalities that may provide limited short-term effects. However, the opposite may also be true – because, unless mobility, strength, motor control, and endurance features are restored to dysfunctional tissues, by means of methods such as MET – normal, pain-free function may be far more difficult to achieve.

Fascial and other mechanisms of MET

Fryer (2013) has summarized the major elements thought to be involved in MET efficacy. Current theories include:

- **Reflex muscle relaxation:** although some studies support the theory that muscle relaxation occurs after isometric contractions, there appears to be only a brief 'post isometric relaxation' effect, with other studies showing – paradoxically – that isometric contractions result in increased, rather than lowered, EMG activity in muscles. It seems probable therefore that *'increased extensibility must occur due to other factors, such as viscoelastic change or increase to stretch tolerance.'*

- **Viscoelastic or muscle property changes:** there is evidence that the addition of an isometric contraction increases the effects of passive stretching, possibly involving the parallel and series elastic components of sarcomeres. Changes in both the series elastic and parallel elastic elements of sarcomeres (as discussed above) take place during the active and passive phases of MET, contributing to muscle elongation, and increased range of motion (Milliken 2003; see Fig. 5.1).

- In addition, processes such as hysteresis (see descriptions in Ch. 1, Box 1.2) may be involved in elastic changes; particularly, it is suggested, in younger individuals (Reid & McNair 2004). While not ruling it out as a contributory factor to increased tissue extensibility, viscoelastic change requires far more research to clarify its role in this process.

- **Stretch tolerance changes:** although the evidence lacks any specific explanation, studies have demonstrated that following MET the increase in the ability to lengthen tissues is due to *'a tolerance of greater stretching force to extend the muscle.'* In other words, after an isometric contraction it is possible to lengthen previously restricted soft tissues more comfortably than before the contraction. If the same degree of force involved in stretching a hamstring after an isometric contraction was used before the contraction, it would not have been as well tolerated. This does not, however, explain the mechanism(s) involved!

Other possible mechanisms and explanations include:

- As described in Chapter 5, hydraulic effects involving the extrusion of water from connective tissue, during contractions and stretching – allow increased freedom of movement for up to 30 minutes – during which time mobilization and/or exercise can be more efficiently achieved (Klingler et al. 2004).

- Fryer and Fossum (2010) suggest that MET stimulates mechanoreceptors that initiate pain-relieving responses, via both ascending and descending pain pathways. Additionally, MET induces mechanical stretching of fibroblasts that increases local blood flow and also alters interstitial osmotic pressure, reducing concentrations of pro-inflammatory cytokines, helping to desensitize pain receptors (Havas et al. 1997).

- Wilson (in Chaitow 2013) has shown that MET has marked pain relieving effects in cases of acute low back pain: MET *not only inhibits the alpha motor neuron, but the technique's gentle stretching also inhibits Ia afferent nerves via post-activation depression. This is due to muscle energy technique's ability to decrease the sensitivity of muscle spindles to stretch. This effect has been shown to last for more than 2 days* (Avela et al. 1999a, b). *This evidence fortifies the argument for the use of MET over other techniques in that the effects are not only longer lasting, but also because MET resolves the pain/spasm cycle by acting on both the efferent and afferent nerves.*

- Natural analgesics, such as endorphins and/or endocannabinoids, appear to be released in response to MET (McPartland 2008).

- As noted in Chapter 5 – it is not possible to manually stretch the sheets of deep dense fascia; for example, in the thoracolumbar fascia. However, using MET makes it possible to reduce the tensional load imposed by hypertonic muscles on such sheets – so reducing the relative stiffness of the fascial planes.

Neurological, mechanical, endocrine, hydraulic – and possibly other – mechanisms appear to contribute jointly to the efficacy of MET.

How and where to acquire skills in MET?

All osteopathic schools teach MET, although not all introduce the more subtle versions, e.g. pulsed MET.

Physical therapists are usually taught elements of MET and are commonly also introduced to METs distant relation – proprioceptive neuromuscular facilitation (PNF) – although this approach has major differences from MET, as described in this chapter.

Other methods that are similar to MET include approaches described by different names (and with little or no reference to the osteopathic origins), such as 'contract-relax' (CR), 'agonist contract-relax' (ACR), contract-relax-agonist contract (CRAC). Whatever the names used, these are all versions of MET, and are widely available as short courses and via books and video instruction.

The protocol list in Box 13.1 summarizes the essentials of MET.

Box 13.1
Protocol summary

Q. What is 'PIR' in relation to MET?
A. Post-isometric relaxation was the theoretical model for the mechanism thought to be involved in MET when the target tissues, the muscle(s) that require 'release', were involved in the isometric contraction. Post-isometric relaxation has been shown to occur, but to be too short-lived to account for the 'relaxation' changes following MET use.

Q. What is 'RI' in relation to MET?
A. Reciprocal inhibition was the theoretical model for the mechanism thought to be involved in MET when the antagonists to the target tissues, the antagonists to the muscle(s) that require 'release', were involved in the isometric contraction. This effect (RI) has been shown to occur, but is too short-lived to account for the 'relaxation' changes following MET use.

continued on next page

Q. Which barrier should be used in MET application?

A. Tissues should be taken to a point just short of the resistance barrier – i.e. to a point before any sense of tension ('bind') is noted.

Q. How strong a contraction should be requested from the patient?

A. Less than one-third of available strength.

Q. For how long should an isometric contraction be maintained?

A. 5 to 7 seconds – or less than a second in pulsed MET – repeated for 10 seconds or so.

Q. Should the isometric contraction involve agonist ('PIR') or antagonist ('RI')?

A. Use of the agonists – the tissues requiring release or lengthening – offers the best results, but pain

Box 13.1 (Continued)

may prevent their use, in which case the antagonists should be employed – or other muscles that might influence the restriction may be used.

Q. Should the direction of the isometric contraction be towards the barrier – or away from the barrier?

A. This is effectively the same as the previous question. If the effort is directed away from the barrier it involves the agonist muscles and 'PIR'. If the contraction effort is towards the barrier it involves the antagonists and therefore 'RI'.

Q. Is breathing cooperation required (respiratory synkinesis)?

A. In basic MET (i.e. not when eccentric stretching is involved), stretching or moving to a new barrier is usual on an exhalation – except in the case of quadratus lumborum because it fires on exhalation.

Q. Should there be a pause following the contraction before movement or stretching is introduced?

A. Yes – a moment of relaxation before the stretch commences is advised.

Q. After the isometric contraction should tissues be taken to the new barrier, or past the new barrier – and if so how far, and for how long?

A. In an acute situation there is no stretch – tissues are taken to a new barrier following the isometric contraction. In chronic settings the movement is to just past barrier, for between 5 and 30 seconds – patient assisted if possible.

Q. How many repetitions should there be of the process described above?

A. 1–2; there seems to be little benefit in repeating the process beyond a second MET application.

Q. Describe a slow eccentric isotonic stretch (SEIS)

A. Tissues are taken towards a mid-range position, in the direction of restriction, and the patient should be requested to maintain that position as the operator slowly stretches the contracting muscles – to a new barrier of resistance, so stretching muscles as they contract. This is also commonly applied to the possibly inhibited antagonists of shortened muscle groups, so toning them.

Q. Describe a rapid isotonic eccentric MET stretch (isolytic)

A. The same as the previous description only performed rapidly in order to deliberately create micro-trauma in the contracting sarcomeres – reducing cross-linkages, fibrosis etc. – to be followed by careful rehabilitation.

Q. Describe pulsed MET

A. Tissues around a restricted joint are firmly held at an easy end-of-range, and a request is made for a small degree of effort towards, or away from, the restriction barrier (or in another direction) that lasts for less than a second. Once the degree and direction of the brief effort has been successfully learned, the patient is asked to produce a series of 10–20 such contractions, rhythmically, against a firm counter-pressure, after which a new barrier is identified and used as a starting point for a further 15–20 mini-contractions.

References

Avela J et al 1999a Reduced reflex sensitivity after repeated and prolonged passive muscle stretching. J Appl Physiol 86:1283–1291

Avela J et al 1999b Reduced reflex sensitivity persists several days after long-lasting stretch-shortening cycle exercises. J Appl Physiol 86:1292–1300

Chaitow L 2013 Muscle energy techniques, 4th edn. Churchill Livingstone Elsevier, Edinburgh

ECOP: Educational Council on Osteopathic Principles 2009 Glossary of osteopathic terminology. American Association of Colleges of Osteopathic Medicine, Chevy Chase, MD

Franke H 2009 The history of MET. In: Muscle energy technique history-model-research. Interview with Fred Mitchell Jr. Verband der Osteopathen Deutschland, Wiesbaden.

Franke H 2013 The history of muscle energy technique. In: Chaitow L (ed) Muscle energy techniques, 4th edn. Churchill Livingstone, Edinburgh

Fryer G 2013 MET: efficacy and research. In: Chaitow L (ed) Muscle energy techniques. Churchill Livingstone Elsevier, Edinburgh

Fryer G, Fossum C 2010 Therapeutic mechanisms underlying muscle energy approaches. In: Fernández-de las-Peñas, C et al (eds) Tension-type and cervicogenic headache: pathophysiology, diagnosis, and management. Jones and Bartlett, Sudbury, MA, pp 221–229

Goodridge J 1981 Muscle energy technique: definition, explanation, methods of procedure. JAOA 81:249–254

Havas E et al 1997 Lymph flow dynamics in exercising human skeletal muscle as detected by scintography. J Physiol 504:233–239

Hoeger B et al 2011 Pain perception after isometric exercise in women with fibromyalgia. Arch Phys Med Rehabil 92:89–95

Hunt G, Legal L 2010 Comparative study on the efficacy of thrust and muscle energy techniques in the piriformis muscle. Osteopatía Scientífica 5(2):47–55

Huxley AF, Niedergerke R 1954 Structural changes in muscle during contraction: interference microscopy of living muscle fibres. Nature 173(4412):971–973

Kappler R 2003 Thrust (high-velocity/low-amplitude) techniques. In: Ward RC (ed) Foundations for osteopathic medicine, 2nd edn. Lippincott, Williams & Wilkins, Philadelphia, pp 852–880

Klingler W, Schleip R, Zorn A 2004 European Fascia Research Project Report. 5th World Congress Low Back and Pelvic Pain, Melbourne, November 2004

Knebl J 2002 Improving functional ability in the elderly via the Spencer technique, an osteopathic manipulative treatment: a randomized, clinical trial. J American Osteopathic Assoc 102(7):387–400

Kuchera WA, Kuchera ML 1992 Osteopathic principles in practice. Kirksville College of Osteopathic Medicine Press, Kirksville, MO

Lederman E 2011 The fall of the postural-structural-biomechanical model in manual and physical therapies: Exemplified by lower back pain. J Bodyw Mov Ther 15:130–152

Lewit K, Simons DG 1984 Myofascial pain: relief by postisometric relaxation. Arch Phys Med Rehabil 65:452–456

McPartland JB 2008 Expression of the endocannabinoid system in fibroblasts and myofascial tissues. J Bodyw Mov Ther 12(2):169

Magnusson S et al 1996 A mechanism for altered flexibility in human skeletal muscle. J Physiol 497(1):291–298

Milliken K 2003 The effects of muscle energy technique on psoas major length. Unpublished MOst Thesis. Unitec New Zealand, Auckland, New Zealand

Mitchell Jr FL, 1998 PKG The muscle energy manual, vol 2. MET Press, East Lansing

Mitchell Jr FL, Mitchell PKG 1999 The muscle energy manual, vol 3. MET Press, East Lansing

Mitchell FL 1958 Structural pelvic function. In: Barnes MW (ed) Yearbook of the Academy of Applied Osteopathy. American Academy of Osteopathy, Indianapolis, IN, pp 71–90

Mitchell Jr FL 2009 Influences, inspirations, and decision points. In: Franke H (ed) Muscle energy technique. History – Model Research, Marixverlag, Wiesbaden

Moore S et al 2011 J Orthop Sports Phys Ther 41(6):400–407

Parmar S et al 2011 The effect of isolytic contraction and passive manual stretching on pain and knee range of motion after hip surgery: a prospective, double-blinded, randomized study. Hong Kong Physiotherapy Journal 29:25–30

Reid D, McNair P 2004 Passive force, angle, and stiffness changes after stretching of hamstring muscles. Med Sci Sports Exercise 36:1944–1948

Ruddy T 1962 Osteopathic rapid rhythmic resistive technic. Academy of Applied Osteopathy Yearbook, Carmel, CA, pp 23–31

Wilson E et al 2003 Muscle energy technique in patients with acute low back pain: a pilot clinical trial. J Orthop Sports Phys Ther 33:502–512

Chapter 14

MYOFASCIAL INDUCTION THERAPY (MIT®)

Andrzej Pilat

Introduction

Myofascial Induction Therapy (MIT®) is a hands-on, full body approach, focusing on restoration of altered function in fascial tissue. In a healthy body, the fascial system maintains movement, fluidity and coordination. Injuries and aging can, however, reduce this tissue dynamic, resulting in fascial restriction, as discussed in Chapters 1 and 2. Adaptation to fascial dysfunction involves both structural and functional responses that are frequently amenable to facilitation via manual methods such as MIT.

MIT is a hands-on evaluation and treatment process in which the practitioner, by applying gentle manual mechanical stress transfer (traction or/ and compression) to a targeted dysfunctional tissue, facilitates the recovery. The term 'induction' relates to the correction of movement facilitation, and not a passive stretching of the fascial system. This is primarily an educational process, in the search for a restored optimal homeostatic level, recovering range of motion, appropriate tension, strength, and coordination. The final aim of the therapeutic process is not establishment of stable hierarchies, but facilitation of optimal and continuous adaptation to environmental demands, with maximum efficiency.

Clinicians familiar with myofascial release (MFR) find similarities between it and MIT. With different nuances, they are based on the same concept of clinical reasoning and complement each other. MIT is characterized as manual tissue remodeling, always avoiding arbitrary stimulus application (altered force intensity and direc-

tion), focusing on the intrinsic natural tissue response.

Definitions

What is fascia?

There are no unified criteria to determine what fascia is (Langevin & Huijing 2009, Schleip et al. 2012). Kumka and Bonar (2012) define fascia as *'an innervated, continuous, functional organ of stability and motion that is formed by 3-dimensional collagen matrices.'* This emphasizes that fascia is not a passive and merely supporting structure, but rather *'a dynamic and mutable system'* (Swanson 2013). This system manifests as different kinds of connective tissue, forming a continuous tensional network, throughout the micro- and macroscopic levels of body architecture (Langevin et al. 2011).

The basic functions of the fascial system (Pilat 2003; see also Ch. 1)

- Suspension
- Support
- Formation of compartments
- Cohesion of body structures
- Protection and autonomy of the muscles and viscera
- Formation of functional units
- Creation and organization of a continuous body communication network
- Participation in posture control
- Absorption and distribution of local stimuli as a synergistic whole:

- o mechanical (pressure, vibration, movement)
- o chemical
- o thermal
- Tissue nutrition
- Facilitation of metabolic exchange
- Participation in wound healing
- Hemodynamic coordination
- Participation in afferent stimuli transmission throughout the network of receptors.

What is fascial dysfunction? (See also Ch. 2)

Fascial system dysfunction is defined as alteration of the highly organized assortment of specialized movements, and as the incorrect transfer of information through the matrix (Pilat 2003). This results in loss of optimal gliding between endofascial fibers and interfacial planes. Accordingly, force transmission may be altered and/or restricted, resulting in anomalous tension and finally movement disorders (Fourie 2008). Mechanical forces distributions are just as important as biochemical signalling in shaping proper cell development, function, and pathologic processes (Ingber 2003).

Which approaches can treat fascial dysfunction?

There are numerous named manual approaches that focus on treatment of fascial dysfunction (Chaitow 2007, Pilat 2003). This section of the book includes a selection of fascia-directed manual approaches, with many of them based on similar conceptual principles. A unification and validation of clinical procedures, via research, is required (Remvig 2007).

What is MIT?

MIT focuses on the body's integrated facilitation processes, including musculoskeletal, neural, vascular, cranial and visceral body components. During the application, the clinician stretches and /or compresses a specific body area to transmit a low intensity mechanical stimulus. This input induces changes that influence the system down to the molecular level (see below, and notes on mechanotransduction in Ch. 1).

The outcome is a reciprocal reaction from the body that involves biochemical changes, signalling, metabolic, and finally physiological responses. This process aims to remodel the matrix quality to facilitate and optimize information transfer to, and within, the fascial system (Wheeler 2004). The objective, and common outcome, of the process is enhanced functionality, with lower energy demands (Pilat 2003, 2011). The reasoning for this process is summarized in Figure 14.1.

What is the validation for MIT?

Fascia is a mechanosensory system as evidenced by a variety of processes (Chiquet et al. 2009) including

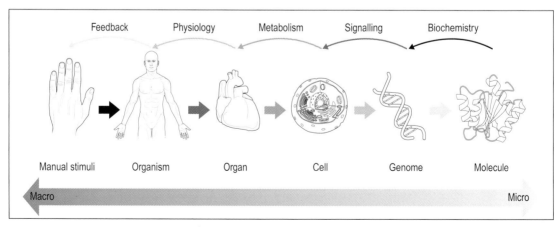

FIGURE 14.1 Schematic analysis of the (MIT®) application mechanism.

three different categories that are sensitive to mechanical forces. Each of these operates on a different scale, potentially influencing the others.

- **Mechanotransduction:** this is a process by which a mechanical input is converted into a biochemical response (Wang et al. 2009).
- **Piezoelectricity:** because collagen (see Ch. 1) is a semi-conductor it is suggested that it is capable of forming an integrated electronic network that enables the interconnection of fascial system components (Ahn & Grodzinsky 2009)
- **Viscoelasticity:** this is a property of fascia that describes the characteristics it displays of viscosity and elasticity, when undergoing deformation, during application of (for example) stretching or shear forces. Elasticity describes a process such as stretching in which the structure returns to normal once the stress ceases; viscosity involves the diffusion of atoms or molecules inside an amorphous material, such as the colloidal extracellular matrix (ECM). The viscoelastic properties of fascia have been observed in numerous studies that have analyzed various fascial structures including the thoracolumbar fascia (Yahia et al. 1993), the fascia lata, plantar fascia, and nasal fascia (Chaudhry et al. 2007).

These three mechanisms can act at different fractions of time, can complement each other, and the system can switch between them at any phase of clinical application (Vaticon 2009).

The fascial system is also innervated (Tesarz et al. 2011) allowing for immunoneuro-endocrine responses, for example:

- Local and global
- Immediate and delayed
- Mechanical and neurophysiological.

Objectives of MIT

The general MIT applications goal is to improve the body's movement ability at all levels. It is a focused process, controlled by the central nervous system, in which the clinician acts as a catalyst (facilitator). The therapeutic action focuses on the provision of resources for optimal homeostatic balance adjustment.

Specific treatments goals are to:

- Mobilize superficial fascial restrictions
- Change the stationary status of the collagenous structures
- Facilitate the release of the sliding matrix properties
- Stimulate physiological orientation in fibroblast mechanics
- Prevent the formation of tissue adhesions
- Arrange superficial fascial planes
- Acquire more efficient circulation of antibodies throughout the matrix
- Improve blood supply (e.g. release of histamine) in the region of restriction
- Improve blood supply to the nervous system
- Increase metabolite flow to and from tissues, facilitating the recovery process.

General MIT treatment recommendations

MIT is recommended mainly for patients with orthopedic, neuro-orthopedic, post-traumatic and degenerative dysfunctions related to the myofascial system (Pilat 2003).

Complementary treatment recommendations

Clinical experience and research, discussed below, note the usefulness of MIT approaches for patients with dysfunctions relating to:

- The nervous system (central and peripheral)
- Pelvic floor disorders
- Circulatory diseases
- Temporomandibular joint (TMJ) dysfunction
- Sports injuries
- Respiratory disorders.

Mechanical characteristics of MIT application

MIT involves gentle force application, in which articular range of motion is never forced. It follows the movement in the direction of reduced tension, towards 'ease'.

These features increase the range of clinical applications, and enable the practitioner to apply the approach to a patient range extending from pediatric to geriatric groups. It may be used promptly in post-traumatic and post-surgical patients.

Although clinical reasoning applied to MIT is mainly linked to the treatment protocols of physical therapists, osteopaths and massage therapy professionals, its application should be useful for all healthcare practitioners with competencies in provision of physical therapy and manual therapy approaches.

Assessment

The goal of MIT treatment is to improve the body's movement capacity and to achieve better body awareness. Body awareness can be adaptive or maladaptive. The objective of assessment is to identify maladaptive dysfunctions caused by different types of trauma influencing the fascial system. Figure 14.2 explains this reasoning. The evaluation of myofascial dysfunction syndrome is performed using the usual assessment procedures conducted in manual therapy, focusing on dysfunctional symptoms. The clinician should perform their usual evaluation, investigating the integrity and harmony of three basic body's areas: physical, autonomic and organic (Pilat 2003).

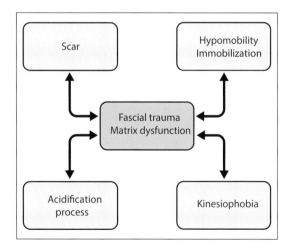

FIGURE 14.2 The most important fascial trauma inputs (based on Pilat 2003).

Assessment process (see also Ch. 4)

The suggested clinical evaluation scheme includes:
- case history taking (anamnesis)
- static evaluation of posture (observation)
- dynamic evaluation of posture
  o global functional tests
  o specific functional tests
- palpatory tests
- additional tests.

Special attention should be addressed to global functional tests when patient performs integrated movements, often similar to everyday activities. The order of procedures is summarized in Figure 14.3. In most assessments a 'before and after' scheme is used. However, assessments that help to observe tissue changes in real time during treatment have been developed. The most important are: EMG (Bertolucci 2008) and sonoelastography (Martínez & Galán del Río 2013).

Through those observations it is possible to record real time changes in fascial structure, allowing accurate clinical decision-making during treatment, and thus improving the outcomes. It also allows the patient to show their progress with treatment. The clinician should consider how the patient interprets the assessment process. Mental influences (expectations, experiences, fears, etc.) can modify the patient's response/behavior.

MIT application mechanisms

During MIT treatment, the clinician applies a low intensity, sustained manual load that initiates a cascade of mechanical and neurophysiological responses. The result may include any of a variety of potentially clinically relevant responses:
- Decreased local and global tissue tension
- Increased tissue resilience
- Increased range of motion
- Increased muscle strength
- Reduction of inflammation
- Improvement of movement coordination
- Decreased pain
- Changes in respiratory rate
- Changes in heart rate

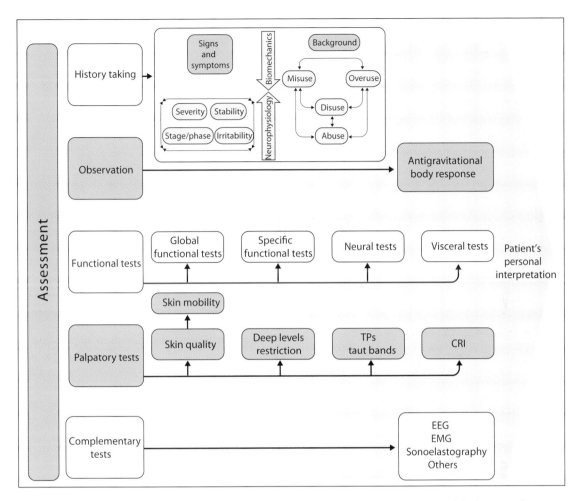

FIGURE 14.3 Diagram of the assessment process (based on Pilat 2003). TPs: trigger points; CRI: cranial rhythmic impulse.

- Sweating
- Peripheral vasodilatation.

The diversity of responses is due to potential interactions among and between individual body systems (action–reaction–interaction), that are coordinated by the peripheral and central nervous systems (integration of mechanical, thermal and/or chemical stimuli), which are then responsible for the clinical outcomes.

Conceptual reasoning

Adaptation, compensation and decompensation are processes associated with overuse, trauma and ageing. Allostatic responses to such adaptive demands – produced in an effort to restore homeostasis – involve hormonal, immunological and neuronal changes (Seeman et al. 1997).

When therapeutic load is applied to tissues in order to encourage harmonious adaptation, deformation of cellular shape occurs, inducing mechanotransduction (see Ch. 1 and below).

In addition, mechanoreceptors, proprioceptors, nociceptors and interoceptors are stimulated during manual loading. The nature of load, its direction, degree, timing etc., determines the influence it will have on tissue responses.

The matrix: cells ecosystem

It is suggested that it is the ECM that carries out the data reception/interpretation/transmission process:

- Cells, the fundamental units of the body are immersed in the ECM, which constitutes its ecosystem.
- The matrix is a biophysical filter that controls the transmission of nutrients, cellular waste products, mediators, and other substances to and from the cells´ environment.
- Cells (such as fibroblasts, adipocytes, osteoblasts, chondroblasts, endothelial cells) are mechanosensitive, as well as mechanoreceptive (Shoham & Gefen 2012).
- The matrix is the medium that conducts the complex mechanotransduction processes in which cells react dynamically, detecting and interpreting signs of mechanical origin, and subsequently converting these into chemical changes and/or modifications in gene expression (Chiquet et al. 2009).

Matrix restriction process

- Anatomical analysis, performed mainly on fresh cadavers, shows fascia to be a highly hydrated structure, which looks like a matrix (Fig. 14.4 and Plate 8).
- Excessive collagen production can induce fibrosis, resulting in loss of matrix smoothness and/or isotropy, with the consequent creation of entrapment areas. This suggests that such entrapment areas may alter body movements in relation to amplitude, velocity, resistance and coordination (Fourie 2008).
- In the presence of long-term restrictions, the fascial tissues become overloaded and suffer dysfunctional consequences.
- These changes first affect the loose connective tissue structures, and then reorganize the specialized tissue (regular or irregular dense connective tissue, such as tendons, ligaments, or capsules), causing excessive density and tissue disorientation.
- Fascial restrictions of shorter duration affect the tissues locally, whereas restrictions of long duration induce a more global dysfunction pattern (Langevin et al. 2005).
- Decreased fascial mobility can alter circulation and cause ischemia, leading to deteriorating of muscle fiber quality. As a result, alterations may appear in the stabilizing functions and coordination of joint movements, resulting an inflammatory process and/or pain along myofascial sequences (Lee 2001).
- Considering that many mechanoreceptors are embedded within fascia, the altered proprioceptive afferents could negatively influence motor control (Vaticon 2009).

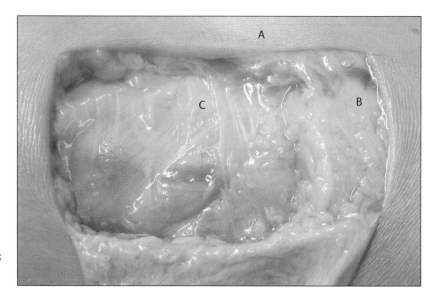

FIGURE 14.4 Fascia as a matrix (note the high level of hydration). This shows the left cubital fossa region on a fresh cadaver dissection. A: skin; B: superficial fascia level; C: deep fascia level. See also Plate 8.

Evidence in support of the effect of manual force application in MIT

Figure 14.5 outlines myofascial induction application processes. This is not a definitive picture but, rather, a proposal to interpret the interactions be-tween very distinct mechanisms that involve the body macro and micro levels.

Basic science research support

- Myofascial force transmission (see Ch. 1) is a widely studied phenomenon that mainly

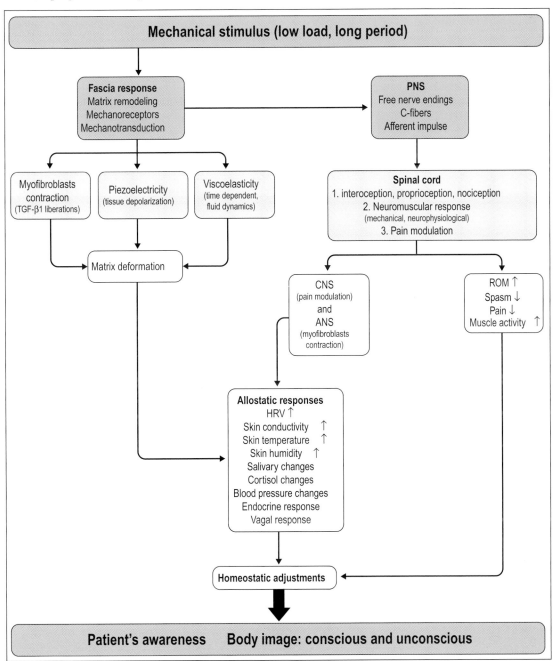

FIGURE 14.5 Diagram of proposed (MIT®) application process.

depends on fascial anatomical continuity, observed during fresh cadaver dissections (Stecco 2004, Schuenke et al. 2012) and surgical procedures (Guimberteau et al. 2010). Mechanical transverse force transmission through the fascia has been extensively studied at microscopic level (Purslow 2010). Special attention is given to the intermuscular fascia where muscle fibers are inserted (see Fig. 14.6).

- Through these connections fibers participate in mechanical action, without direct insertion into the bone (van der Wal 2009). Motion analysis should thereby be focused not only on biomechanics, which are based on the topographic anatomy (*where*), but mainly on

questions related to the function (*how*). For this reason the expression *musculoskeletal architecture* appears with increasing frequency in research related to body movement. Perhaps the dynamic model that comes closest to these requirements is the **tensegrity** model, proposed by Ingber (Ingber 1997, Pilat & Testa 2009). This suggests a system of shared tensions at multiple body levels; that also explains the global reactions of the fascial system in response to mechanical stimulus.

- Different studies have shown that dynamic and active responses of the cell's cytoskeleton, receiving mechanical forces from the ECM, induces tissue remodeling at both the cellular and sub-cellular levels (Wang et al. 2009).

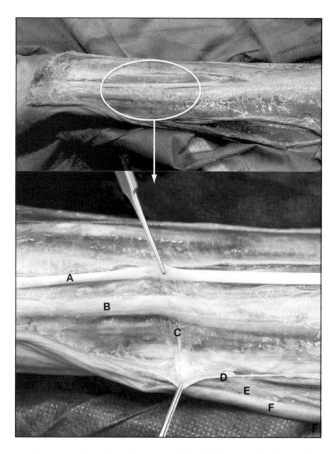

FIGURE 14.6 Fascial intermuscular connections. Anterior aspect of the left forearm. A: palmaris longus muscle tendon; B: flexor carpi radialis muscle; C: lateral intermuscular fascial connection; D: deep forearm fascial level; E: superficial forearm fascial level; F: skin.

- The presence of interstitial connective tissue and its importance in force modulation deserves emphasis. Specialized connective tissue structures are related not only to muscle structure (endomysium, perimysium, epimysium) but also to other body systems: circulatory (arterial, venous, lymphatic) and the nervous system. Remodeling of interstitial connective tissue may have an important biomechanical, vasomotor and neuromodulatory effects.
- Dynamic matrix remodeling – contracture has been widely studied in relation to scar formation (Tomasek et al. 2002). The application of mechanical input changes the biomechanical behavior of fascia in relation to the properties of the ECM (stiffness and viscosity; Chiquet et al. 2003) and in cellular and subcellular tissue level responses (mechanotransduction process; Langevin et al. 2011). The key structures in this process are integrins, the molecular bridges between the matrix and the cytoskeleton through which the cell 'senses' its environment and responds to it according to its needs. Cells that are essential for matrix dynamics are fibroblasts and its phenotype transformation to myofibroblasts (Tomasek et al. 2002). The contractile nature of these cells appears to give them the ability to rapidly alter fascial tension, through contraction and relaxation (Nekouzadeh et al. 2008). Cellular activation subsequently alters gene expression, protein synthesis, and modifies the ECM (Langevin et al. 2011).

Fascia as mechanosensitive structure

A strong link between fascia and the autonomic nervous system has been identified (Haouzi et al. 1999); for example, involving a network of mechanoreceptors, the so-called interstitial mechanoreceptors (group III and IV free nerves endings), each of which has two subgroups with low and high levels of mechanosensitivity related to cell architecture.

- Group III muscle afferents are found, for example, in perimuscular fascia and the adventitia of muscle blood vessels, and respond to deforming stimuli such as pressure and stretch (Lin et al. 2009). Neural action

potential firing through nerve terminals is linked to specific mechanical deformation and ECM interactions (Yi-Wen et al. 2009). Stimulation of group III and IV muscle afferents has reflex effects on both the somatic and autonomic nervous systems, including an inhibitory effect on alpha motoneurons, an excitatory effect on gamma motoneurons, and an excitatory effect on the sympathetic nervous system (Kaufman et al. 2002).

- Through the mechanoreceptors, the fascial system is in a continuous process of internal communication (Vaticon 2009):
  o somato – somatic
  o somato – visceral
  o viscero – visceral
  o viscero – somatic.

The questions to be asked are, can this theoretical framework be clinically confirmed, and if so, is it clinically relevant?

Below is a brief summary of a selection of clinical studies.

Scientific evidence related to the results of the myofascial approach

Research related to pathology

- Marshall et al. (2009) concluded that myofascial release helps reduce the severity and intensity of muscle pain in people with chronic fatigue syndrome.
- Hicks at al. (2009) report that human fibroblasts secrete the soluble mediators of myoblast differentiation and that myofascial release can regulate muscle development.
- An objective form for evaluating the effect of MIT applications in muscular lesions with dynamic sonoelastography was reported by Martínez and Galán del Río (2013).
- Useros and Hernando (2008) concluded that myofascial induction has beneficial effects in patients with brain damage, with special emphasis on automatic posture control.
- In patients with unilateral spatial neglect (an alteration of the head's position with respect to the median line), Vaquero Rodríguez (2012)

observed significant results for the sensitivity variable in the experimental group treated with MIT, as compared with those treated with Bobath therapy.

- Fernández-Lao et al. (2011) applied myofascial release technique in breast cancer survivor patients. The authors observed that myofascial release led to an immediate increase in salivary flow rate, suggesting a parasympathetic effect of the intervention.
- Vasquez (2011) presents the effectiveness of MIT in treating swimmers´ shoulder, with respect to articular balance and pain.
- Arguisuelas Martínez et al. (2010) demonstrated the effects of lumbar spine manipulation and thoracolumbar MIT on erector spinae activation patterns.

Clinical research in healthy subjects

- Arroyo-Morales et al. (2008a) stated that the heart rate variability and blood pressure recovery after a physically stressful situation were improved by myofascial release compared with sham electrotherapy treatment.
- Arroyo-Morales et al. (2008b) reported that application of an active recovery protocol using whole-body myofascial treatment reduces EMG amplitude and vigor when applied as a passive recovery technique after a high-intensity exercise protocol.
- Toro et al. (2009) state that the application of a single session of manual therapy (including MIT) produces an immediate increase of heart rate variability and a decrease in tension, anger status, and perceived pain in patients with chronic tension-type headache.
- In a randomized single-blind placebo-controlled study, Arroyo-Morales et al. (2009) reported that MIT might encourage recovery from a transient immunosuppression state induced by exercise in healthy active women.
- Henley et al. (2008) demonstrated quantitatively that cervical myofascial release shifts sympathovagal balance from the sympathetic to the parasympathetic nervous system.

- In a study involving 41 healthy male volunteers who were randomly assigned to experimental or control groups, Fernandez et al. (2008) reported significantly decreased anxiety levels in healthy young adults after the application of myofascial induction treatment. Additionally, significantly lower systolic blood pressure values were observed, as compared with baseline levels.
- Heredia-Rizo et al. (2013) demonstrated that MIT (sub-occipital muscle inhibition technique) immediately improved the position of the head with the subject seated and standing. Additionally, it immediately decreased the mechanosensitivity of the greater occipital nerve.
- Fernández-Pérez et al. (2013) observed major immunological modulations with an increased B lymphocyte count 20 minutes after the craniocervical application of MIT.

MIT approach protocol

MIT application involves a selection of procedures that optimize function and balance inside and within the fascial system, reducing pain and enhancing function. The applications of MIT, as suggested below, are based on the clinical experience of the author (Pilat 2003, 2009, 2011), supported by the theoretical framework discussed above. The MIT process may be combined with other manual therapy strategies, or as an exclusive treatment procedure.

Clinical procedure principles

All procedures (protocols) should be individualized according to the assessed dysfunction and the patient's individual physical and emotional condition, culture, age and gender.

- A first stage requires identification of the body region affected by symptom-producing myofascial dysfunction. This region should be identified during the initial assessment process described above. See also Chapter 4 and Figure 14.3.
- The conceptual basis of the MIT application process is outlined in Figure 14.5.

Suggested treatment protocols (Fig. 14.7)

- **Superficial (local) technique procedures** address the surface and/or local restrictions detectable through direct palpation, involving different *strokes*. A stroke is a short-term passively applied movement (with or without sliding over the skin), which changes the matrix quality and collagen's stationary attitude, facilitating its local sliding ability. Depending on the body´s region and on each patient´s morphology, the movement can be applied digitally, or by knuckle, forearm or elbow.
- The main goal is the correction of subcutaneous restrictions (related to the superficial fascia) and also those that affect muscles, tendons, or ligaments that can be felt directly below the skin. In these procedures the therapeutic movement direction should always run towards the restriction (Pilat 2003).
- **Deep local technique procedures** are the most important and most effective tools used in MIT. These techniques address the local deep fascia restrictions (undetected through direct palpation), which can appear in multiple directions and planes.

After performing the functional assessment process (see Fig.14.3) the basic procedures are as follows (Pilat 2003):

o Given that fascia responds biomechanically to compression and traction input (Chaudhry et al. 2007), these two mechanical strategies can be used when applying MIT.

o The clinician applies a slow, three-dimensional compression and/or traction (keeping in mind the idea that the body is like a glycerine-filled balloon, which can be compressed or stretched), causing the tissue to become tense. This is referred to as the first restriction barrier.

o The arbitrary displacement of engaged tissues should be avoided.

o The patient is asked to maintain a state of active passivity.

o The applied pressure is constant during the first 60– 90 seconds. This is the time required for releasing the first restriction barrier, according to the viscoelastic response (Chaudhry et al. 2007, Pilat 2003).

o During the first phase of the technique, the therapist barely causes the tissue to move.

o After overcoming the first restriction barrier, the therapist follows the movement in the direction of least resistance pausing at each new barrier.

o In each application, the therapist must overcome between three and six consecutive barriers; the minimum time required to obtained release and pain decrease is usually 3–5 minutes (Borgini et al. 2010). Depending on the severity of the dysfunction, the process may take up to 25–30 minutes.

o The tension applied to the tissue should be constant, although the pressure (force)

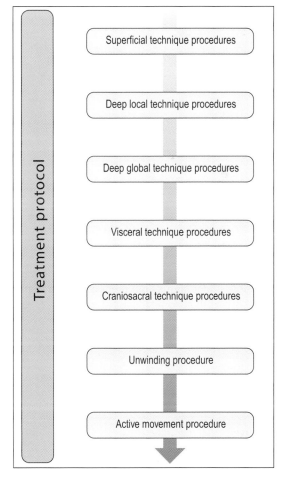

FIGURE 14.7 Suggested order of protocol application.

Exercise

Example of MIT® deep local technique self-application

For a correct application of deep techniques, the therapist must clearly differentiate the elastic movement (arbitrarily conducted by him/her) from the facilitated movement that occurs in response to the tissue remodeling process, described above. The following exercise is an example of learning facilitated movement strategy.

Sit in a chair and relax. Gently embrace your cheeks with your hands and without allowing slipping over the skin, move the tissues gently in all directions and at different speeds. Explore the amplitude and final resistance as you reach the end of range. This is the elastic movement.

Subsequently, embrace your jaw as shown in Figure 14.8. Close your eyes, breathe deeply and relax your shoulders. For about 3 minutes apply a very gentle traction toward the floor. If you notice movement, follow it. There should be no increase in force throughout the exercise. The sense of movement that you will feel is the facilitated movement. After this – retest amplitude and resistance as you again move tissues in all directions. What has changed?

applied may need to be modified after overcoming the first barrier. For example, pressure should be reduced if there is an increase in pain and/or excessive response/reaction to the therapeutic stimulus (tremor, fibrillation etc.)

o   The tissue release response is usually local (in the area of application). However, it is possible that spontaneous movement in other body regions may occur.

• **Deep global technique procedures.** The difference between this and the previously described method relates to the tissue reaction the clinician is seeking. The local tissue changes are still important, especially at the start of treatment. However, responses in tissue tension in other (any) body regions may be anticipated; for example, the application of the initial manual mechanical load to the cervical area may initiate, over time (several minutes), tissue responses (i.e. quality changes) in any body region. The response need not to be linear (i.e. a chain reaction); for example, involving the patient's hand. In this case, the arm and forearm are the zone of transmission of activity

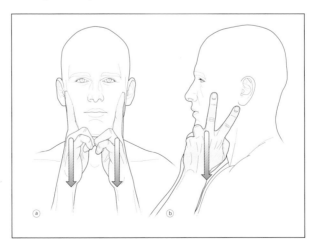

FIGURE 14.8 Example of MIT® deep local technique self-application.

(without any body movement observed in these) – to the hand. Tensegrity principles (tension adjustment of the entire system) are operating (Pilat & Testa 2009). Usually, body areas that have the oldest and largest restrictions react first.

The general principles described above are valid for the treatment of each body structure. However, specific dysfunctions require individual therapeutic strategies (see Pilat 2003, 2009, 2011).

Training

MIT training does not require previous experience in manual therapy. The learning process consists of three areas: theory, practice and manual palpation skills. The third is considered to be the most complicated and requires a prolonged learning period together with extensive clinical experience. The theoretical framework based on evidence opens a wide and increasing range of clinical applications. However, clinical evidence remains limited requiring unified research criteria, including:

- More objective evaluation processes
- Classification of strategies (local vs global approach)
- Unification of parameters as to force, timing, intensity and frequency of application
- Identification and analysis of responses in different body systems
- Identification and classification of no responders
- Analysis of long-term results.

References

Ahn AC, Grodzinsky AJ 2009 Relevance of collagen piezoelectricity to 'Wolff's Law'. Med Eng Phys 31:733–741

Arguisuelas Martínez MD et al 2010 Effects of lumbar spine manipulation and thoracolumbar myofascial induction technique on the spinae erector activation pattern. Fisioterapia 32(6) pp250–255

Arroyo-Morales M et al 2008a Effects of myofascial release after high-intensity exercise. J Manipulative Physiol Ther 31(3):217–223

Arroyo-Morales, M et al 2008b Psychophysiological effects of massage-myofascial release after exercise. JACM 14;10 pp1223–1229

Arroyo-Morales M et al 2009 Massage after exercise – responses of immunologic and endocrine markers: a randomized single-blind placebo-controlled study. Journal of Strength & Conditioning Research 23:638–644

Bertolucci F 2008 Muscle repositioning: a new verifiable approach to neuro-myofascial release? J Bodyw Mov Ther 12 (3): 213–224

Borgini E et al 2010 How much time is required to modify a fascial fibrosis? J Bodyw Mov Ther 14:318;325

Chaitow L 2007 Positional release techniques. Elsevier, Edinburgh

Chaudhry H et al 2007 Viscoelastic behavior of human fasciae under extension in manual therapy. J Bodyw Mov Ther 11:159–167

Chiquet M et al 2003 How do fibroblasts translate mechanical signals into changes in extracellular matrix production? Matrix Biol 22(1):73–80

Chiquet M et al 2009 From mechanotransduction to extracellular matrix gene expression in fibroblasts. Biochimica Biophysica Acta 1793: 911–920

Fernandez AM et al 2008 Effects of myofascial induction techniques on physiologic and psychologic parameters. JACM 14:807–811

Fernández-Lao C et al 2011 Widespread mechanical pain hypersensitivity as a sign of central sensitization after breast cancer surgery. Pain Med 12:72–78

Fernández-Pérez AM et al 2013 Can myofascial techniques modify immunological parameters? JACM 19(1):24–28

Fourie WJ 2008 Considering wider myofascial involvement as a possible contributor to upper extremity dysfunction following treatment for primary breast cancer. J Bodyw Mov Ther 12(4):349–355

Guimberteau JC et al 2010 The microvacuolar system: how connective tissue sliding works. J Hand Surg Eur Vol 35(8):614–22

Haouzi P et al 1999 Responses of group III and IV muscle afferents to distension of the peripheral vascular bed. J Appl Physiol 87(2):545–553

Henley et al 2008 Osteopathic manipulative treatment and its relationship to autonomic nervous system activity as demonstrated by heart rate variability. Osteopathic Medicine and Primary Care 2:7

Heredia-Rizo AM et al 2013 Immediate changes in masticatory mechanosensitivity mouth opening, and head posture after myofascial techniques in pain-free healthy participants. J Manipulative Physiol Ther 36 (5):310–318

Hicks M et al 2009 Human fibroblast (HF) model of repetitive motion strain (RMS) and myofascial release. In: Huijing PA et al (eds) Fascia research II, basic science and implications for conventional and complementary health care. Elsevier GmbH, Munich, p 259

Ingber DE 1997 Tensegrity: the architectural basis of cellular mechanotransduction. Ann Rev Physiol 59:575–599

Ingber DE 2003 Mechanobiology and diseases of mechanotransduction. Ann Med 35(8):564–577

Kaufman MP et al 2002 Discharge properties of group III and IV muscle afferents. Adv Exp Med Biol 508:25–32

Kumka M, Bonar B 2012 Fascia: a morphological description and classification system based on a literature review. Can Chiropr Assoc 56(3)

Langevin HM 2006 Connective tissue: a body-wide signaling network? Med Hypoth 66: 1074–1077

Langevin H, Huijing P 2009 Communicating about fascia: history, pitfalls, and recommendations. Int J Ther Massage Bodywork 2(4):1-6

Langevin HM et al 2005 Dynamic fibroblast cytoskeletal response to subcutaneous tissue stretch ex vivo and in vivo. Am J Physiol Cell Physiol 288:747–756

Langevin HM et al 2011 Fibroblast cytoskeletal remodeling contributes to connective tissue tension. J Cell Physiol 226(5):1166–1175

Lee D 2001 An integrated model of joint function and clinical application. 4th Interdisciplinary World Congress on Low Back and Pelvic Pain, Montreal

Lin YW et al 2009 Understanding sensory nerve mechanotransduction through localized elastomeric matrix control. PLoS One 4(1): e4293. doi:10.1371/journal.pone.0004293

Marshall R et al 2009 Evaluating the effectiveness of myofascial release to reduce pain in people with chronic fatigue syndrome (CFS). In: Huijing, PA, Hollander, P, Findley, TW, Schleip R (eds) Fascia research II, basic science and implications for conventional and complementary health care. Elsevier GmbH, Munich, p305

Martínez Rodríguez RF 2013 Mechanistic basis of manual therapy in myofascial injuries. Sonoelastographic evolution control. J Bodyw Mov Ther 17(2):221–234

Martínez Rodríguez R, Galán del Río F 2013 Mechanistic basis of manual therapy in myofascial injuries. Sonoelastographic evolution control. J Bodyw Mov Ther 17(2): 221–234

Nekouzadeh A et al 2008 Stretch-activated force shedding, force recovery, and cytoskeletal remodeling in contractile fibroblasts. J Biomech 41:2964–2971

Pilat A 2003 Inducción Miofascial. MacGraw-Hill, Madrid

Pilat A 2009 Myofascial induction approaches for patients with headache. In: Fernández-de- las-Peñas C, Arendt-Nielsen L, Gerwin RD (eds) Tension type and cervicogenic headache: patho-physiology, diagnosis and treatment. Baltimore: Jones and Bartlett, Sudbury, MA, pp 350–367

Pilat A, Testa M 2009 Tensegridad: el sistema craneosacro como la unidad biodinámica. Libro de Ponencias XIX Jornadas de Fisioterapia EUF ONCE, Madrid, pp 95–111

Pilat A 2011 Myofascial induction. In: Chaitow et al (eds) Practical physical medicine approaches to chronic pelvic pain (CPP) & dysfunction. Elsevier, Edinburgh

Purslow P 2010 Muscle fascia and force transmission. J Bodyw Mov Ther 14:411–417

Remvig L 2007 Fascia research. Myofascial release: 5.4.5 – 140: an evidence based treatment concept. Elsevier Urban & Fischer, New York

Schleip R, Jäger H, Klinler W 2012 What is 'fascia'? A review of different nomenclatures. J Bodyw Mov Ther 16(4):496-502

Schuenke M D et al 2012 A description of the lumbar interfascial triangle and its relation with the lateral raphe: anatomical constituents of load transfer through the lateral margin of the thoracolumbar fascia. J Anat 221(6):568–576

Seeman TE et al 1997 Price of adaptation – allostatic load and its health consequences. MacArthur studies of successful aging. Arch Intern Med 157(19):2259-2268 doi: 10.1001/archinte.1997.00440400111013

Shoham N, Gefen A 2012 Mechanotransduction in adipocytes. J Biomech 45(1):1–8

Stecco L 2004 Fascial manipulation for musculoskeletal pain. Piccin, Padova

Swanson RL 2013 Biotensegrity: a unifying theory of biological architecture with applications to osteopathic practice, education, and research. J Am Osteopath Assoc 113 (1):34–52

Tesarz J et al 2011 Sensory innervation of the thoracolumbar fascia in rats and humans. Neuroscience 194:302–308

Tomasek JJ et al 2002 Myofibroblasts and mechano-regulation of connective tissue remodelling. Nature Rev Mol Cell Biol 3:349–363

Toro C et al 2009 Short-term effects of manual therapy on heart rate variability, mood state, and pressure pain sensitivity in patients with chronic tension-type headache: a pilot study. J Manipulative Physiol Ther 32:527–535

Useros AI, Hernando A 2008 Liberación miofascial aplicada en un paciente adulto con daño cerebral. Biociencias 6:1–7

van der Wal JC 2009 The architecture of connective tissue as parameter for proprioception – an often overlooked functional parameter as to proprioception in the locomotor apparatus. Int J Ther Massage Bodywork 2(4):9–23

Vaquero Rodríguez A 2012 Influence of myofascial therapy applied to the cervical region of patients suffering from unilateral spatial neglect and head deviation with respect to the median line. CSIC (ICNR 2012) Covering Clinical and Engineering Research on Neurorehabilitation. Editorial Springer. Part I: 371–374

Vásquez C 2011 Effectiveness of the myofascial induction technique in the swimmer´s shoulder with respect to the articular balance and pain. Cuest Fisioter 40(3):177–184

Vaticon D 2009 Sensibilidad miofascial libro de ponencias XIX. Jornadas de Fisioterapia EUF ONCE, Madrid, pp 24–30

Wang N, Tytell J, Ingber DE 2009 Mechanotransduction at a distance: mechanically coupling the extracellular matrix with the nucleus. Science 10:75–81

Wheeler AH 2004 Myofascial pain disorders: theory to therapy. Drugs 64:45–62

Yahia LH et al 1993 Viscoelastic properties of the human lumbodorsal fascia. J Biomed Eng 15:425–429

Yi-Wen L et al 2009 Understanding sensory nerve mechanotransduction through localized elastomeric matrix control. PLos One 4(1):e4293

NEUROMUSCULAR TECHNIQUE (NMT) AND ASSOCIATED SOFT TISSUE MANIPULATION MODALITIES

Leon Chaitow

What is NMT? - Introduction

In an earlier text describing neuromuscular technique (NMT), the following introduction was used (Chaitow 2011), as it is again here without apology, as it encapsulates the essence of the subject:

'Imagine a palpation technique that becomes a means of therapeutic intervention by virtue of the addition of increased pressure.

Imagine also a palpation technique that, in a non-invasive manner, meets and matches the tone of the tissues it is addressing and sequentially seeks out changes from the norm in almost all accessible (to finger or thumb) areas of the soft tissues.

Imagine this approach as systematically providing information regarding tissue tone, induration, fibrosity, oedema, discrete localized soft tissue changes, areas of altered structure, adhesions or pain – and being able to switch from a painless and pleasant assessment mode, to a treatment focus that starts the process of normalizing the changes it uncovers.

This is neuromuscular technique (NMT).'

Box 15.1
Major NMT methods and modalities

The soft tissue manipulation methods and modalities listed below are all considered to be 'neuromuscular therapies' and are complementary to the following versions, both of which are outlined in this chapter:

- Neuromuscular Technique (Lief's European version)
- Neuromuscular Therapy (American version)

Most of the approaches listed below alphabetically are featured as separate chapters in this book. All others in the list (in bold typeface) are briefly defined in Box 15.2.

- **Active Release Technique® (ART)**
- Bowen Technique - see Chapter 6
- Connective tissue manipulation – see Chapter 7
- Fascial Manipulation® – see Chapter 9
- **Harmonic technique**
- **Integrated neuromuscular inhibition technique (INIT)**
- Massage – see Chapter 19
- Muscle energy technique – see Chapter 13
- Myofascial release – see Chapter 14
- Rolfing (Structural Integration) – see Chapter 17
- Scar release – see Chapter 18
- **Specific (scar/adhesion) release techniques**
- Strain–counterstrain/positional release – see Chapters 10, 11 and 16
- Trigger point release techniques – see Chapter 20.

Two versions

This chapter describes *Neuromuscular technique* (European version) as well as *Neuromuscular therapy* (American version) – both of which are soft tissue assessment and treatment methods, developed in the 1930s in the UK, and separately in the USA – as well as a variety of adjunctive, soft tissue manipulation methods complementary to both versions of NMT, examples of which are listed in Box 15.1.

Aims of NMT and allied approaches

NMT refers to specialized diagnostic (assessment mode) or therapeutic (treatment mode) manually applied methods.

When used therapeutically, NMT aims to produce modifications in dysfunctional tissue, encouraging a restoration of normality, with a primary focus of deactivating focal points of dysfunctional activity, e.g. myofascial trigger points, as well as paying attention to causative or maintaining features – such as postural or overuse patterns.

Additional NMT attention is towards normalizing imbalances in hypertonic and/or fibrotic tissues, either as an end in itself, or as a precursor to joint mobilization/rehabilitation. In doing so, NMT aims to elicit physiological responses involving mechanoreceptors, Golgi tendon organs, muscle spindles and other proprioceptors, in order to achieve the functional improvements.

Insofar as they integrate with NMT, other means of influencing such neural responses may include all or any of the approaches listed in Box 15.1.

NMT attempts to:

- Offer reflex benefits
- Deactivate myofascial trigger points and other sources of pain
- Prepare for other therapeutic methods, such as rehabilitation exercises or manipulation
- Relax and normalize tense, fibrotic, soft tissues
- Enhance lymphatic and general circulation and drainage

- Simultaneously offer the practitioner diagnostic information
- Include re-education (enhanced posture, breathing, ergonomics etc.) in all therapeutic approaches
- Assist in rehabilitation.

NMT takes account of issues commonly involved in causing or intensifying pain and dysfunction – including:

- **Biochemical features:** nutritional imbalances and deficiencies, toxicity (exogenous and endogenous), endocrine imbalances (e.g. thyroid deficiency), ischemia, inflammation, and where appropriate refers for medical advice/attention
- **Psychosocial factors:** stress, anxiety, depression, etc. and where appropriate referrals for medical advice/attention
- **Biomechanical factors:** posture, including patterns of use, hyperventilation tendencies, as well as locally dysfunctional states such as hypertonia, trigger points, neural compression or entrapment, and where appropriate referrals for medical advice/attention.

NMT sees its role as attempting to normalize or modulate whichever of these (or additional) influences on musculoskeletal pain and dysfunction can be identified, in order to remove or modify as many etiological and perpetuating influences as possible without creating further distress or requirement for excessive adaptation.

NMT recognizes self-regulation as the primary agent in recovery, and sees its role as identification and modulation, or removal, of factors that may retard recovery. As an essential adjunct to that role, it sees a requirement to advise on prevention and modification of factors that may lead to adaptation exhaustion.

NMTs origins

European version (Lief's) NMT

Stanley Lief DO, DC, the founder of the British College of Osteopathic Medicine and developer of the European version of neuromuscular technique was greatly influenced in the 1930s by an Ayurvedic practitioner, **Dr Dewanchand Varma**, whose manual treatment method involved an early form of what was to become NMT, which he called 'pranotherapy'.

Varma (1935) discussed the ways in which 'energy pathways' could be obstructed 'by adhesions,' in which the superficial soft tissues harden – 'so that the nervous currents can no longer pass through them'.

Varma mentions changes in the skin when such obstructions occur, saying: 'If the skin becomes attached to the underlying muscle, the current cannot pass, the part loses its sensibility.'

Discussions in Chapter 2 that describe current thinking and evidence relating to 'densification' and reduced sliding potential of superficial fascia correlate well with Varma's description of the changes he found in these tissues.

Varma's form of manual soft tissue manipulation was designed – as he explained – to 'release' these palpable obstructions. Varma's methods were adapted and incorporated by Lief into what became known as NMT; however, with a quite different therapeutic focus – aimed at normalizing soft tissue dysfunction, releasing restrictions and easing pain.

Varma suggested a two-stage treatment protocol comprising, as it does in the current use of NMT, an assessment phase that seamlessly merges with treatment delivery, as what is being palpated becomes the target for therapeutic attention, as required. The actual manipulation of the tissues in Varma's model was performed by first 'separating' skin from underlying tissue, followed by a gentle 'separation' of the muscle fibers, a process which required: '... highly sensitive fingers, able to distinguish between thick and thin fibers, and ... highly developed consciousness and sensitivity, attained by hours of patient daily practice on the living body.'

These skills are still required for successful use of NMT. See the NMT palpation exercise later in this chapter in order to compare Varma's descriptions with those in the exercise.

Boris Chaitow DC, co-developer with Lief of NMT, has written (personal communication 1983):

This unique manipulative formula [NMT] is applicable to any part of the body, for any physical and physiological dysfunction, and for both articular and soft tissue lesions.

To apply NMT successfully it is necessary to develop the art of palpation and sensitivity ...the whole secret is to be able to recognise the 'abnormalities' in the feel of tissue structures.

The pressure applied by the thumb (in general), should involve a 'variable' pressure, i.e. with an appreciation of the texture and character of the tissues ...The level of the pressure applied should not be consistent because the character and texture of tissue is always variable. These variations can be detected by an educated 'feel.' ...This variable factor in digital pressure constitutes probably the most important quality any practitioner of NMT can learn, enabling him to maintain more effective control of pressure, develop a greater sense of diagnostic feel, and be far less likely to irritate or bruise the tissue.

The clinical relevance of Boris Chaitow's words deserve emphasis for anyone learning or using NMT, since variation of applied digital pressure, during the application of NMT, is probably the most important single feature that distinguishes it from other forms of manual therapies. Refining the ability to 'meet and match' the tension of the tissues being evaluated is a key feature of Lief's NMT.

Peter Lief DC (1963), the son of the developer of NMT, has observed that: 'It sometimes takes many months of practice to develop the necessary sense of touch, which must be firm, yet at the same time sufficiently light, in order to discern the minute tissue changes that constitute the palpable neuromuscular lesion.'

Brian Youngs (1963), who worked as an assistant to Stanley Lief, described what the palpating fingers are seeking and finding and – because NMT diagnosis and treatment are virtually simultaneous – what they are aiming to achieve:

The palpable changes in soft tissues – as listed by Lief – can be summarized by the word 'congestion'. This ambiguous word can be interpreted as a past hypertrophic fibrosis. Reflex cordant contraction of a muscle region reduces the blood flow – and in such relatively anoxic regions of low pH and low hormonal concentration, fibro-blasts proliferate and increased fibrous tissue is formed. This results in an increase in the thickness of the existing connective tissue partitions – the epimysia and perimysia – probably infiltrating deeper between the muscle fibres to affect the normal endomysia.

Thickening of the fascia and subdermal connective tissue occurs if these structures are similarly affected by a reduced blood flow ...Fibrosis seems to occur automatically in areas of reduced blood flow... depending upon the constitutional background. Where tension is the aetiological factor, fibrosis seems inevitable.'

The description by Young of the myofascial environment of ischemia and congestion is, of course, precisely the background out of which myofascial trigger points evolve. It should be no surprise, therefore, that NMT is seen as an ideal treatment approach for identifying and deactivating trigger points (see notes on integrated neuromuscular inhibition technique (INIT) later in the chapter.)

Youngs suggested that Lief's NMT may offer beneficial effects, including:

- Restoration of muscular balance and tone and consequent pain reduction and enhanced function
- Encouragement of normal trophicity in muscular and connective tissues by altering the histological picture from a pathohistological to a physiologic–histological pattern, with more normal vascular and hormonal responses
- Potentially providing visceral benefits by reducing levels of somatovisceral reflex activity
- Improving circulation and drainage relating to areas of stasis.

American version NMT

The original work that evolved into the American version of NMT took place in the late 1970s and early 1980s, based largely on the methods devised and taught by Raymond Nimmo DC (1959) – known as 'receptor-tonus technique'.

Nimmo's research into the pathological influences and relevance, as well as the therapeutic implications of treating what he termed 'noxious pain points', paralleled the work of his contemporary, Janet Travell MD, in relation to her research into myofascial trigger points (Travell & Simons 1999).

Nimmo's approach to these pain generators was modified and expanded by others (Vannerson & Nimmo 1971), building on the writings and research of Travell and Simons (1999).

American version NMT now incorporates systematic approaches to health enhancement, with attention to biochemical, biomechanical and psychosocial causative and maintaining factors.

Despite major evolutionary differences, the two versions of NMT are currently very similar. Both utilize a full range of soft tissue manipulation modalities (see list in Box 15.1) as well as evidence-based rehabilitation methodologies. Both versions also focus on the full range of somatic dysfunction and pain, and the causes of these – with the American version possibly paying more attention to myofascial pain than Lief's model.

NMTs evolution – a combined training and a new profession

Neuromuscular physical therapists, trained in both versions of NMT, have formed an Association of Neuromuscular Therapists, and are now recognized health care providers in the Republic of Ireland. This, together with the establishment of a Masters level degree course in Neuromuscular Therapy, validated by the University of Chester in the UK, marks a major point in the continued evolution of NMT in Europe.

In the USA, members of organizations such as The National Association of Myofascial Trigger Point Therapists are strong advocates of NMT.

Validating studies

Stecco et al. (2013) offer a compelling description of the origins of myofascial pain.

They note that aponeurotic fascia (such as the thoracolumbar fascia) is made up of layers of dense fascia where forces load are absorbed, dispersed and transmitted from myofascial insertions (as described in Ch. 1). These richly innervated layers are separated by looser connective tissue that encourages gliding between deep fascial layers, due to the presence of hyaluronic acid (HA).

They also note that epimysial fascia (surrounding muscles) contains free nerve endings and is directly connected to muscle – creating functional continuity between muscles, joints and deeper fascial structures: *'The collagen fibers of the epimysial fasciae is occupied by the matrix or ground substance, rich in proteoglycans, and in particularly hyaluronic acid (HA).'*

Following injury (overuse, misuse etc.), fatty infiltration occurs, HA decreases, viscosity and acidification increases, sliding function reduces, and 'free nerve endings become hyperactivated', resulting in local inflammation, pain and sensitization. These changes can be reversed by reducing stiffness, density and viscosity – and improving pH – all potentially possible via manual therapies (as described in Ch. 5).

Therefore: *'Dysfunction of fascia – [involves] – alteration of the loose connective tissue (LCT) comprising adipose cells, glycosaminoglycans, and HA. ...an alteration of the quantity or quality of the component of the LCT may change the viscosity and therefore the function of the lubricant that the LCT facilitates.... We suggest this syndrome [myofascial pain] be defined as "densification of fascia" .... [and that]... this is different from the functional alterations observed from morphological alterations such as frank fibrosis.'*

Regarding NMT's efficacy in achieving reversal of such changes, research validation is slowly appearing, for example:

- **Myofascial trigger points:** Nagrale and colleagues (2010) demonstrate the efficacy of NMT methods that were incorporated into a focused trigger point protocol – INIT (described in Box 15.2; Chaitow 1994).
- **Jaw pain:** Spanish researchers (Ibáñez-García et al. 2009) show that NMT (Lief's method) and strain–counterstrain (Ch. 16) are equally, and significantly, effective in the management of latent trigger points in the masseter muscle.
- **Chronic neck pain:** Escortell-Mayor et al. (2011) treated patients with chronic neck pain ('mechanical neck disorder') either with NMT and complementary soft tissue approaches or by means of electrotherapy (TENS). A

significant degree of short-term pain relief was noted in both groups with approximately 30% maintaining their improvement at 6-month follow-up.

- **Shoulder impingement pain:** using a combination of trigger point release (Ch.20) and neuromuscular techniques, Hidalgo-Lozano et al. (2011) were able to demonstrate that manual treatment of active trigger points (TrPs) reduced spontaneous pain and increased pain tolerance in patients with shoulder impingement. They note that: *'current findings suggest that active TrPs in the shoulder musculature may contribute to shoulder [pain] complaint and sensitization in patients with shoulder impingement syndrome.'*
- **Whiplash:** Fernández-de-las-Peñas et al. (2005) report that the soft tissue techniques used in their protocol comprised neuromuscular technique in paraspinal muscles, muscle energy techniques (Ch. 13) in the cervical spine, myofascial release (Ch. 14) in the occipital region, and myofascial trigger point manual therapies (Ch. 20), as required. *'The manipulative protocol developed by our research group has been shown to be effective in the management of whiplash injury. The biomechanical analysis of a rear-end impact justifies some of the manipulative techniques [...] myofascial trigger points in trapezius muscles, suboccipital muscles, scalene muscles and sternocleidomastoid muscles, commonly play an important role in the treatment of people suffering from post-whiplash symptoms.'*
- **Plantar heel pain:** Renan-Ordine et al. (2011) compared the benefits of self-stretching with the same stretching methods accompanied by NMT, in treatment of 60 patients with plantar heel pain. One group of patients performed calf and foot stretches, and had hands-on therapy (NMT) provided by a physical therapist, while the other group only performed stretches. The treatment performed by the physical therapist focused on treating trigger points that felt 'knotty' and which were significantly painful when pressed. The researchers

found greater improvements in patients who both performed the stretches and who also received hands-on therapy. The scale of benefit was clinically important for both improved physical function as well as for bodily pain. Importantly, there was also a significant increase in pain threshold levels within the NMT group, supporting the suggestion of the general pain modulating effects of this form of therapy.

A number of these studies demonstrate the practical, clinical way in which NMT may be successfully used alongside complementary modalities, most of which are outlined in different chapters in this book. The other listed modalities in Box 15.1 are briefly defined in Box 15.2.

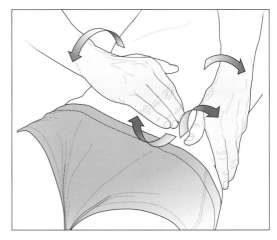

FIGURE 15.1   Specific release technique (described in Box 15.2).

Box 15.2

Adjunctive/complementary (to NMT) soft tissue methods

Box 15.1 lists the major methods that are used alongside NMT, both European and American versions. Most of these topics are covered in separate chapters – with those that are not, briefly described and defined below.

Active Release Technique® (ART)

Active Release Technique® is a modality with similarities to traditional 'pin and stretch' techniques. ART involves the practitioner isolating a contact point close to the region of soft tissue dysfunction, after which the patient is directed to move in ways that produce a longitudinal sliding motion of soft tissues (nerves, fascia, ligaments, muscles) beneath the anchored contact point. Alternatively the movements may be initiated by the practitioner, or may involve both passive and active movements,

Several studies have evaluated the efficacy of ART in different settings, for example:

• Increased pain threshold (Robb & Pajaczkowski 2010)
• Increased hamstring flexibility (George 2006)
• Carpal tunnel syndrome (George et al. 2006)
• Quadriceps strength (Drover et al. 2004).

Harmonic technique (and oscillation)

Harmonic technique involves the induction of cyclical motion in different body regions in an attempt to bring about a state of resonance in body tissues. The method differs from rhythmic articulation where the practitioner imposes a rhythm on the patient's tissues. In harmonic technique, the practitioner tunes in to and uses the patient's own free oscillation frequency to induce the cyclical motion

A study of the method found that the motion induced in the lumbopelvic complex, using a modified harmonic technique – involving rhythmic rocking – displayed properties of harmonic motion (Waugh 2007). The advantages of this approach in relation to fascial function is suggested by evidence of enhanced HA production when oscillating motions are induced, as explained in Chapter 1.

Integrated neuromuscular inhibition technique (INIT)

INIT is a validated sequence of modalities used in treatment of myofascial pain (Chaitow 1994). Following identification of an active myofascial trigger point (TrPt), a sequence is introduced :

1.   Rhythmic intermittent compression of the

TrPt until sensitivity reduces, followed by

2. The application of counterstrain positioning of the tissues (see Ch.16), followed by

3. An isometric contraction of the tissues housing the trigger point and subsequent stretching of those local tissues (see Chs 13 & 20).

4. Finally, an isometric contraction of the entire muscle (not just the local area) is used as a precursor to stretch of the muscle.

Studies have validated the method when compared with other trigger point deactivation approaches (Nagrale et al. 2010).

Specific ('scar/adhesion') release techniques (Fig. 15.1)

Lief described and used methods that could be applied to tight, fibrosed, contracted soft tissue areas of the body, where scarring or adhesion formation is inhibiting normal tissue function (Newman Turner 1984).

Method:

1. Having located an area of contracted tissue, the therapist's middle finger (of the right hand in this description) locates a point of strong restriction and these tissues are drawn towards the practitioner to the limit of pain-free movement.

2. The therapist then abducts the right elbow as the shoulder is internally rotated, adding torsional load to the already extended and compressed tissues.

3. The middle finger (right hand) and its neighbors should by now be flexed and fairly rigid, and be imparting force in three directions i.e. downwards (towards the floor), towards the practitioner, and with a slight rotational addition.

4. The tip of the flexed thumb of the left hand is then placed no more than ¼ inch (0.5cm) adjacent to the middle finger of the right hand, exerting downward pressure (towards the floor) and away from the therapist – as the left elbow is abducted and the shoulder internally rotated, in order to provide a counter-pressure to the forces being created by the right hand.

5. The fulcrum created by the tensions created by the right hand fingers pulling one way, and the left thumb pushing the other, while also being torsioned against each other, builds a combination of tensional forces in several directions at the same time.

6. After all slack has been removed, a very rapid clockwise movement of the right hand and anticlockwise movement of the left hand produces a high-velocity soft tissue 'springing' release – as the elbows snap towards the trunk and the palms of the hands turn rapidly upwards. The amount of force imparted should not produce pain.

7. The sequence can be repeated several times to start a process of change in the connective tissues – usually accompanied by erythema.

8. Variations of hand placement and directions of imposed force offer alternatives.

NMT palpation exercise

Note: The NMT palpation exercise described in detail below derives from the Lief European tradition, and would be preceded, accompanied, or followed, by other palpation methods, such as those described in Chapter 4 (STAR assessment; skin function palpation).

Although described as a 'palpation' exercise, it is important to grasp that palpation and treatment are not seen as separate operations in NMT – one flows to and from the other, backwards and forwards.

As areas of local interest are identified they are explored and, if necessary, treated using slightly firmer pressure than the palpation level, or one or other of the range of complementary methods listed at the start of this chapter.

During the NMT palpation exercise described below, try to focus on as many of the following features as possible, as your contact fingers or thumb moves through and across the tissues being explored:

• **Temperature changes:** Hypertonic muscle will probably be warmer than chronically fibrosed tissue, and there may be variations within a few centimeters.

- **Tenderness:** Ask for feedback whenever there seems a 'different' feel in the tissues being palpated.
- **Edema:** Pay attention to any impression of swelling, fullness, 'bogginess' or congestion
- **Fiber direction:** Try to establish the orientation of tissues, their likely attachment sites, and the vectors of force that daily living imposes on them.
- **Localized contractures:** Local, sometimes very small, areas, may display evidence of reflex or trigger point activity with the presence of taut bands or minute contracture 'knots' that are exquisitely painful on pressure, and which may refer pain to distant areas (see Ch. 20).

Ask yourself constantly as you assess:

- What tissues am I feeling?
- What is the significance of what I can feel in relation to the individual's condition (posture, for example) or symptoms?
- How does what I can feel relate to any other areas of dysfunction I may have noted elsewhere?
- Is what I can feel acute or chronic?
- Is this a local problem, or part of a larger pattern of dysfunction?
- What do these palpable changes mean?

NMT palpation protocol

A light lubricant is always used in NMT to avoid skin friction.

The examination/treatment table should be at a height that allows the therapist to stand erect, legs separated for ease of weight transference, with the assessing arm fairly straight at the elbow.

This allows the practitioner's bodyweight to be transferred down the extended arm through the thumb, imparting any degree of force required, from extremely light to quite substantial, simply by leaning on the arm (see Fig. 15.2). This may present a problem for practitioners whose thumbs are too flexible or unstable. A solution is for them to use only the finger contact as described below.

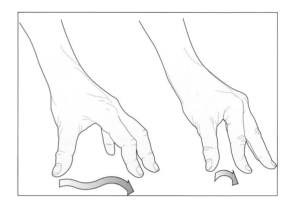

FIGURE 15.2 NMT thumb stroke – the stationary fingers provide a fulcrum as the moving thumb weaves through the tissues, assessing and treating.

For finger palpation the main contact is usually made with the tip of the middle or index finger, ideally supported by a neighboring digit (see Fig. 15.3).

For the thumb stroke it is important that the fingers of the assessing/treating hand act as a fulcrum, and that they lie ahead of the contact thumb, allowing the stroke being made by the thumb to move across the palm of the hand, in the direction of the ring or small finger, as the stroke progresses.

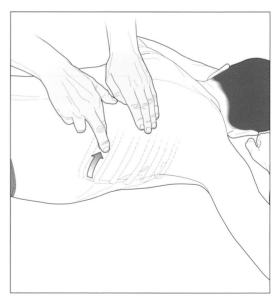

FIGURE5 15.3 NMT finger stroke intercostal assessment, with non-active hand supporting and distracting tissue to prevent bunching.

For balance and control, the fingers should be spread (as in Fig. 15.2), the tips of fingers providing a point of balance, a fulcrum or 'bridge', in which the palm is arched in order to allow free passage of the thumb towards one of the fingertips, as the thumb moves in a direction that takes it away from the practitioner's body.

Each thumb stroke, whether diagnostic or therapeutic, covers approximately 4–5 cm before the thumb stops, as the fingers/fulcrum is then moved, as the thumb stroke continues searching through the tissues.

In contrast, finger strokes move towards the practitioner, commonly with the other hand acting to prevent tissues from bunching or mounding.

Variable pressure essential

The very essence of either the thumb or finger contact involves application of *a variable degree of pressure* that allows the palpating contact to 'insinuate' its way through whatever fibrous, indurated or contracted structures it meets. In the palpation mode of NMT these strokes 'meet and match' tissue tensions, so that the therapist becomes aware of changes in tissue resistance, a fraction ahead of the thumb or finger contact, as it teases its way through the tissues.

This variability of pressure represents a major difference between European and American NMT, with the latter tending to employ strokes that glide across or through the tissues being assessed, in a firm manner, with little pressure variation. In European NMT, degree of resistance or obstruction presented by the palpated tissues determines the degree of effort required.

Tense, contracted or fibrous tissues are never simply overcome by force, instead, the fibers are 'worked through', using a constantly varying amount of pressure, as angles of application modify. If reflex pressure techniques are being employed, a much longer stay on a point will be needed, but in normal diagnostic and therapeutic use the thumb continues to move as it probes, decongests and generally treats the tissues.

All significant findings – whether relating to the quality of the tissues, or of responses from the patient, particularly in relation to sensitivity or pain, should be recorded on a chart. A degree of vibrational contact, as well as variable pressure, allows the contact to have an 'intelligent' feel that does not risk traumatizing or bruising tissues, even when or if heavy pressure is used.

In deeper NMT palpation, or when a shift occurs from palpation to treatment, the pressure of the palpating fingers or thumb may need to increase sufficiently to make contact with structures, such as the paravertebral musculature, without provoking a defensive response.

The changes that might be sensed during palpation could include immobility/rigidity, tenderness, edema, deep muscle tension, fibrotic and interosseous changes.

Apart from fibrotic changes, characteristic of chronic dysfunction, all these changes can be found in either acute or chronic problems.

American NMT: the palpation glide

Effleurage (gliding stroke) forms an important component of the American version of NMT (see Fig. 15.4).

Gliding strokes warm the superficial fascia and are thought to enhance drainage. As with the European assessment methods described above, the gliding process helps to identify contracted bands, along with nodules and tender points. Gliding repeatedly

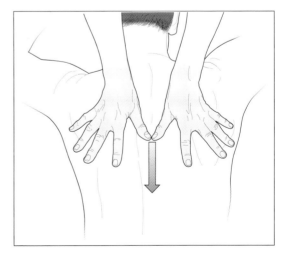

FIGURE 15.4 NMT glide stroke: the fingers support and steady the hands as the primary tools – the thumbs – assess and treat palpation findings.

on these may reduce their size and tenacity. Clinical experience suggests that gliding on the tissues several times, then working somewhere else and returning to glide again, may produce optimal results. The direction of application of glides may be either with or across the direction of the muscle fibers, or more usually, a combination of both. Following the course of lymphatic flow is particularly suggested if tissues are congested.

Therapeutic objectives: palpation becomes treatment

NMT – both versions – aims to produce modifications in dysfunctional tissue, encouraging a restoration of normality, with a primary focus of deactivating focal points of reflexogenic activity such as myofascial trigger points. NMT therefore utilizes physiological responses involving neurological mechanoreceptors, Golgi tendon organs, muscle spindles and other proprioceptors, in order to achieve the desired responses.

An alternative focus is towards normalizing imbalances in hypertonic and/or fibrotic tissues, either as an end in itself or as a precursor to joint mobilization.

Similarly, it should be obvious that the very nature of NMT evaluation makes it an ideal tool for searching for superficial fascial restrictions, characterized by loss of gliding potential, as explained in earlier chapters, and of assisting in restoration of normal function.

The clinical examinations that uses NMT – as described above – should move seamlessly from the gathering of information, into application of treatment objectives. The process of discovery leads to therapeutic action as the practitioner searches for evidence of tissue dysfunction, and then applies appropriate techniques, turning 'finding into fixing'. This transition from examination to treatment and back to examination is a characteristic of NMT.

Use of complementary modalities

Insofar as they integrate with NMT, other modalities, including positional release (strain–counter-

strain) and muscle energy methods, are seen to form a natural set of allied approaches. Traditional massage methods that encourage a reduction in retention of metabolic wastes are included in this category of allied approaches.

Conclusion

Emerging as it does from an amalgam of traditional Asian massage methods ('pranotherapy'), through a prism of osteopathic assessment approaches (see notes on STAR palpation in Ch. 4), while being influenced by physical therapy palpation techniques (see notes on skin assessment methods, also Ch. 4) – with distinct influences from research into myofascial pain – modern NMT has both an interdisciplinary and a trans-Atlantic flavor.

Now validated in a number of studies, NMT can be seen to be a useful assessment and treatment approach to almost all other soft tissue approaches – as well as evolving to become the major therapeutic tool of an emerging profession.

References

Chaitow L 1994 Integrated neuromuscular inhibition technique. British Journal of Osteopathy 13:17–20

Chaitow L 2011 Modern neuromuscular techniques, 3rd edn. Churchill Livingstone Elsevier Edinburgh, pp 35

Drover J et al 2004 Influence of active release technique on quadriceps inhibition and strength: a pilot study. J Manip Physiol Ther 27(6):408–413

Escortell-Mayor E et al 2011 Primary care randomized clinical trial: manual therapy effectiveness in comparison with TENS in patients with neck pain. Man Ther 16(2011):66–73

Fernández-de-las-Peñas C et al 2005 Manual treatment of post-whiplash injury. J Bodyw Mov Ther 9:109–119

George J 2006 The effects of active release technique on hamstring flexibility: a pilot study. J Manipulative Physiol Ther 29:224–227

George J et al 2006 The effects of active release technique on carpal tunnel patients: a pilot study. Journal of Chiropractic Medicine 5(4):119–122

Hidalgo-Lozano A et al 2011 Changes in pain and pressure pain sensitivity after manual treatment of active trigger points in patients with unilateral shoulder impingement: A case series. J Bodyw Mov Ther (2011)15:399–404

Ibáñez-García J et al 2009 Changes in masseter muscle trigger points following strain-counterstrain or neuro-muscular technique. J Bodyw Mov Ther 13(1):2–10

Lief P 1963 British naturopathic. British Naturopathic Journal 5(10):304–324

Nagrale et al 2010 Efficacy of an integrated neuromuscular inhibition technique on upper trapezius trigger points in subjects with non-specific neck pain. J Man Manip Ther 18(1):37–43

Newman Turner R 1984 Naturopathic medicine: treating the whole person. Thorsons, Wellingborough, UK

Nimmo R 1959 Factor X. The receptor (1):4. Reprinted in: Schneider M, Cohen J, Laws S (eds) 2001 The collected writings of Nimmo and Vannerson, pioneers of chiropractic trigger point therapy. Self-published, Pittsburgh

Renan-Ordine R et al 2011 Effectiveness of myofascial trigger point manual therapy combined with a self-stretching protocol for the management of plantar heel pain: a randomized controlled trial. J Orthop Sports Phys Ther 41(2):43–51

Robb A, Pajaczkowski J 2010 Immediate effect on pain thresholds using active release technique on adductor strains: pilot study. J Bodyw Mov Ther 15(1):57–62

Stecco A et al 2013 Fascial components of the myofascial pain syndrome. Curr Pain Headache Rep 17:352

Travell J, Simons D 1999 Myofascial pain and dysfunction: the trigger point manual, vol 1, 2nd edn. The lower body. Williams & Wilkins, Baltimore

Vannerson J, Nimmo R 1971 Specificity and the law of facilitation in the nervous system. The receptor 2(1). Reprinted in: Schneider M, Cohen J, Laws S (eds) 2001 The collected writings of Nimmo and Vannerson, pioneers of chiropractic trigger point therapy. Self-published, Pittsburgh

Varma D 1935 The human machine and its forces. Health for All, London, 1935

Waugh J 2007 An observational study of motion induced in the lumbar–pelvic complex during 'harmonic' technique: a preliminary investigation. Int J Osteopath Med 10(2–3):65–79

Youngs B 1963 The physiological background of neuromuscular technique. British Naturopathic Journal and Osteopathic Review 5:176–178

Chapter 16

POSITIONAL RELEASE TECHNIQUES (INCLUDING COUNTERSTRAIN)

Leon Chaitow

Introduction

The symptoms of musculoskeletal pain and restricted range of motion – the shorthand for which is somatic dysfunction – seldom arise in joints themselves, unless there is frank pathology or traumatic damage. Instead, such pain and restriction are largely imposed and maintained by muscles that traverse or attach to such joints.

Features of somatic dysfunction often include abnormal proprioceptive activity, involving muscle spindles that appear unable to reset – so helping to maintain joint dysfunction. The term 'positional release techniques' (PRT) describes those methods that have one common feature in their methodology – the disengagement of dysfunctional tissues from their restriction barriers – involving a movement of the affected structures towards comfort or 'ease', rather than towards restriction or 'bind' – a process that allows spindles to rest and reduces nociceptor sensitivity (Bailey & Dick 1992).

Muscle spindles are located between muscle fibers and are extremely sensitive to position, load, and motion, potentially at least giving a partial explanation as to why a period of relative absence of stimuli – while being held at 'ease' – allows a reduction in hypertonicity.

PRT methods therefore involve indirect approaches that aim to restore tissue to normal physiological function, using two or three planes of movement to place tissues into a '*position of ease*' or comfort.

Note:

- Indirect and direct approaches are defined in Chapter 5 (Box 5.1)

- The barrier phenomenon is discussed in Chapter 1, and in other chapters, particularly Chapters 13 (Muscle energy techniques) and 18 (Scars)
- Examples of PRT approaches that are covered in detail in separate chapters include:
  o Chapter 10, Fascial unwinding
  o Chapter 11, Balanced ligamentous tension
  o Chapter 14, Myofascial induction therapy (some aspects of this approach are indirect, some are direct).

In this chapter three further PRT related modalities – each with a different fascial connection – are outlined:

- Strain–counterstrain (SCS), also known simply as *counterstrain*
- Functional positional release (FuPR).
- Facilitated positional release (FPR)

SCS definition

'*Strain–counterstrain is a soft tissue manipulation technique in which the practitioner seeks to locate and alleviate nonradiating tender points in the patient's myofascial structures. The practitioner positions dysfunctional tissue at a point of balance in a direction opposite the restrictive barrier. The position of ease is held for 90 seconds, after which the patient is gently returned to the original position where the tender point is rechecked*' (*Mosby's Dictionary of Complementary and Alternative Medicine* 2005).

Barnes study

It is suggested that you revisit Chapter 5 and the description of the Barnes' hysteresis report (Barnes et al. 2013). This was the study in which several hundred individuals with neck pain were treated using one of four methods:

- Balanced ligamentous tension – Chapter 11
- Muscle energy technique – Chapter 13
- High velocity manipulation – discussed in Chapters 2 and 5
- Counterstrain (SCS) – as outlined in this chapter.

Soft tissue 'stiffness' in the dysfunctional regions, involving muscle and fascia, was measured before and after treatment using a durometer. The levels of changes in stiffness – defined as hysteresis, as explained in Chapter 5 – was recorded, with the greatest change being noted following SCS.

Strain–counterstrain

Strain–counterstrain (SCS), also known simply as 'counterstrain', is a treatment method developed in the USA by osteopathic physician Lawrence Jones (1997).

The method requires identification of a localized area in dysfunctional tissues that is painful on light pressure – known in SCS methodology as a 'tender point'. For those familiar with Traditional Chinese Medicine these equate with so called 'ah shi' (spontaneously tender) points.

Tender points have been defined and described as small (between 3 mm and 10 mm in diameter), tense, tender, and edematous zones, located deep in muscle, tendon, ligament, or fascia (Jones 1997). They are considered to be sensory manifestations of neuromuscular or musculoskeletal dysfunction (Korr 1975).

Tender points are not necessarily trigger points, although at times they may manifest characteristics of both, being both sensitive as well as producing referred or radiating pain.

Jones (1997) postulated that in most situations of somatic dysfunction what is being treated is a situation involving a persistent neuromuscular noxious stimulus, and that use of SCS decreases or eliminates irritation, and allows self-regulating mechanisms to operate.

SCS – basic method

Just sufficient pressure should be applied to the tender point to create moderate discomfort – at which time the patient is instructed to ascribe to it a value of '10'.

The patient, or the area involved, is then moved into a position of ease, where the palpated discomfort reduces by at least 70% – and where it is held for up to 90 seconds, before slowly being returned to a neutral position.

The so-called *'position of ease'* has been frequently identified as being in a position that exaggerates any perceived tissue distortion; for example, shortened soft tissues would be placed into an even shorter position, so painlessly exaggerating their shortness and apparently allowing neurological 'resetting' (see discussion of mechanisms, below).

Another observation of possible clinical interest is that the 'position of ease' may be seen to virtually replicate the position in which an initial strain occurred.

The essence of SCS, therefore, is the model in which tissues affected by dysfunction will have been taken to a position where a 70% or more reduction in palpated pain in a monitored tender point has been achieved. The position of comfort/ease would then be maintained for approximately 90 seconds, before being gently released (D'Ambrogio & Roth 1997).

Importantly: after identifying and compressing the tender point in order to achieve a *'position of ease'*, light digital contact should be maintained throughout the 90-second holding time, without pressure, apart from periodic checking for the response to pressure, to ensure the ease position has not been lost. After 90 seconds, and passively and slowly taking the tissues back to their neutral position, the point may be rechecked at which time it should feel less tense and be less tender.

The patient should be warned to avoid active use of the area for a day or so and that increased soreness is normal if experienced for 24 to 48 hours.

Box 16.1

Modified strain–counterstrain (SCS) protocol

The SCS protocol described here is based on the work of D'Ambrogio and Roth (1997) and in this example relates to elbow pain:

1. After completing a visual analog scale (VAS) for pain intensity on digital pressure applied to the predetermined tender point (TeP) site, pressure was again applied (fingertip or thumb) to evaluate tissue tension. At the same time the patient was asked to confirm tenderness. The patient was also asked to relax throughout the process.

2. The practitioner introduced movements of the arm in several planes, while monitoring with the contact digit the primary TeP site for relaxation of the myofascial tissues. The range of movements used to influence the elbow joint involved a selection from: compression or distraction; flexion or extension; supination or pronation; translation (anterior and posterior); and wrist flexion or wrist extension. The practitioner sought verbal confirmation of a reduction in pain intensity when applying approximately $3kg/cm^2$ pressure with either the fingertip or the thumb to the TeP.

3. With minimal movements in all directions the practitioner refined the patient's positioning to maximize the reported reduction of pain at the TeP, as well as the palpated sense of tension or stiffness. The subject's arm was then held in the combined ease position for approximately 90 seconds.

4. The subject was then instructed to 'remain relaxed and not to try to help' as the practitioner slowly returned the upper limb to a neutral position.

5. After the intervention the subject completed another VAS for pain intensity at the TeP before post-intervention outcomes measurement.

SCS as a prescriptive approach

Over a period of many years, Jones and his associates (1995, 1997) compiled lists of specific tender point locations relating to almost every possible strain of most joints and many muscles. The accuracy of the locations were 'proven' by clinical experience, as well as an increasing amount of research evidence (see below).

Jones also provided prescriptive guidelines for achieving 'ease' for any tender points – usually involving a 'folding' or crowding of the tissues in which the tender point had been identified. The benefits noted (see studies below) included a rapidly achieved – and usually lasting – reduction of pain and inflammation, as well as increased mobility and strength.

A reduction in the time required before clinical effects are perceived when using SCS – from the recommended 90 seconds to less than 20 – has been shown to result from the addition of a facilitating load into the tissues, based on the methods of facilitated positional release, which is described below (Chaitow 2009, Schiowitz 1990).

Modifications to the prescriptive model designed and developed by Jones and his colleagues have evolved in recent years. One such modification is that described by Goodheart (1984).

Goodheart's SCS guidelines

Goodheart suggested that instead of relying on charted maps of points, as compiled by Jones and colleagues, therapists should seek – via palpation (see Chs 4 & 15) – tender points in muscles antagonistic to those that are active when pain or restriction is identified or reported. If pain or restriction occurs during movement, the muscles antagonistic to those active at the time will be those housing tender point(s).

Example:

- If someone is locked in painful forward bending, pain will be experienced during extension when trying to stand upright.

- Irrespective of where the pain is felt on extension, tender points will be found in the muscles antagonistic to those working when the pain is experienced i.e. a tender point will be located in the flexor muscles (possibly in rectus abdominis or in psoas) in this example.
- A number of local tender areas may be identified on palpation of the target muscles, with one of these, usually the most tender, being selected to act as a monitor during application of SCS. If there is uniformity of discomfort in a number of possible tender points, it is suggested that the most medial and most proximal of these should be chosen as a monitoring point.
- The selected tender point is then used as a monitor to guide the practitioner as tissues are positioned and fine-tuned, until initial tenderness (on digital pressure) reduces from the starting pain score of 10 to 3 or less.
- This is then maintained, as described above, for 90 seconds, with the palpating finger in touch but not compressing the point, before slowly taking it back to the starting position.
- In other words, the prescriptive Jones' model has been modified by Goodheart's insights as to where to locate suitably tender 'points' – avoiding the need for relying on a virtual cookbook of tender-point charts.

Facilitated positional release

Facilitated positional release (FPR) is an indirect myofascial release method where the tender point, or area of dysfunction, is gradually maneuvered ('fine-tuned') until a relatively pain-free neutral position is achieved, on all planes. At this time a further facilitating influence (either torsion, distraction, shear force or compression) is introduced, in order to release joint or soft tissue restriction further, reducing tissue tension, lowering perceived discomfort – without any increase in discomfort elsewhere (Schiowitz 1990, Jonas 2005).

The addition of facilitation offers a major clinical benefit in that the holding time in the ease position reduces markedly, from 90 seconds to under 20.

Combining SCS with FPR (see Fig. 16.1)

- Locate and palpate an appropriate tender point – usually located in shortened structures that would be active in producing the opposite movement to one that is either painful or restricted
- Use minimal monitoring pressure on the tender point, and request the 'patient' to value the resulting discomfort as a '10'
- Reposition tissues using minimal force to achieve maximum ease/comfort as reported 'pain scores' reduce
- Add a facilitating compressive, distracting, or other force that:
  o decreases discomfort in the palpated point further – ideally to less than 30% of initial sensitivity, and
  o does not create any additional discomfort
- Release after 20 seconds and return slowly to a neutral position
- Recheck the tender point after you return to neutral, it should feel less tense and should be less tender
- Warn the patient they may experience increased soreness for 24 hours as tissues adapt to the change.

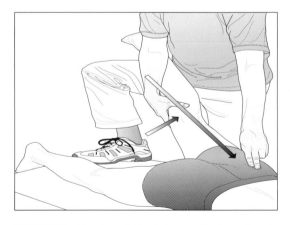

FIGURE 16.1 A tender point in gluteus medius is monitored as the ipsilateral leg is used to achieve reduction in tender point sensitivity. The facilitating force involves long-axis compression towards the hip – reducing tender-point discomfort to below 30%, without creating additional discomfort

General SCS guidelines for achieving tender-point ease

- For tender points on the front of the body, flexion, side-bending and rotation should usually be towards the palpated point, followed by fine-tuning, in order to reduce sensitivity by at least 70%
- For tender points on the back of the body, extension, side-bending and rotation should usually be away from the palpated point, followed by fine tuning in order to reduce sensitivity by 70%
- The closer the tender point is to the midline the less side-bending and rotation should be required, and the further from the midline the more side-bending and rotation should be required, to achieve an ideal ease position
- Additional facilitating forces such as compression or distraction, should not create new discomfort, and should enhance 'ease/comfort' – which should be reflected in the reported reduction in pain 'score'.

If these guidelines are not effective in reducing tender point sensitivity, try other variations in positioning – in other words, these are not absolute rules, merely suggestions.

Mechanisms that may explain SCS effects

A number of explanations have been offered and described that either individually or in combination, may account for the clinical results obtained using SCS (see a selection of studies later in the chapter). Some of the more fascia-related explanations are expanded on below:

- **Neurological changes** involving muscle, fascial and joint mechanoreceptors including Ruffini corpuscles, Golgi tendon organs, muscle spindles etc. (Jones 1995) and pain receptors (Howell et al. 2006). See Chapter 5 for discussion of neural influences deriving from load variations on tissues, under the subheading: *Neural influences and fascial structures*, as well as Box 1.3 in Chapter 1.

- **Proprioceptive theory:** this is the most commonly discussed explanation for the efficacy of SCS. It suggests that a disturbed relationship between muscles and their antagonists may emerge following strain (see below).
- **Altered fibroblast responses** – involving the shape and architecture of cells i.e. mechanotransduction effects – leading to reduced inflammation (Standley & Meltzer 2008) influenced by fluid dynamics (see below).
- **Ligamentous reflexes** (Solomonow 2009, Chaitow 2009; see below).
- And possibly others?

Proprioceptive theory

Wong (2012) has summarized the hypothesised process as follows:

'According to the Proprioceptive Theory rapid stretching injury stimulates muscle spindles causing reflexive agonist muscle contraction that resists further stretching. However, a reflexive counter-contraction resulting from pain induced withdrawal quickly reverses the aggravating movement thereby exciting antagonist muscle spindles. The resulting neuromuscular imbalance, perpetuated by opposing muscle spasms each unable to release due to ongoing muscle spindle excitation (Korr 1975), can affect myofascial mobility and force transmission around neighboring joints and muscles (Kreulen et al. 2003, Huijing and Baar 2008). Underlying muscle imbalance can persist long after the strain heals (Goering 1995) with lasting motor impairment evident long after pain symptoms subside (Sterling et al. 2003).'

It is suggested that the position of ease/comfort in SCS procedures then allows overactive agonist muscle spindle activity to reset, after which antagonist muscle spindle activity also returns to normal, restoring function (Bailey & Dick 1992).

Fibroblast (and fluid dynamic) responses to SCS

Explanations are offered in Chapter 1 regarding mechanotransduction and associated processes, in which a variety of cellular effects are noted in response to mechanical load applications. Of particular interest are the effects of altered degrees and types of strain and load on fibroblasts – plentifully present in fascial structures.

- Dodd et al. (2006) report that: *'Human fibroblasts respond to strain by secreting inflammatory cytokines, undergoing hyperplasia, and altering cell shape and alignment ...and that biophysical* [tissue changes] – *whether resulting from injury, somatic dysfunction, or* [soft tissue manipulation, such as SCS] – *affects range of motion, pain, and local inflammation.'*

- In 2007 Standley and Meltzer observed that: *'Data suggests that fibroblast proliferation and expression/secretion of pro-inflammatory and anti-inflammatory interleukins may contribute to the clinical efficacy of indirect osteopathic manipulative techniques.'*

- Standley and Meltzer (2008) report on various clinically applied fascial methods (counterstrain, as well as myofascial release, see Ch. 14) used to treat somatic dysfunctions. These methods produced positive clinical outcomes such as reduced pain, reduced analgesic use, and improved range of motion. They note that *'it is clear that strain direction, frequency and duration, impact important fibroblast physiological functions known to mediate pain, inflammation and range of motion.'*

- Meltzer et al. (2010) note that traumatized fascia disrupts normal biomechanics of the body, increasing tension exerted on the system and causing myofascial pain and reduced range of motion. They found that resulting inflammatory responses by fibroblast cells can be reversed by changes in load on the tissues, delivered either by either counterstrain or myofascial release (see Ch. 14) and that such changes may take only 60 seconds to manifest.

- Wong (2012) highlights the possible fluid dynamic nature of the effects of SCS: *'decreased interleukin (IL-6) levels, important for mediating inflammatory healing after acute injury (Kopf et al. 1994), suggest SCS may affect local circulation (Standley & Meltzer 2007).*

Clinically, Achilles tendonitis patients reported decreased swelling after SCS (Howell et al. 2006) but research is needed to understand potential circulatory effects of SCS.'

Ligamentous reflexes (and water)

Solomonow (2009) spent many years researching the functions of ligaments. He identified their sensory potential and major ligamentomuscular reflexes that have inhibitory effects on associated muscles, and states: *'If you apply only 60–90 seconds of relaxing compression on a joint ... an hour plus of relaxation of muscles may result. This may come not only from ligaments, but also from capsules and tendon'* (personal communication 2009).

A possible clinical application of this ligamentous feature may be seen when joint crowding is induced as part of facilitated positional release and/or strain–counterstrain protocols. Such effects would be temporary – 30 to 60 minutes – but this would be sufficient to allow enhanced ability to mobilize or exercise previously restricted structures.

Coincidently, crowding (compression) of soft tissues would have an effect on the water content of fascia, leading to temporary (20–30 minutes) of reduced stiffness of fascial structures – with similar enhanced mobility during that period. See *Water and stretching* discussion in Chapter 5.

Wong (2012) summarizes current thinking regarding ligamentomuscular reflexes and SCS:

'Ligamentous strain inhibits muscle contractions that increase strain, or stimulates muscles that reduce strain, to protect the ligament (Krogsgaard et al. 2002). For instance, anterior cruciate ligament strain inhibits quadriceps and stimulates hamstring contractions to reduce anterior tibial distraction (Dyhre-Poulsen & Krogsgaard 2000). Ligamentous reflex activation also elicits regional muscle responses that indirectly influence joints (Solomonow & Lewis 2002). Research is needed to explore whether SCS may alter the protective ligamento-muscular reflex and thus reduce dysfunction by shortening joint ligaments or synergistic muscles (Chaitow 2009).'

Cautions

SCS usage should be avoided in cases involving:
- Open wounds
- Recent sutures
- Healing fractures
- Hematoma
- Hypersensitivity of the skin
- Systemic localized infection.

SCS studies

Wong (2012) has reviewed and evaluated current research into SCS:

'Descriptive cases HAVE documented SCS applications for foot (Jones 1973), knee (Pedowitz 2005), lower back (Lewis & Flynn 2001), shoulder (Jacobson et al. 1990), and myofascial disorders (Dardzinski et al. 2000). Some studies combined SCS with other treatments for disorders including complex regional pain syndrome (Collins 2007), cervicothoracic pain (Nagrale et al. 2010), lateral epicondylalgia (Benjamin et al. 1999), and cavus foot (Wong et al. 2010).'

Examples:
- 49 volunteers aged 19–38 years, with hip weakness and corresponding tender points (TP)... [after four SCS treatments over 2 weeks] ... all groups reported reduced pain and increased strength 2–4 weeks following the intervention (Speicher et al. 2004)
- Lewis and Flynn (2001) used strain–counterstrain to successfully treat patients with low back pain: *'The SCS intervention phase for each case took approximately one week and consisted of 2 to 3 treatment sessions to resolve perceived "aberrant neuromuscular activity".'*
- In treatment of Achilles tendonitis, Howell et al. (2006) noted that following treatment incorporating SCS: *'subjects indicated significant clinical improvement in soreness, stiffness, and swelling ...Because subjects' soreness ratings also declined immediately after treatment, decreased nociceptor activity may play an additional role in somatic dysfunction, perhaps by altering stretch reflex amplitude.'*

- Dardzinski et al. (2000) reported: *'SCS techniques should be considered and evaluated further as adjunctive therapy for patients previously unresponsive to standard treatment for myofascial pain syndrome.'*
- Wynne et al. (2006) found that: *'Clinical improvement occurs in subjects with plantar fasciitis in response to counterstrain treatment [SCS]. The clinical response is accompanied by mechanical, but not electrical, changes in the reflex responses of the calf muscles.'* See notes on SCS and plantar fasciosis in Chapter 2, and Figure 2.2.
- *'Symptoms of a 30-year-old distance runner with ITBFS were reduced with the help of OMT, specifically SCS. This technique allows for relief of pain at a tender point by moving the affected body part into its position of greatest comfort, aiding in the reduction of receptor activity. The tender point was located from 2cm proximal to the lateral femoral epicondyle. There is no prior documentation of the osteopathic manipulation of this specific tender point. Thus, this case report reflects an initial identification of a distal iliotibial band tender point, and a new therapeutic modality for ITBFS'* (Pedowitz 2005).

Functional positional release (FuPR)

Functional positional release (FuPR) technique has the same clinical objective as counterstrain and FPR – identification of a position of ease in relation to pain or restriction, acute or chronic, irrespective of whether dysfunction involves muscles, fascia or joint complexes.

However, unlike counterstrain, FuPR does not use pain reduction as a guide to finding the desired position of ease – instead it relies on a reduction in palpated tone in stressed (hypertonicity/spasm) tissues, as the body (or part) is being positioned or fine-tuned, using/testing all available directions of movement. Hoover (1969), the osteopathic developer of functional technique, used the term *'dynamic neutral'* to describe what was being achieved as disturbed tissues were positioned in a state of 'ease'.

FuPR methodology (Bowles 1981)

The practitioner's hand palpates the affected tissues (molded to them, without invasive pressure), in order to 'listen' to, and assess changes in tone, as the other hand guides the patient, or part, through a sequence of positions aimed at increasing the sense of palpated 'ease' as 'bind' is reduced.

A sequence of evaluations is carried out, each involving different directions of movement (flexion/extension, rotation right and left, side-bending right and left etc.), with each evaluation starting at the point of maximum ease discovered during the previous evaluation, or at the combined position of ease of a number of previous evaluations.

In this way one position of ease is 'stacked' on to another until all directions of movement have been assessed for ease. The precise sequence in which the various directions of movement are evaluated is not relevant, as long as all possibilities are included.

Only very limited ranges of motion might be available in some directions during this assessment, and the whole procedure should be performed very slowly. When a position of maximum ease – involving the combined 'positions of ease' in multiple directions – is arrived at, this is held for up to 90 seconds, to allow a process of self-regulation and resetting to reduce hypertonicity and pain to start.

The final position of palpated maximum ease (reduced tone) in the distressed tissues should correspond with the position that would have been found if pain was being used as a guide, as in counterstrain methodology. Despite the gentleness of the methods there is almost always a reaction involving stiffness and possibly discomfort on the day following treatment, as adaptation processes accommodate to changes.

Examples of FuPR

Note: Both facial unwinding (Ch. 10) and balanced ligamentous tension (Ch. 11) are examples of functional technique.

Post-surgical use of FuPR

In order to determine the effects on cardiac hemodynamics, O-Yurvati et al. (2005) documented the effects of FuPR applied to traumatized thoracic tissues, as part of a broader osteopathic intervention, following coronary artery bypass graft (CABG):

- 10 subjects undergoing CABG were compared, pre-treatment versus post-treatment, involving measurements of thoracic impedance, mixed venous oxygen saturation and cardiac index
- Immediately following CABG surgery, FuPR was provided to *anesthetized and pharmacologically paralyzed patients* to alleviate anatomic dysfunction of the rib cage, caused by median sternotomy, and to improve respiratory function.

As shown in Figure 16.2, this FuPR treatment approach involved the practitioner placing one hand under the supine patient, to rest/palpate tissues between the scapulae. Simultaneously, the other hand was placed anteriorly, directly over the surgically traumatized tissues. Just sufficient pressure was exerted to allow the superficial skin and fascia to be moved in the directions being tested:

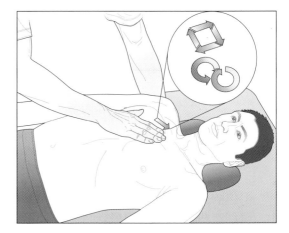

FIGURE 16.2 Each hand – independently – stacks positions of ease onto each other as all directions are assessed for 'ease'. The final combined position of ease is held for 90 seconds during which circulatory, proprioceptive and viscoelastic effects are thought to induce a self-regulating process.

- Each hand independently evaluated tissue preference directions – superior/inferior?
- Lateral to the left/lateral to the right?
- Clockwise/anticlockwise?

Each evaluation commenced from the 'ease' position of the previous evaluation(s).

Once the final ease position was identified by each hand independently, the tissues were maintained in those positions for 90 seconds before a slow return to the starting position. Results suggested improved peripheral circulation and increased mixed venous oxygen saturation after the treatment. These increases were accompanied by a significant improvement in cardiac index.

FuPR variation: integrated neuromuscular release

Integrated neuromuscular release is a form of FuPR involving a segmental, anteroposterior approach that aims to correct muscular, fascial and neural imbalances. *'Osteopathic manipulative treatment has been concerned, purposefully or not, with manipulation of the fascia'* (Danto 2003)

- With the patient seated, the practitioner's hands are placed anteriorly and posteriorly. Independently, they perform evaluations of tissue direction preferences, in the same way described above in the post-surgical example (Fig. 16.3).
- Each direction sequence is asking the same question – in which direction do the tissues move most freely – with each change in direction commencing from the position(s) of ease previously identified?
  - o Superior/inferior?
  - o Lateral to the left/lateral to the right?
  - o Clockwise/anticlockwise?
- In this way the palpated tissues are taken into their preferred directions of motion towards a combined 'ease' position, at which time compression is added – a feature of facilitated positional release (FPR). This is held for 60–90 seconds, or longer if changes in the tissues are being sensed – pulsation, rhythmic motion, etc.– before a slow release.

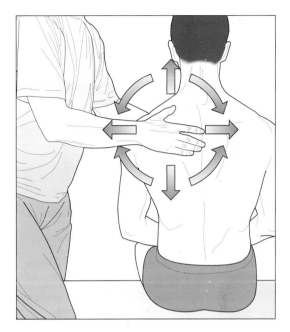

FIGURE 16.3 In the same manner as in Fig. 16.2, each hand – independently – stacks positions of ease onto each other as all directions are assessed for 'ease'. The final combined position of ease is held for 90 seconds during which circulatory, proprioceptive and viscoelastic effects are thought to start a self-regulating process.

Conclusion

Positional release methods are safe, easy to apply and have been validated clinically. They clearly have a fascial connection whether via fibroblast influences or ligamentous reflexes and they combine efficiently with most other manual modalities.

References

Bailey M, Dick L 1992 Nociceptive considerations. J Am Osteopathic Assoc 92(3):334: 337-341

Barnes P et al 2013 A comparative study of cervical hysteresis characteristics after various osteopathic manipulative treatment (OMT) modalities. J Bodyw Mov Ther 17:89-94

Benjamin S et al 1999 Normalized forces and active range of motion in unilateral radial epicondylalgia. J Orthop Sports Phys Ther 29:668-676

Bowles C 1981 Functional technique – a modern perspective. J American Osteopathic Association 80(3):326-331

Chaitow L 2009 Editorial. J Bodyw Mov Ther 13(2):115-116

Collins CK 2007 Physical therapy management of complex regional pain syndrome in a 14-year-old patient using strain counterstrain: a case report. J Man Manip Ther 15(1):25-41

D'Ambrogio K, Roth G 1997 Positional release therapy. Mosby, St Louis

Danto JB 2003 Review of integrated neuromusculoskeletal release and the novel application of a segmental anterior/posterior approach in the thoracic, lumbar, and sacral regions. J Am Osteopath Assoc 103(12):583-96

Dardzinski J et al 2000 Myofascial pain unresponsive to standard, treatment: successful use of a strain/counterstrain technique with physical therapy. J Clin Rheumatol 6(4):169-174

Dodd J et al 2006 In-vitro biophysical strain model for understanding mechanisms of osteopathic manipulative treatment. J Am Osteopath Assoc (106)3:157-166

Dyhre-Poulsen P, Krogsgaard MR 2000 Muscular reflexes elicited by electrical stimulation of the anterior cruciate ligament in humans. J Appl Physiol 89:2191-2195

Goering EK 1995 Physical manipulation. In: Strain-counterstrain. Jones Strain-Counterstrain, Indianapolis

Goodheart G 1984 Applied kinesiology workshop procedure manual, 21st edn. Detroit, Privately published

Hoover H 1969 Collected papers. Academy of Applied Osteopathy Year Book

Howell JN, et al 2006 Stretch reflex and Hoffmann reflex responses to osteopathic manipulative treatment in subjects with Achilles tendinitis. J Am Osteopath Assoc 106(9): 537-545

Huijing PA, Baar G 2008 Myofascial force transmission via extramuscular pathways occurs between antagonistic muscles. Cells Tissues Organs 188(4):400-414

Jacobson E et al 1990 Shoulder pain and repetition strain injury to the supraspinatus muscle: etiology and manipulative treatment. J Am Osteopath Assoc 89(8):1037-1040

Jonas WB 2005 Mosby's dictionary of complementary and alternative medicine. Elsevier Mosby, St Louis

Jones LH 1973 Foot treatment without hand trauma. J Am Osteopath Assoc 72:481-489

Jones LH 1995 Strain-counterstrain. Jones Strain-Counterstrain, Indianapolis

Jones LH 1997 Strain and counterstrain. Academy of Applied Osteopathy, Colorado Springs

Kopf M et al 1994 Impaired immune and acute-phase responses in interleukin-6-deficient mice. Nature 368:339

Korr I 1975 Proprioceptors and somatic dysfunction. J Am Osteopath Assoc 74(7):638-650

Kreulen M et al 2003 Biomechanical effects of dissecting flexor carpi ulnaris. J Bone Joint Surg Br 85 (6):856–859

Krogsgaard M et al 2002 Cruciate ligament reflexes. J Electromyogr Kines 12:177-182

Lewis T, Flynn C 2001 Use of strain-counterstrain in treatment of patients with low back pain. J Man Manip Ther 9(2):92-98

Meltzer K et al 2010 In vitro modeling of repetitive motion injury and myofascial release. J Bodyw Mov Ther 14:162

Mosby's Dictionary of Complementary and Alternative Medicine 2005 Elsevier Mosby, St Louis

Nagrale A et al 2010 The efficacy of an integrated neuromuscular inhibition technique on upper trapezius trigger points in subjects with nonspecific neck pain: a randomized controlled trial. J Man Manip Ther18:37-43

O-Yurvati A et al 2005 Hemodynamic effects of osteopathic manipulative treatment immediately after coronary artery bypass graft surgery. JAOA105(10):475-481

Pedowitz R 2005 Use of osteopathic manipulative treatment for iliotibial band friction syndrome. J Am Osteopath Ass105(12):563-567

Schiowitz S 1990 Facilitated positional release. American Osteopathic Association 90(2):145–156

Solomonow M 2009 Ligaments: a source of musculoskeletal disorders. J Bodyw Mov Ther 13(2) 136-154

Solomonow M, Lewis J 2002 Reflex from the ankle ligaments of the feline. J Electromyogr Kines 12:193-198

Speicher T et al 2004 Effect of strain counterstrain on pain and strength in hip musculature. J Man Manip Ther 12(4):215-223

Standley P, Meltzer K 2007 Modeled repetitive motion strain and indirect osteopathic manipulative treatment in regulation of human fibroblast proliferation and interleukin secretion. J Am Osteopath Assoc 107:527-536

Standley P Meltzer K 2008 In vitro modeling of repetitive motion strain and manual medicine treatments: Potential roles for pro- and anti-inflammatory cytokines. J Bodyw Mov Ther 12:201–203

Sterling M et al 2003 Development of motor system dysfunction following whiplash injury. Pain 103:65-73

Wong C et al. 2010 Deformity or dysfunction? Osteopathic manipulation of the idiopathic cavus foot: a clinical suggestion. N Am J Sports Phys Ther 5(1):27-32

Wong CK 2012 Strain counterstrain: current concepts and clinical evidence. Man Ther17:2-8

Wynne M et al 2006 Effect of counterstrain on stretch reflexes, Hoffmann reflexes, and clinical outcomes in subjects with plantar fasciitis. J Am Osteopathic Assoc 106(9):547-556

Chapter 17

ROLFING® STRUCTURAL INTEGRATION

Jonathan Martine

Introduction

Structural integration (SI) is a system of manual therapy and sensorimotor education that aims to enhance economy of function, and promote ease of coordinated movement (Jacobson 2011). Presently, there are over 19 schools recognized by the International Association of Structural Integrators (IASI) who certify practitioners of *structural integration*. *Rolfing®* Structural Integration was created by Ida Pauline Rolf, PhD (1896–1979) and the Rolf Institute of Structural Integration (RISI) was created by Dr Rolf and her original teachers in 1971. (Dr Rolf's work is now known by her original title, structural integration. Rolfing® Structural Integration refers to the work of graduates and members of the Rolf Institute® of Structural Integration, Dr Rolf's original school. The Little Boy logo and the terms *Rolfing®, Rolf Movement®* and *Rolfer™* are service marks of the Rolf Institute.) While there are unique aspects to each SI school, the essential elements are consistent in the curricula presented in each program.

In order to disseminate her work to others and to make the education process accessible, she developed a series of 10 sessions, which came to be known as the Ten-Series. It is suggested that the Rolf Ten-Series offers a systematic approach to reorganizing the body and its movement in relationship to the force of gravity and its environment (Maitland 1995).

Founded in 2002, IASI was founded as a grassroots organization from within the profession, to set standards, develop certification criteria, ensure continuation of a professional identity, and promote structural integration's continued growth as a respected profession in the healthcare field (http://www.theiasi.net). The author will draw from his experience as a practicing Certified Advanced Rolfer™ and Faculty at the RISI in this chapter.

Overview

Rolfing SI, developed by Ida P. Rolf PhD, aims to organize the body in relationship to gravity. It purports to improve structural and functional integrity as a whole, rather than treating specific symptoms. The effectiveness of SI is based upon foundational principles that distinguish it from other manual and movement modalities as outlined below. Catalyzed by her initial formal education as a biochemist, and her desire to find answers for her family health problems, Dr Rolf explored many healing arts and movement practices. Her extensive search included osteopathy and hatha yoga, and was influenced by Alfred Korzybski and his work in General Semantics, as well as the movement awareness methods of Elsa Gindler, Charlotte Selver, Jeanette Lee, and Moshe Feldenkrais (Jacobson 2011).

Dr Rolf also referred to the concept of 'tensegrity', coined by Buckminster Fuller and related his ideas to the body. In a tensegrity structure, tensional integrity is maintained by compressive structures or struts – like bones – held in, and suspended apart, by tensional units such as tendons and ligaments (Myers 2001).

Through her study Dr Rolf realized three key concepts:

1. The body functions most efficiently when its segments (head, torso, pelvis, legs and feet) are organized allowing its central axis to align more closely to the gravitational vertical.
2. Fascia is the organ of form in the body: surrounding, supporting, dividing, protecting and connecting every bone, ligament, tendon, muscle, nerve, vessel, tube and organ.
3. The body is a plastic medium, changeable at any time in our life. The forces that create our body's shape are also the forces that reinforce inefficient alignment. Through hands-on manipulation, educating optimal movement patterns for daily activities and increasing body awareness in relationship to the environment, functional efficiency can be improved or restored.

Rolfing SI achieves its outcomes through a combination of hands-on manipulation and movement education, designed to differentiate structures, improve performance, and increase body awareness. The standard protocol of 10 sessions systematically realigns the body and aims to restore efficient movement (see details later in the chapter).

Traditionally the mechanism of Rolfing's structural and functional change was believed to be the physical separation and 'ungluing' of fascial adhesions, leading to improved alignment. Recent influences from the field of neuroscience suggest that the mechanical changes deriving from Rolfing's manual manipulation may be expanded to include changes in the brain's 'mapping' of the body and the space it occupies (Frank 2008).

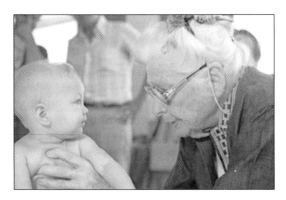

FIGURE 17.1 Dr Rolf working with child

Research evidence of clinical effectiveness and proposed therapeutic mechanisms are limited. Recent quasi-experimental and descriptive case studies have examined SI and low back pain, chronic pain, neck motion and pain levels, spastic cerebral palsy in young children, and systemic lupus erythematosus (SLE). A summary of the relevant research can be further examined by reading Jacobson's paper (2011). Details will follow later in the chapter.

Objectives of Rolfing® structural integration

According to Dr Rolf, all bodies have some degree of disorder and compensation in their structure; therefore she believed that everyone from children to adults, would benefit from receiving Rolfing SI (RSI). Those who have a history of injury, stress or repetitive strain, and who notice that the effects of their injuries are interfering with everyday life, may consider RSI, as well as those looking for a way to ease pain and chronic stress, or improve performance in their professional and daily activities.

RSI is commonly offered in private practice setting as an approach to health. This treatment can also be found as an adjunct to other therapies in medical offices, physical therapy clinics, holistic and complementary health practices. Because of its focus on body awareness, Rolfing SI is also utilized in psychotherapy settings to assist the process of identifying and accessing habitual patterns. Increased body awareness may also serve physical therapy patients, yoga practitioners, and those practicing movement modalities such as martial arts, Pilates and dance. In addition, there are many competitive athletes and sports teams (amateur and professional) that call on the services of Rolfers to assist in maintenance during their seasons, as well as recovery from injury.

Although Dr Rolf originally intended SI to be a method by which healthy individuals could improve posture and function, it is increasingly utilized for the treatment for musculoskeletal pain and dysfunction. This trend has prompted Workmen's Compensation boards and insurance companies in several states in the US, including

Colorado, California, Virginia, Alaska and Arizona, to acknowledge SI by reimbursement when billed as a type of massage therapy.

Dr Rolf taught practitioners that when the body is held with its segments (head, torso, pelvis and legs) in random alignment, muscular tension is required to hold the body upright. In addition, the body will respond to repetitive motion, stress, strain, accidents and injuries by reinforcing the fascia, depositing fibrous tissue and adhering adjacent layers, and thus reinforcing repeated movement while limiting others. In order to return the body to its most efficient functioning, the segments need to be aligned around a central axis, or line, in relation to gravity.

Research: mechanisms and hypotheses

Research evidence of clinical effectiveness and proposed therapeutic mechanisms are limited. An extensive summary of these studies, by Eric Jacobson PhD, was published in the *Journal of Alternative and Complementary Medicine* in 2011. He found that hypothesized mechanisms for changes in structural alignment and functional efficiency include improved biomechanical organization, which leads to reductions in mechanical stress and nociceptive irritation, a perception of improved efficiency and coordination that effect greater sense of overall well-being, and improvements in sensory processing and vagal tone (Jacobson 2011):

'Limited evidence exists for improvements in neuromotor coordination, sensory processing, self-concept and vagal tone, and for reductions in state anxiety. Preliminary, small sample clinical studies with cerebral palsy, chronic musculoskeletal pain, impaired balance, and chronic fatigue syndrome have reported improvements in gait, pain and range-of-motion, impaired balance, functional status, and well-being' (Jacobson 2011).

Further studies are summarized here. An article by Deutsch et al. (2000) reported on 20 individuals who participated in an inpatient rehabilitation program complementing a 10-session SI series.

Those, who had chronic pain in the low back, cervical region and extremities, demonstrated significant decreases in pain reports and improvements of posture and functional mobility (Deutsch & Anderson 2008).

Ball offers more recent investigations of efficacy and potential application for SI as part of a treatment plan suggesting anecdotal efficacy in addressing symptoms of SLE. Two SLE patients reported reduced pain, fatigue/exhaustion, and anxiety, and enhanced functional mobility, autonomy, emotional state, and quality of life following a series of SI-based interventions (Ball 2011).

James studied cervical spine dysfunction in 31 patients over 3 years who were receiving RSI. The results of the investigation suggest RSI reduces pain and increases cervical movement. (James et al. 2009).

A preliminary study of young children with spastic cerebral palsy suggests using SI as a complementary technique to loosen and realign muscles and joints could facilitate improved motor function (Hanson et al. 2012).

These studies suggest the need for broader-based clinical studies of motor control, non-motor benefits such as body function, participation in activity, and quality of life. Dr Rolf referred to general mechanisms to explain the positive effects of her work in reducing chronic musculoskeletal pain and improving perceived effort in movement. Anecdotally reported psychological effects include increased self-confidence, being more proactive with less reactive behavior, increased tolerance for emotional experience, increased stability under emotional stress, and reductions in anxiety and depression (Jacobson 2004, Anson 1998). The most common anecdotally reported physical effects are improvements in: posture, ease in movement, flexibility, pain reduction, improved balance and increased overall relaxation.

Jacobson concluded, 'Evidence for clinical effectiveness and hypothesized mechanisms is severely limited by small sample sizes and absence of control arms. However, in view of the rapidly increasing availability of SI and its use for treatment of musculoskeletal pain and dysfunction, more adequate research in warranted' (Jacobson 2011).

Neurophysiologic mechanisms

Neurophysiologic mechanisms have not been directly assessed in clinical trials, yet much of the recent fascial research and neuroscience discoveries points towards potential explanations for changes in postural alignment and perceived functional ease following Rolfing treatments. According to Schleip, the fascial web, densely populated with various mechanoreceptors, is a body-wide mechanosensory organ informing us as to where we are in space and what our bodies are doing (Schleip 2003). The information collected and carried through the fascial web communicates with the self-regulating and self-organizing functions of the neuromotor system.

Currently, Rolfing SI utilizes two aspects of structural education: one primarily aimed at increasing tissue pliability and one more concerned with eliciting perception and coordination. Dr Rolf believed that hands-on manipulation was responsible for a large part of the postural change that occurs from SI. More recently this concept has been expanded. Physical contact augmented by directed dialogue and sensory exploration between client and practitioner could also serve to define the individual body parts to the brain, increasing afferentation and thus immediately changing motor pathways. The maps initiated by touch inform the brain of the internal and surface space, while maps of 'peripersonal space' define the brain's perception of the space around the body, extending to the reach of the appendages and surface of the skin, head to toe (Frank & Blakeslee 2009). Mechanoreceptors, stretch reflexes, proprioception, and our common senses of vision, taste, hearing, smell and touch all inform our ability to move normally. The vestibular mapping gives us a sense of our location in relationship to gravity. These maps change in relationship to experience and are thought of as plastic. Once differentiated physically and identified as separate, the body parts are related through integrating awareness of habitual patterns, allowing new possibilities for movement. The process leads to increased capacity for discrete movement and efficient coordination based upon the reorganization of muscles with these changes then becoming represented in the brain's motor regions.

Lesion vs inhibition

Rolfers aim to address the obstacles that may limit efficiency and free in movement. Such restrictions may be held physically as adaptations resulting in tight, restricted soft tissue, produced by repeated patterns of movement as in habitual patterns of use. To differentiate structural from movement restrictions, the terms 'lesions' and 'inhibitions' are used. RISI instructor Hubert Godard has explained posture as the potential for movement (Caspari 2005). 'Lesions', according to this model, are fixations in the fascia or joints that show up as restrictions when testing client's passive ranges of motion, which are best addressed by physical manipulation on the biomechanical level. 'Inhibitions', however, need to be addressed on the coordinative or perceptive level, utilizing the senses to influence the neuromuscular pathways and muscle firing sequences. Godard considers each of our movements to be initiated by largely unconscious Anticipatory Postural Activity (APA or pre-movement). APA sets the conditions for movement in place, and is a function of where we are in space and in relationship to the forces of gravity (Caspari 2005).

'Inhibitions' commonly arise from our body image (defined by our subjective experience, beliefs, attitudes and personal history) rather than from the body schema (a non-conscious system of neural processes that constantly regulate posture, movement and peripersonal space) (Caspari 2005).

In Rolfing SI, inhibitions are considered to be held in the APA and not simply restriction in the soft tissues or joints. When an inhibition restricts movement, the practitioner needs to address the client's perception through developing a mutual vocabulary of sensations. A sense of weight in our limbs, our contact with the ground, an awareness of the felt sense of space around and above the body and defining a felt sense of embodiment, are used to orient the client and expand body awareness.

Rolf's suggested protocol

Dr Rolf's Ten-Series is fundamental to the curricula in the 19 Structural Integration schools acknowledged by IASI. Movement and perceptual/orienting exercises have been developed by the various schools to reinforce and expand the structural goals of the sessions and to continue her inquiry.

One example of the ongoing developments in the SI world is Rolf Movement Integration (RMI). This is a system of movement awareness training applied as a complement to Rolfing SI, or an isolated treatment. Rolfers trained in this approach draw from a variety of techniques to create an individualized process of reeducating the body though training the senses (Bond 2007). During Rolfing SI sessions, the RMI may be woven into the process to assist in deepening understanding of habitual movement patterns, integrating the fascial manipulation, and reinforcing new movement and perceptual channels.

Self-applied postural exercise

The following postural exercise is based upon Rolfer and RISI Rolf Movement Faculty member Mary Bond's supported sitting exercise, from her book *The new rules of posture* (2007).

Many jobs require us to spend time working at desks, so knowing how to sit with greater ease and support is certainly useful and beneficial to one's health and well-being. Begin by finding a chair with a firm, flat surface that is tall enough to have your hips above your knees as your feet rest on the floor. Sit on the chair as if it was a bench or stool, don't lean against the chair back.

Begin by noticing the contact of your ischial tuberosities on the chair if you assume a typical C-curve or slouch posture that may be familiar at the end of a long day. Your weight will fall to the back edge of these bones, your coccyx will tuck under, narrowing the ischia and contracting the pelvic floor. Your feet and legs now have less contact as your base of support has shifted back. Now your lumbar spine will be posterior, placing pressure on the sacroiliac joints. Your body is now supported by a small area between your ischia and the sacrum.

If you scan your upper body you may notice your shoulders have rounded forward, your sternum has dropped, compressing the rib cage on to your abdomen. Notice if you try to turn your head, this head-forward position restricts the range of motion. The shortened front line will also compress the intestines while restricting breath as well. If you were to simply sit up or pull your shoulders back to appear upright without adjusting the base of support it would be difficult to sustain this posture.

To come out of the slouch, roll your pelvis forward so you feel the pubic bone drop and the pelvic floor widens in the back. About 60% of your weight will now rest through your pelvis, and 40% into your legs and feet. Allow your spine, chest and shoulders to adjust to the change in your foundation and the curve in your low back. The spinal undulation generates a lifting of your chest and throat taking pressure off the abdomen and diaphragm. You may notice more ease in breathing now, as well as increased range of motion in your head and neck as you turn to look over your shoulder.

Healthy upright posture requires a broad base of support, weight resting both through the ischia, anchoring the sacrum, and forward of the ischial tuberosities, into the legs and feet. A slight lumbar lordosis will follow as the pelvis tilts and this in turn elevates the chest, sternum, head and neck. To accommodate this upright stance, muscles and fascia must be adaptable in the legs, hips, spine, chest, back and neck. Difficulty or fatigue in maintaining this posture may indicate a need for exercise, bodywork or both.

The context

A Rolfer's primary focus is to balance opposing tensions within the fascial network. The *palintonic ideal in Rolfing* refers to optimal posture and movement as a function of appropriate spatial relationships – for example, back/front, side/side, top/bottom, and inside/outside balance. Palintonic comes from the Greek word 'palintonos' meaning 'unity in opposition' (literally, 'stretched back and forth') (Maitland 1995). Palintonic balance is established by a combination of structural manipulation that informs the mapping of sensory and motor pathways, and a conscious practice of awareness and sensing (Fig.17.2).

Through specific sequences relating to regions of the body and the specific fascial layers, the sessions move from superficial layers to deeper fascial layers and alternate from shoulder girdle to pelvic girdle, inviting adaptability and support. Support is seen as access to a more complete sense of ground connection, transmission of weight through the body, and an associated lifting up through the structures to the top of the head. This grounding is added to the dimension of orientation to the environment, or space that the body occupies. As individuals experience these polarities, a sense of two-directional attention or *palintonicity* may emerge. As one feels the ground and also bring attention to the environment through the common senses of sight, sound, and the special sense of kinesphere (the area that the body is moving within, and how attention is being paid to it), a more complete picture of the world emerges. Individuals may experience a shift in perceived structural order; for example, alignment of the head, shoulder girdle and thorax may occur as both a sense of yielding downward to the ground through the feet, legs and pelvis is noted, as well as a lengthening upward in front of the spine, through the head to the space above the head.

The Ten-Series

The SI standard protocol or the therapeutic 'recipe', consists of 10 sessions of 60–75 minutes each, scheduled between 1 and 3 weeks apart. Each session begins with an assessment of static posture and basic movements like walking, sitting, standing and breathing. During the session, the RSI practitioner will use fingers, knuckles, soft fist and the flat of the elbow to loosen and differentiate the fascial layers, as verbal cuing and dialogue is used to orient the client to their present habits and sensation. Rolfers utilize a spectrum of touch expressing a range including direct manipulation with focus on input to the body, to a contact biased towards listening touch with more focus on perceiving tissue status and response, rather than a manipulative focus. Throughout the intervention, contrast in sensation is commonly used to compare the felt sense and quality of motion during performance of these basic movements.

The goals of each of Dr Rolf's original 10 sessions and those of several other systems of SI have been detailed in a series of articles by Myers (2004a, 2004b, 2004c; and see Ch. 3). While there are unique aspects in each program, the essential elements of Dr Rolf's vision of the body are present and consistent with each variation.

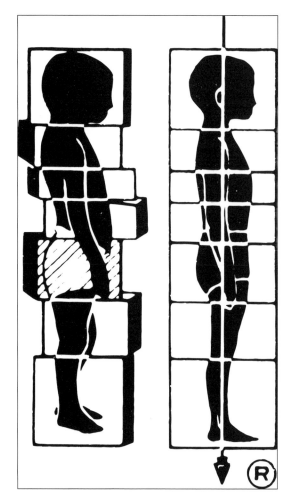

FIGURE 17.2 Little Boy logo: the Rolf Institute's logo suggests the palintonic principle.

Sessions 1–3, opening the superficial fascia

- The first three sessions focus on the superficial fascial layer being contacted with the goal of increasing pliability and differentiation to address lesions and inhibitions. The client is encouraged through the specific attention to this layer to experience their body in three-dimensional space. The first session establishes a sense of the vertical direction releasing the arms, shoulders, torso, diaphragm, and hips to allow full expression of the breath. Specific direction, pace and angle of application is required to target the superficial layers. The oblique 'shearing' of this outside layer is used as an assessment of differentiation, as well as the initiation of release and mobilization. For instance, a kyphotic thorax with a head and shoulders forward postural holding may present with shortened pectoral fascia extending from the clavicle to the sternum, abdominal fascia to the pubic bone. This superficial front fascial continuity is released to allow the anterior excursion of breathing.

- The second session offers a stable foundation by balancing the foot and lower leg muscles, inviting a sense of left and right, or bilateral, support. The crural fascia is released or loosened from the deeper investing fascia and then the functional compartments in the lower leg are mobilized with slow sustained pressure. Clients' movements are used at the hinges: phalangeal metatarsal joints, ankle and knee, as the practitioner holds the joints towards neutral alignment, giving a proprioceptive feedback and identifying the areas that require lengthening to allow for efficient movement. Antagonistic groups are 'balanced' by releasing functional groups then inviting the length into opposing fasciae. Ankle retinaculum and plantar fascia are stretched and mobilized with oblique gliding strokes. Individuals may be invited to experience the connections across segments – foot, ankle, knees, and hips – as soft tissue and joints are held towards neutral alignment. This tracking is thought to assist proprioceptive and kinesthetic integration.

- Finally, the third session evokes a sense of front-to-back depth by utilizing a positional strategy with the client lying on one side, giving access to the structures from the lateral leg, hip, torso, neck and head inclusively. The third session offers a 'side view' for an understanding of how the head, shoulder girdle, and hips are related to one another when standing; for instance, the fan of superficial fasciae from trochanter to the anterior superior iliac spine, along the crest of the ilium, to the sacroiliac joint, is mobilized from the epimysium of the gluteals. Similar spreading and mobilizing is done along the lateral side of the body, defining the front-to-back relationship. Detailed myofascial release is performed to release the axillary fasciae, the rotator cuff, and pectoral fascia. The lateral 'line' (see Ch. 3) is extended into the neck as trapezius, posterior to the transverse processes, and sternocleidomastoid and superficial 'bandaging' fascia anteriorly are released.

Each session has specific goals and builds upon the previous ones to gradually align the body, invite new options for movement and explore the present experience of a lived body. The first three sessions prepare the body for the next unfolding as the focus turns to the deeper structures that support and stabilize the pelvis and spine.

Sessions 4–7: relating to the core

- Sessions 4–7 are referred to as 'core' sessions and begin by examining the spatial order of the pelvis as it relates to the legs and torso. Individuals with low back restriction and dysfunction often find that these sessions assist in supporting appropriate balance of mobility and stability. Sessions 4–6 explore the pelvis to leg relationship from lateral, medial, anterior and posterior directions. Session 7 completes the organization and balance of the deeper core structures with focus on shoulders, neck, head, and jaw.

- The territory of session 4 extends from the inside arch of the foot, following the inner leg across the knee to the lower aspect of the pelvis. Fascial continuities from the inner leg and adductors to the inferior ramus are differentiated with slow pressure releasing the septa between the hamstrings and quadriceps. The goal is soft tissue pliability and spatial differentiation spanning front to back at the base of the pelvis, leg and foot. The fascial connections of the adductors to obturator internus and pelvic floor offer a base for the contents of the pelvis to rest into oppositional tension and support. The adductor fascial attachments are released and 'spread' along the inferior ramus, while slow, sustained digital contact on the medial side of the ramus allows release of the fascial continuity to the obturator internus and pelvis floor. A sense of the pelvis supported by the head of the femur invites a felt sense of weight transfer through the sacroiliac joint around the pelvic arcuate line, to the inner legs, relating the legs to the front of the spine.

- Session 5 then follows the legs to the pre-vertebral space by balancing the layers of the abdomen from the muscular corset to the spinal erectors, and lumbodorsal fascia to peritoneum, and, finally, the iliopsoas. Balancing involves both manipulation and re-patterning movements. With the individual positioned supine, knees flexed and feet on table, the abdominal obliques and transversus abdominus fasciae are differentiated with fingers with a gathering and lifting action along the lateral edge of the rectus abdominus. Deeper celomic sacs and the peritoneum are differentiated to access the psoas. Contact of the psoas is combined with pelvic tilting, allowing the lumbar spine to drop towards the table into flexion, eccentrically releasing the psoas. This coordination of practitioner contact and client movement assists the releasing of the psoas and feeds length to the erectors and posterior back fasciae.

- The palontonic balance of these structures offers a pathway to weight transfer and movement along the front of the spine, to the iliac fossa and over the superior ramus to the lesser trochanter. The objective is that the experience of inner space now includes the front of the spine, inside and lateral sides of the abdomen, top of the diaphragm and bottom of the pelvic floor.

- Session 6 completes the *core* work around the pelvis relating the posterior body from plantar surface of the foot to the upper thorax, inclusively. The details include relating the foot to the posterior lower leg, balancing the fasciae that move the heel and provide spring to the sole of the foot. Next, the fasciae of the calf and posterior thigh are released with deeper strokes to mobilize large fascial sheets and also local restrictions of layers and septa. Fascial release accompanied by movements of the client's ankle and foot aim to increase tissue pliability and balancing rotations between tibia and femur, and femur to pelvis. Finally, the fasciae influencing the sacrum and spine are differentiated and released with slow deep contact, often with elbows or a soft fist, to invite balanced tension and tone of the associated muscles. This completes the biomechanical and proprioceptive orientation of the sacrum to the spine, and sacrum to pelvic girdle.

Each session concludes with manual mobilization accompanied by movement relating the areas that have been worked on to the neck and spine. These integrating approaches provide additional flexibility and stability to the spine so that the vertebrae relate to the change invited in other areas (Jacobson 2011).

The final core session, the 7th, relates and differentiates the shoulders to neck, neck to head, and the cranium to jaw, comprising specific stretching and differentiation of deeper layers of muscles in the motor cylinder associated with movement to the visceral compartment anterior to the transverse processes. Muscles of mastication are mobilized with slow stretching below the mandible into the temporal fascia and inside the mouth with contact on the roof and floor of the mouth. Tissue pliability and balanced tone in this area allows for enhanced function as blood flow, nervous signals, and orienting through suboccipital reflexes, are improved.

Session 8–10: integration and closure

Integration is emphasized throughout the remaining three sessions, as sessions 8–10 provide an opportunity for the practitioner to blend previously established awareness, and to encourage accurate pre-movement and perception-based coordination in order to address remaining *lesions and inhibitions*.

Although specific soft tissue manipulations, such as stretching, separating and lengthening, may offer great relief, in order to restore optimal function individuals need to also increase awareness and alter negative perceptual habits. The integrative sessions explore connections of the lower and upper extremities to the spine in sessions 8 and 9; while session 10 reinforces optimal biomechanical flow of extremities to the spine, increasing uniform, full body tonus. This may include changes to habits through movement, perceptual and coordination training, as well as finding new ways to respond emotionally and perceptually to daily activities and demands.

Session 10 serves as a closure for this initial process. Clients are encouraged to allow time for integration and assimilation of their increased awareness and new movement options. Following this interval, they may return for 'tune-up' sessions to address imbalances from daily activities and injuries or simply to explore refinement of coordination.

RISI, an ongoing inquiry

Faced with new insights gained from neuroscience and fascia and back pain research, RISI has continued to examine the stories we use to explain the results of our work. Is Rolfing a manual therapy? Is it an avenue of transformation through increasing embodiment and proprioception? Is it perceptual-based change that informs the postural change? All these questions seem relevant and shed new light on the initial inquiry that Dr Rolf began.

'While Rolfing® is often defined and associated with the field of manual therapy; anyone with first hand experience would know that this a limited view. Rolfing is actually more accurately categorized as a philosophy since it is an inquiry into the nature of human embodiment' (Bond 2007).

References

Anson B1998 Rolfing: stories of personal empowerment. North Atlantic Books, Berkeley, CA

Ball T 2011 Structural integration–based fascial release efficacy in systemic lupus erythematosus (SLE): two case studies. J BodywMov Ther 15:217–225

Bond M 2007 The new rules of posture: how to sit, stand and move in the modern world. Healing Arts Press, Rochester, VT

Caspari M 2005 The functional rationale of the recipe. Structural Integration 03 33(1): 4–24

Deutsch, J Anderson E 2008 Complementary therapies for physical therapy a clinical decision-making approach. Elsevier, St Louis

Deutsch , Derr LL, Judd P, Reuven B 2000 Treatment of chronic pain through the use of Structural Integration (Rolfing). Orthop Phys Ther Clin North Am 9:411–427

Frank K, Blakeslee S 2009 The confluence of neuroscience and structural integration. Structural Integration 37: 2: 26–29

Frank K 2008 Body as a movement system, a premise for structural integration. Journal of Structural Integration pp 14–23

Hanson A, Price K, Feldman H 2012 Myofascial structural integration: a promising complementary therapy for young children with spastic cerebral palsy. J Evid Based Complementary Altern Med 2:131–135

International Association for Structural Integrators, PO Box 8664, Missoula, MT 59807. Available online at www.theiasi.org. Accessed 20 April 2013

Jacobson E 2004 'Getting Rolfed': structural bodywork, biomechanics and embodiment. In: Oths KS, Servando ZH (eds) Healing by hand: bonesetting and manual medicine in global perspective.: Altamira Press, Walnut Creek, CA:171–193

Jacobson E 2011 Structural Integration, an alternative method of manual therapy and sensorimotor education. Journal of Alternative and Complementary Medicine, 17(10): 891–899

James H, Casteneda L, Miller M, Findley T 2009 Rolfing structural integration treatment of cervical spine dysfunction. J Bodyw Mov Ther 13:229–238

Maitland J 1995 Spacious body: explorations in somatic ontology. North Atlantic Books, Berkeley

McHose C, Frank K 2006 How life moves: explorations in meaning and body awareness. North Atlantic Books, Berkeley

Myers T 2001 Anatomy Trains: myofascial meridians for manual and movement therapists. Churchill Livingstone, Edinburgh

Myers T 2004a Structural Integration: developments in Ida Rolf's 'recipe'. Part 1. J Bodyw Mov Ther 8:131–142

Myers T 2004b Structural Integration: developments in Ida Rolf's 'recipe'. Part 2. J Bodyw Mov Ther 8:189–198

Myers T 2004c Structural Integration: developments in Ida Rolf's 'recipe'. Part 3. J Bodyw Mov Ther 8:249–264

Rolf Institute of Structural Integration 2013 Research on Rolfing. Boulder, CO. Available online at http://rolf.org/about/Research. Accessed 24 June 2013

Schultz R, Feitis R 1996 The endless web: fascial anatomy and physical reality. North Atlantic Books, Berkeley

Schleip R 2003 Fascial plasticity – a new neurobiological explanation. J Bodyw Mov Ther 7(1):11–19 (Part 1), 7(2):104–116 (Part 2)

Chapter 18

MANAGEMENT OF SCARS AND ADHESIONS

Willem Fourie

Introduction

The treatment of scars and adhesions cannot be described as a set modality. Treatment could rather be defined as a *'management strategy'* using combinations of different massage and manual techniques to constitute a therapeutic approach aimed at improving tissue quality and mobility.

Techniques would include combinations of effleurage, petrissage, manual lymphatic drainage, fascial release techniques, fascial unwinding, friction techniques, myofascial release and more, and could collectively be called *'scar tissue massage/ mobilization/manipulation.'*

Some sources trace the use of manual techniques in the treatment of wounds and scars back to one of the founders of modern surgery and pioneer in surgical techniques, Ambroise Paré (1510–1590), a French barber surgeon. He used, among other techniques, massage to relieve joint stiffness and promote wound healing after surgery on the battlefields (http://www.therapycouch.com/ MT.Theory.History.htr). From these almost crude beginnings, the treatment and care of damaged tissue has grown into a management programme based on better understanding of anatomy, physiology, pathology, tissue healing responses and available therapeutic modalities.

Extensive medical literature has been published on the subjects of tissue healing, scarring, adhesions and its development and prevention, but evidence to support the use of manual scar management remains inconclusive (Shin & Bordeaux 2011). Non-surgical techniques to help prevent and treat abnormal scars include laser therapy, intralesional agents, cryotherapy, radiation, pressure therapy, occlusive dressings, topical agents and scar massage. Although various scar massage techniques can be used, none has been validated to date. Their use is thus based on the experience of various teams and does not yet have scientific basis (Roques 2002, Atiyeh 2007). Although the concrete benefits of manual techniques on scars are hard to document, reported benefits include improved relationships with the patient, improved skin quality, relieved sensitivity, increased cutaneous hydration, improved scar quality, and better acceptance of the lesion by the patient (Roques 2002). Shin and Bordeaux (2011) also add hastening the release and absorption of buried sutures and aiding the resolution of swelling and induration as potential positive effects of scar massage (Shin & Bordeaux 2011).

Although scar management has been shown to produce positive results in patients, as many practitioners may have observed, there remains a major need for well-designed clinical trials that use objective criteria in order to establish evidence-based recommendations for or against the use of manual scar treatments in the care of surgical and other wounds.

This chapter offers an overview of principles involved in the planning and use of a scar tissue and adhesion treatment programme. Wound care is a multidisciplinary process, starting with the acute phases under the care of a medical team, and continuing through various stages of rehabilitation and treatment of the damaged tissue, to full recovery. Many therapeutic disciplines will be involved in the programme at different stages of the process. The rest of this chapter discusses the extent of the problem, background knowledge needed by the practitioner, how to evaluate and treat scar tissue, and methods for approaching special scenarios.

Overview

For normal day-to-day use sensation, mobility, stability and freedom from disabling pain and anxiety are all prerequisites for quality of life. A failure within or breakdown of any of the above may compromise normal functioning, not only of the affected part, but may even influence function globally. The body is a functional unit – if one part is injured, the entire unit suffers. Maintenance of our well-being depends on the body's ability to guide any injury through an appropriate sequence of repair, without complications.

Nature has given us a highly effective survival tool by restoring tissue integrity via granulation scar tissue in response to damage. While non-surgical tissue trauma such as infection, chemotherapy, radiation and cancer may damage tissue and initiate the healing cascade, a common trigger to tissue healing and scarring is still injury and surgery. Although all wounds pass through the same mechanism of repair towards full recovery, the final cosmetic and functional result may differ considerably. The ideal is for a scar to first close the wound and establish tissue stability; and secondly, to blend cosmetically with surrounding tissue, allowing for pre-injury function.

For open wounds (including surgical wounds) and severe internal tears (ruptured tendon or ligament), wound closure and tissue strength are critical and a certain amount of scarring is necessary and inevitable. When scar tissue fills defects in loose, flexible tissue, it will change to duplicate the same tissue characteristics as far as possible in the final stages of healing (Bouffard et al. 2008). Impaired mobility within loose, flexible tissue may contribute to chronic pain and tissue stiffness as well as abnormal movement patterns within the musculoskeletal system (see notes in Chs 5 and 13 of the use, post-surgically, of eccentric loading during the remodeling stages).

What is the problem?

After an injury or surgery, successful healing of the part does not necessarily correlate with a return to full pre-injury/intervention function. A repaired tendon may develop normal tensile strength after surgery, but will be a functional failure if it does not glide within its tendon sheath. Similarly, a healed surgical incision on the surface with compromised movement between muscles, contracture of a joint capsule or adhesions between visceral organs may also be classified as functional failures – often ending in a dysfunctional unit. An important requirement for any post-injury or post-surgical management strategy is the maximization of *function* without disruption of the wound healing and tissue repair processes.

The extent of the problem

Post-surgical scarring and adhesions result from injured tissue (following incision, cauterization, suturing or other means of trauma) fusing together to create abnormal connections between two normally separate surfaces of the body (Ergul & Korukluogl 2008). Outcomes differ depending on the injured tissue, type of injury, genetic factors and the presence of systemic disease, and the impact on function may range on a continuum from inconsequential to debilitating with considerable clinical consequences. For example:

- After a laparotomy, almost 95% of patients are shown to have adhesions at later surgery (Ellis 2007). Intestinal obstruction, chronic abdominal and pelvic pain and female infertility are also reported.
- Previous abdominal surgery has been shown to be a factor in lower backache, myofascial pain syndromes (Lewit & Olsanska 2004).
- Minimally invasive surgical procedures (e.g. arthroscopy) are reported as contributing to increased risk of developing knee osteoarthritis (Ogilvie-Harris & Choi 2000).
- Previous surgical scars can be associated with surgical difficulties and postoperative complications in primary total knee arthroplasty (Piedade et al. 2009).
- Adhesions, tissue fibrosis and loss of tissue glide between structures can be identified as the source of pain and restriction of movement and function in up to 72% of patients after surgery for breast cancer (Lee et al. 2009).

Not only do severe injury, aggressive surgery (e.g. cancer surgery) and burns potentially lead to a poor cosmetic outcome or disfigurement, but there is also a heavy economic burden on the medical care system. This could be as direct costs of care, or as future re-admissions and surgery as a result of the original procedure or injury. In the US, adhesion-related health costs exceed one billion dollars annually (ASRM Committee 2013).

A key problem is how to define and develop a sensible postoperative programme to optimise final functional outcomes after injury or surgery. The development of such programmes starts with an understanding of what a scar is, how it is formed, and its possible involvement in dysfunction.

What do we need to know?

To develop a scar and adhesion treatment strategy the following needs to be understood:
* The entire healing process and its phases
* The way tissue responds to injury and knowledge of healing outcomes
* Factors influencing the repair process at different stages
* An anatomic understanding of the tissue layers between the surface and the deeper layers of the body
* A good working knowledge of massage and manual tissue techniques.

Phases of wound healing

It is beyond the scope of this chapter to describe the healing process in detail. For detailed descriptions, refer to some of the references in this chapter (also see notes on wound repair in Ch. 2).

Scar formation is our primary method of restoring tissue integrity. All wounds, whether the result of surgery or trauma, progress through the same sequence and repair process, but may, however, vary markedly in the final cosmetic and functional result. Normal, uncomplicated healing and its time frames will be discussed.

Superficial wounds heal without scar tissue formation by simply regenerating the damaged epithelium. The healing of deeper wounds is an organized and predictable process consisting of three overlapping phases: **inflammation, proliferation and maturation/remodeling** (Myers 2012).
* The first response to injury is **inflammation**, allowing the body to control blood loss and fend off bacterial invasion. It also recruits the cells needed to restore the injured area. This phase usually lasts from 48 hours to 6 days, depending on the extent of the damage. During this phase, the wound has no tensile strength and has a poor response to mechanical stress.
* During the **proliferative phase**, new tissues are built to fill the gap left by damaged and debrided tissues. As a result, epithelial integrity is restored, and the wound is considered **closed**. This is an active healing phase starting from about day 5, reaching a peak around day 14 and lasting up to several weeks. There is now a slow increase in tensile strength with fibroblasts and collagen aligning along lines of stress.
* **Maturation and remodeling** starts at around day 21 and may last up to 2 years after wound closure. During this time scar tissue is reorganized from haphazard fiber arrangement to being oriented along the lines of tissue stress, until reaching maximum strength and function. During this phase tensile strength and mechanical behaviour of the scar continue to improve (Lederman 1997). Unfortunately, even after remodeling, scar tissue is less elastic than the original tissue and may only achieve a maximum of approximately 80% of the original tissue strength (Myers 2012). A wound is considered **healed** after it is resurfaced, and has achieved maximal attainable tissue strength.

Different healing outcomes

'Friendly' scars close the wound, create stability, blend cosmetically with the surrounding tissue and allow structures to resume their pre-injury function. Problem or 'unfriendly' scars fall into two categories:

- Failure to heal within the expected time frame due to the absence of inflammation, reduced inflammation (delayed healing) or chronic inflammation due to foreign bodies, malnutrition, infection, repetitive mechanical trauma or insufficient scar formation (dehiscence)
- Excessive repair including hypertrophic scarring (overproduction of immature collagen), keloids, or contractures (pathological shortening of scar tissue resulting in deformity; Myers 2012).

A **scar** is the fibrous tissue that replaces normal tissues which a burn, wound, surgery, radiation, or disease has destroyed (Andrade & Clifford 2008). Scar tissue is never as strong as normal, uninjured skin or tissue.

Hypertrophic scarring is due to the overproduction of immature collagen during the proliferative and remodeling phases of wound healing. This is more likely to occur in wounds that cross the lines of tension in the skin, in wounds with a prolonged inflammatory phase (large or infected wounds) or in burns because of their lengthy proliferative phase (Myers 2012).

A **contracture** is the pathological shortening of scar tissue resulting in deformity (Myers 2012). The term 'contracture' is usually used to indicate a loss of joint range of movement as a result of connective tissue and muscle shortening. Underlying contracture formation are adhesions or excessive cross-links.

Adhesions/fixations are related to the scarring process and develop secondary to the normal healing process. It is the process of adhering or uniting two surfaces or parts, especially the union of the opposing surfaces of a wound (*Stedman's Medical Dictionary* 1972). Unlike scarring, adhesions are characterized by a loss of mobility of tissues that normally glide or move in relation to each other and once matured, may even be stronger than the tissue to which they adhere (Lederman 1997). Adhesions can contribute to impaired muscle, joint, and connective tissue integrity (Andrade & Clifford 2008). Secondary to an adhesion, a continuous state of mechanical irritation can affect many systems that are far removed from the involved site. The impact of the adhesion of normally sliding surfaces on normal organ or musculoskeletal function could range on a continuum from inconsequential to debilitating.

Fibrosis is defined as the thickening and scarring of connective tissue. Fibrosis, as a process, is less linear than scarring, which typically occurs step by step in sequence. Fibrosis usually involves the connective tissues and structures of an entire region.

Factors influencing outcomes

Examples of factors that may influence the rate of wound healing or change the outcomes of certain stages include:

- **Wound characteristics** such as the mechanism of onset, location, dimensions, temperature, wound hydration, necrotic tissue and infection
- **Local factors** include local blood circulation, sensation and mechanical stress in the wound area
- **Systemic factors** include age, inadequate nutrition, comorbidities, medication and behavioural risk-taking like smoking and alcohol abuse
- **Inappropriate wound management.**

Management protocols must be flexible enough to promptly recognize complications and risks in order to adjust the timing and application of therapeutic intervention.

The anatomy of tissue layers

When palpating tissues, therapists will encounter a succession of tissue layers. Using the different characteristics of these layers such as hardness, density, texture, and mobility, the therapist can distinguish between layers summarized below. For a full description of tissue layers, please refer to Chapter 1.

The body is arranged in several layers:
- The **skin** formed by the epidermis and dermis
- The **superficial fascia** consisting of two or more adipose, loose connective tissue layers separated by a membranous layer(s) of collagen and elastic fibers
- The **deep fascia** that envelops the large muscles of the trunk and forms fascial sleeves in the limbs
- The **muscle** and its **epimysial fascia** beneath the deep fascia of the limbs
- The **peritoneum** is a thin layer of irregular connective tissue that lines the abdominal cavity. It further consist of two layers:

o The **parietal peritoneum** as the outer lining of the abdominal cavity
o **Visceral peritoneum** covering the viscera and organs contained therein.

How do we evaluate and treat?

Guidelines

The practitioner needs to keep two basic guidelines in mind during the evaluation and treatment of scars and adhesions. Touch needs to be graded and it should be understood where and how tissue stops under one's palpating fingers or hands.

Depth and grading of touch

An advantage of manual techniques is that the hand is a sensitive instrument which establishes a feedback relationship with the manipulated tissue. When treating wounds and scarring, the therapist should be clear of how deep and firmly to work. A grading scale of 1–10 could be used (Fourie & Robb 2009).

- **Grade 1 to 3:** Very light, mild and non-irritating. It can be compared to moving the eyelid on the eyeball without irritating the eye. No discomfort.
- **Grade 4 to 6:** Moderate to firm. This is where most massage techniques are performed. There may be mild discomfort, but with no irritation or damage to tissue.
- **Grade 7 and 8:** Firm, deep and uncomfortable pressure with discomfort, but is tolerable. Potential exists for tissue bruising. Trigger point work would be performed at this level.
- **Grade 9 and 10:** Deep, very uncomfortable or painful with a strong potential for tissue damage. It is often described as 'surgery without anaesthesia'. An example of this grade would be deep transverse friction.

The barrier phenomenon

Similar to joints, soft tissue has a specified range of available movement. Within this range of movement, normal soft tissue has three barriers, or resistances, that can limit movement – the physiological barrier, the elastic barrier, and the anatomical barrier (Andrade & Clifford 2008).

- Physiological range is necessary for smooth, unrestricted movement of underlying structures during normal movement – it determines the available active range of movement.
- The elastic barrier is the resistance one feels at the end of the passive range of movement when taking the slack out of the tissue (engaging the tissue).
- The anatomical range (barrier) refers to where tissue can be stretched beyond the physiological range before coming to a stop without discomfort or pain (the final passive range of movement).
- The distance between physiological and anatomical limits constitutes a 'safety' zone protecting the body from damage should external forces be applied.

At the physiological barrier minimal resistance to stretch or shift is encountered. When resistance is met with no further tissue movement possible, the anatomical barrier is reached. Under normal conditions this barrier has a soft, elastic end-feel and can be moved easily accompanied by a sensation that no unnecessary tension or pain is present in the target tissue.

In a *pathological* barrier, the anatomical (passive) tissue range is reached prematurely and occurs when soft tissue dysfunction is present. This barrier characteristically has a tense, restrictive feel, with an abrupt, hard or leathery end-feel. Normal physiological movement may still be present with no apparent movement restriction, but there will be reduced protection when the tissue is strained. Restrictive barriers may occur in skin, fascia, muscle, ligament, joint capsule, or a combination of these tissues (Andrade & Clifford 2008). Pathological barriers can limit available range of motion in tissue or alter the position of the mid-range, thereby changing the quality of available movement in joints or between structures.

Evaluation

Scar evaluation aims to determine the **quality, extent and depth** of the 'premature or pathological' tissue barrier.

- **Quality** refers to the perceived **end-feel** – a normal soft, elastic or an abnormal solid, abrupt end-feel.
- The **extent** of the barrier refers to **where** in the available range resistance is encountered, and the size of the involved area.
- The **depth** of the tissue barrier may be subjective but an attempt should be made to distinguish between **which tissue layers** restrictions are felt: superficial between dermis and deep fascia, deep restrictions between muscles, organs or between a tendon and its sheath.

Assessment of fascial glide:

- **Skin and superficial fascia** – manually glide the skin **over** the deep fascia. Move hand and skin as a unit to the end of available tissue glide using a pressure grading of 2–4.
- **Deep fascia and myofascial interfaces** – move one deep structure **over** another. Change hand or finger position accordingly and glide tissue at a firm pressure grading of 4–6.
- **Deep muscle and soft tissue on bone interfaces** – modify hand and/or finger position to test for specific directional restrictions with fingertip or thumb pressure at a pressure grade of 6–8. Discomfort may be experienced by the patient and should therefore be done with care.

This is an assessment of tissue **movement**, not of painful areas within the soft tissue. Palpation is for tissue mobility, flexibility and freedom of tissue glide. The position and direction of tight, hypomobile or inflexible tissue should be documented.

Assessment of scar movement:

- **Longitudinal** along the length of the scar
- **Transverse** across the long axis of the scar
- **Rotation** clockwise and anti-clockwise
- **Lifting** the scar vertically away from deeper layers.

Treatment

Treatment is guided by both the **source** of a restriction and extent of the resultant dysfunction. Primary treatment is directed at the restricted tissue glide (local source of the problem) before rehabilitating the abnormal condition that the patient presents with (the dysfunction). Depth, site and extent of restricted tissue gliding should be clearly ascertained.

Principles

- Treatment is directed at the mechanical restriction identified through evaluation.
- The goal is to move the tissue barrier towards a normal end-feel and amplitude.
- Treatment is approached in a layered fashion from superficial to deep; clearing one layer or compartment of restrictions before moving to a deeper or adjacent layer.
- Techniques are performed at or just before the palpable tissue barrier at varying angles to the restriction.
- Gentle touch grading is used during the early stages. For mature, chronically adhered scars more forceful treatment at higher touch grading may be necessary.

How to treat

To safeguard against wound breakdown and increased inflammation, gentle treatment should be used in the early stages of healing. However, when using higher touch grades for longstanding scars and adhesions, care must be taken to avoid triggering a **new** inflammatory response.

Approaches to engage and move the tissue barrier (Lewit & Olsanska 2004):

- Engage the barrier directly and wait with a sustained pressure until the tissue releases and the barrier shifts after a short delay.
- Use a sustained stretch of the scarred tissue. Stretch could be uni- or multidirectional.
- Apply slow rhythmic mobilizations towards and into the tissue barrier. Movement direction could be perpendicular to, at an angle to, or away from the tissue barrier.

Manipulating tissues

There are many ways of effectively applying manual techniques in the treatment of troublesome scar tissue and adhesions. In reality only a limited number of ways of treating tissues exist, with most of the scar tissue treatment techniques being variations of these (Lederman 1997, Chaitow & DeLany 2008).

Variations of possible direct tissue loading approaches are (from Chaitow & DeLany 2008):

1. **Tension loading** where traction, stretching, extension and elongation is involved. The objective is to **lengthen** tissue by encouraging an increase in collagen aggregation.

2. **Compression loading** to shorten and widen tissue by increasing the pressure thus influencing fluid movement. Compression not only affects circulation, but also influences neurological structures and encourages endorphin release.

3. **Rotation loading** effectively elongates some fibers while simultaneously compressing others. This produces a variety of tissue effects. 'Wringing' techniques or 'S' bends are examples of rotation loading.

4. **Bending loading** is in effect a combination of compression and tension with both a lengthening and circulatory effect on the target tissues. 'C'-shaped bending or 'J'-stroke movements are commonly employed.

5. **Shearing loading** translates or shifts tissue laterally in relation to other tissue. All techniques attempting to slide a more superficial soft tissue layer **on or across** a deeper tissue layer or structure is included here.

6. **Combined loading** involves the combination of variations of all the loading approaches above leading to complex patterns of adaptive demands on the targeted tissue. For example, the multidirectional combining of a stretch with a side bend is more effective than either a stretch or a side bend alone.

Additional factors to consider include:

- How hard? The degree of force being used (refer to grading above).
- How large? The size of the area force is being applied to.
- How far? Refers to the amplitude of the applied force. At the beginning of the range, in the middle of the range, full range large amplitude, or at the end of the range small amplitude (refer to the barrier phenomenon above).
- How fast? The speed with which the force is being applied – fast or very slow. The speed will influence pain and autonomic receptor responses.
- How long? Could refer to the length of a treatment or the length of time a force is being maintained.
- How rhythmic?
- How steady? Does the employed force involve movement or is it static?
- Active, passive or mixed? Is the patient active in any of the processes?

Basic techniques

Manual techniques used on scars and adhesions mostly have no prescribed style or sequence, but are based on the principles outlined above. The goal of treatment is to loosen the collagen fiber linkages that have developed within the scar and the adherences between it and its surrounding tissues. Effective treatment applies direct pressure to specific points and directions of resistance i.e. **concentrating effective force on local areas.** For effective, concentrated force application, the therapist's fingers or hand should not glide over the skin's surface. No, or very little, lubrication should therefore be used.

Examples of basic techniques:

1. **Gross stretch (Fig. 18.1):** this is the most superficial scar technique using tension loading. Using finger or full hand contact:
   - Take up all the tissue slack.
   - Apply a gentle stretch along the length of the scar.
   - Hold, wait for release and stretch again.
   - Change hand position and repeat the stretch perpendicular to the original stretch.
   - Repeat the stretch sequence diagonal to the previous position.
   - Continue to stretch across the scar in a radiating pattern until no further stretch is possible.

Note: this technique should only be applied along the length of the scar in the early phases of healing as perpendicular shearing forces should be avoided.

2. **Gentle circles (Fig 18.2):** the fingers move the skin **over** the deep fascia. Tissue movement takes the form of an engaged shearing nature, combining tension, shearing and compression loading:
   - Rest the fingers on the part to be treated (next to the scar). The heel of the hand

FIGURE 18.1 Gross stretch of the scar and surrounding tissue. (a) Stretching along the long axis – elongating the scar. (b) Gliding scar and surrounding tissue along the long axis. (c) and (d) Stretching in opposite directions. Extra care should be taken in immature scars.

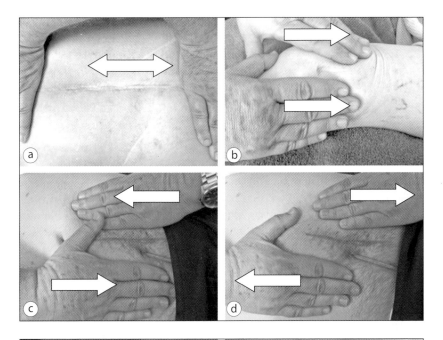

FIGURE 18.2 Gentle circles next to or on the scar. (a) Circular movement with fingertips engaging the tissue barrier directly. (b) Two-handed circles stretching away from the scar and barrier. (c) One-handed circle engaging the barrier directly. (d) Gentle circles on the scar – moving the scar in a circular motion.

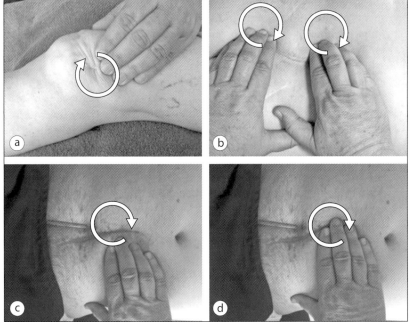

may rest on the body for better control (Fig.18.2a & c).

- Starting at the 6 o'clock position, push the skin clockwise in a circle with the middle three fingers.
- Slowly move the skin towards the scar to engage and shear the tissue barrier in a circular movement with even pressure and speed.

- Change hand position, repeat the circle and release.
- Treat the full length of the scar and repeat several times in a session if needed.

Alternatively, start the circle at the 12 o'clock position and pull away from the scar (Fig. 18.2b), or place the fingers on the scar (Fig. 18.2d) to move the scar over the deeper layers in a circular movement.

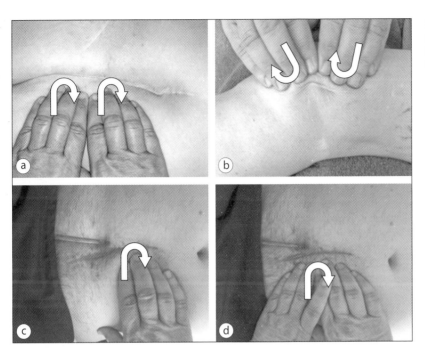

FIGURE 18.3 Direct engagement and shifting of the tissue barrier – firm upside down 'J' strokes.

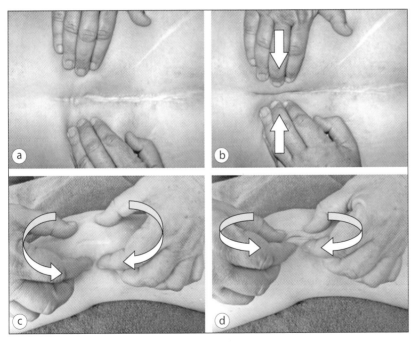

FIGURE18.4 Sliding towards and 'under' the scar attempting to 'lift' the scar. (a) and (b) Sliding towards the scar and attempting to glide 'under' the scar. (c) and (d) Taking the scar between fingers and thumbs attempting to lift the scar vertically away from the surface. This should be done gently with adherent scars.

3. **Firm upside down 'J' (Fig. 18.3):** similar to the previous technique in terms of starting position and depth. Tissue movement is of a combined loading nature:
   • Direct the stroke perpendicular towards the scar from about an inch (2.5cm) away.
   • Movement is slow, firm and deliberate into the tissue barrier.

• When the barrier is engaged, the fingers shear away towards the left or right and the tissue is allowed to return to its nonstretched position.
• Repeat until the tissue barrier has moved, or discomfort subsides.

This technique could be used very gently in early healing stages (Fig.18.3c & d; touch grading

1–3), or firmly (touch grading 8) on mature scars (Fig. 18.3a & b).

4. **Vertical lifts (Fig. 18.4):** vertical lifts are used to treat any scar that can be gripped between thumbs and fingers and uses tension loading.
    *   Grip an area of the scar gently, but firmly.
    *   Apply a vertical stretch perpendicularly off the surface of the body.
    *   Hold, wait for a release and increase the stretch.
    *   Repeat the lift sequence from different angles until no further stretch is available.

5. **Skin rolling (Fig. 18.5):** a tension loading technique used to treat restricted mobility of the skin and superficial fascia.
    *   Using as broad a contact surface as possible, grasp the skin and superficial fascia between thumb and fingertips.
    *   Lift the tissue and while maintaining a stretch on the tissue, roll the superficial tissue along the surface in a slow wave.
    *   Glide the thumb or fingers along the tissue as you simultaneously gather and release tissue while maintaining the grasping and lifting motion.

This technique can be used as an assessment, introductory technique, treatment or re-assessment.

6. **Wringing or 'S' bends (Fig. 18.6):** when used for scar or adhesion treatment, this is a modified pettrisage technique using compression and shearing with varying amounts of drag, lift and glides repetitively to release and mobilize tissue.

An impairment-based approach is recommended for treatment of restrictive scars and adhesions, regardless of the modality used. The selection of technique, direction and depth of application, are based on the level of dysfunction revealed during the assessment. This approach gives the therapist the flexibility to adapt treatment to the person, rather than treating the 'diagnosis'. Furthermore, treatment can be modified in line with the patient's improvement or lack of progress based on the tissue response (Fourie & Robb 2009).

Treatment is discontinued when the release has been completed in all directions and layers.

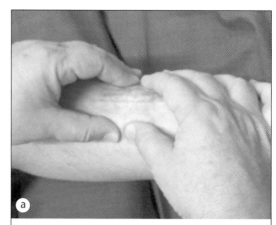
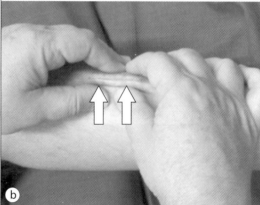
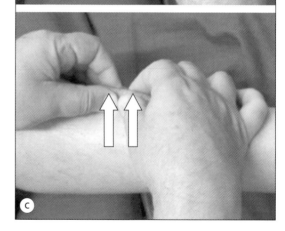

FIGURE 18.5 Skin rolling.

This may not happen in a single treatment and may even take several months – especially in long-standing chronic scars. Care should be taken to

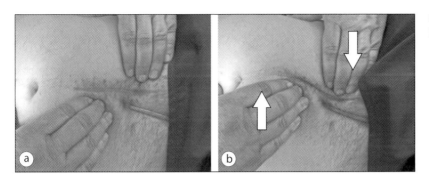

FIGURE 18.6 Wringing or 'S' bends.

avoid creating wound breakdown or an inflammatory response to tissue mobilization.

Are there special concerns?

Broad outlines and guiding thoughts on early wound massage, burns, breast scarring and the abdomen will briefly be discussed. At all times these special groups should be treated with consent from the patient and the supervising medical practitioner or medical team.

Early intervention

Intervention may start early after an injury or surgery. Treatment should progress with care as the inflammatory phase is dominant and the wound has no strength to resist straining forces. Dressings and sutures may be in place and some level of muscle spasm, pain and swelling (edema) may be present. The aims of treatment should be the control of edema and swelling and the prevention of potential adhesions while gently guiding the wound towards full recovery.

Inflammatory phase

Edema is part of the normal inflammatory response that occurs after injury and surgery and can be defined as excess fluid in the interstitial space (Villeco 2012). Such swelling may compromise the diffusion of waste and nutrients between the blood capillaries and the cells. During the inflammatory phase (days 2–6), edema is liquid, soft and easy to

mobilize. This fluid should be managed through the principles of compression, elevation, cold, and gentle active movement. Gentle massage techniques to stimulate the lymphatic system proximal to the injured area may be used. No tissue barriers should be engaged or stretched and a touch grading of 3 should not be exceeded.

Proliferative phase

As scar production is accelerated during the proliferative phase (2–6 weeks), organized adhesions start to form between structures and edema, if present, becomes more viscous. The excess fluid is now called exudates (Villeco 2012). The wound is now closed, and there is a gradual increase in tensile strength.

• Lymphatic massage and other techniques that stimulate an intact lymphatic system should be the focus of the therapy program.

• Gentle techniques (as described above) engaging the subcutaneous layers can now be introduced, together with active motion and tendon gliding exercises to minimize adhesions between the developing scar and surrounding tissue.

Burn scars

Burn injuries cause destruction of the skin, as well as a host of other physiological changes that can affect every body part (Myers 2012). Skin thickness varies in different anatomical areas and individual burns are not uniform in depth. This may complicate classification of the degree of damage as well as the final selection of tissue mobilization technique.

A single burn scar may have areas of partial thickness (epidermis and dermis) damage with minimal scarring, through to areas of full thickness (epidermis, dermis and subcutaneous tissue) destruction with severe hypertrophic scarring. Differing degrees of damage will need individual intervention strategies and will vary greatly in final outcome.

Burn scars may need 6 to 24 months to mature. The scar tissue is fragile and prone to breakdown from friction, shearing, and trauma. Hypertrophic scarring and keloids are possible complications of the remodeling phase of burn wound healing (Myers 2012). Scar mobilization may help remodel scar tissue quality and appearance. More severe scars may benefit from more aggressive interventions.

Indication and aims of massage and manual intervention are:
- Development of a good quality scar
- Reduction or prevention of contractures from forming
- Reduction of pruritis (itching)
- Reduction of swelling – burned and grafted extremities commonly have lingering edema that can result in pain (due to compression on underlying structures) and joint stiffness
- Pain reduction and management
- Reduction of hypersensitivity of the skin
- Treatment of the underlying soft tissues (i.e. muscles, fascia)
- Prevention of dysfunction of compensatory patterns
- Preparation of the tissue for stretching and strengthening exercises
- Assistance in management of psychological symptoms.

Starting during the remodeling phase, scar tissue should be gently cleaned and a moisturizer should be applied to prevent dryness, cracking, and skin breakdown. This may result in better relief of itching, pain, and anxiety. Scar mobilization may further help remodel tissue quality and appearance. Gentle scar mobilization using a moisturizing agent may be used to help remodel scar tissue. These interventions may be started with care as soon as the wound is closed (Myers 2012). Care should be taken to limit shearing forces as blisters may occur if scars are exposed to friction or shear forces.

As scar tissue matures, techniques could be applied with more loading, greater amplitude and for longer periods as tissue allows. Techniques could include stretching, wringing, 'S' bending, 'J' strokes targeting specific tight areas, skin rolling and even careful friction-type tissue mobilizations. Monitoring scar tissue response to massage techniques (especially vigorous techniques such as frictions) is particularly important with burn scar tissue as it is compromised and can be susceptible to breakdown (Kania & Boersen-Gladman 2013).

Once matured, burn scars may still contribute to abnormal movement patterns and tissue tension in normal parts of the body for many years. Healthy muscle and fascia around and underneath a burn scar also need to be addressed. Spasms, tightness and adhesions frequently happen due to damage from the initial trauma and tension on the surrounding tissue as the scar progresses through its healing phases. To alleviate this, a full selection of massage and fascial release techniques could be used.

Breast scarring

The breast is a glandular structure of the superficial fascia layer, separated from the deep fascia of pectoralis major by the retromammary space. It does not have active internal supports, such as muscles, and its fascial membranes take all the stresses of gravity and body movements. Further to this, breasts do not have usable planes of dissection, so surgical cuts have to be made bluntly through the tissues. As a result there can be a greater tendency for puckering and pulling as the scar dehydrates and contracts within its tissue host. There is also a greater tendency for large planes of adherence to develop within breast tissue itself, or adherence to the underlying pectoralis major muscle. This can lead to less compliant, more irritating types of scarring with established scars having a non-functional, matted fiber pattern.

A significant number of women may have lingering problems with edema, pain and uncomfortable scar formation, which can be aesthetically and symptomatically troubling (Curties 1999). Scar tissue in the breast may develop into a long-term pain focus, even after minor surgical procedures, such as a biopsy or draining a breast abscess. When there is an area of tissue scarring or adherence present, forces can be exerted unevenly through the neck and shoulder girdle.

Ideally, the therapist could begin working on optimizing fiber orientation once collagen deposition is well started but the scar has not consolidated (10–14 days). However, in the majority of cases the practitioner only starts treating the scar after it has become well established. Since breasts do not have inherent muscles, the exertion of 'good' directional forces does not occur. These forces help a developing scar to adjust its collagen fiber direction to the lines of force normal to the body part. Bras further tend to hold breasts tightly to the chest wall while their scars are forming. As a result, breast scars are very susceptible to spreading and bulging or, alternatively, to becoming strongly thickened and reinforced, with established scars having a non-functional, matted fiber pattern.

Aims of scar management on the breast or a mastectomy site is the same as for other body parts – reduction and control of edema and the re-orientation of collagen fibers within the scar. Treatment of scar tissue and adhesions should be aimed at firstly the breast tissue itself, and secondly at movement between breast and chest wall. Direct or indirect fascial techniques can also be employed to great effect. A less aggressive approach is advised to limit stresses on supporting fascial membranes.

Abdominal scarring and visceral adhesions

Almost all patients develop adhesions after transperitoneal surgery. Adhesions (a fixed connection between tissues which normally slide relative to each other) can form between viscera and/or intra-abdominal/pelvic organs. Adhesions between omentum and the wound are most common (Van Goor 2007). The normal range of motion of the tissues is inhibited by the abnormal relations of the visceral (or other) fascia, potentially disrupting the proper physiological functioning of the organs (Hedley 2010).

The circumstances which give rise to the adhesion of normal sliding surfaces are multiple and include the following causes:

- Inflammation from infections or other types of disease processes
- Inflammation and scarring caused by surgical intervention
- The sequelae of prior limitations upon movement cycles
- Intentional therapeutic adhesions.

Risks and extent of adhesions further depend on factors such as: type of incision, number of previous laparotomies, damaged visceral or parietal peritoneum and intra-operative complications at initial laparotomy (Van Goor 2007).

Treatment strategies for this group of patients may be divided into treatment of:

- Abdominal wall scarring
- Peritoneal and/or visceral adhesions.

Abdominal wall

The goal of scar work is to restore tissue elasticity. Under guidance of the patient's surgeon, early scar work could be undertaken, aiming to:

- Stimulate lymphatic absorption. In order to resolve local swelling and induration, manual lymphatic drainage techniques could be used, directing fluids towards the closest lymph nodes.
- Hasten the release and absorption of buried sutures.
- Maintain freedom of tissue glide between dermis and underlying tissue layers. As the wound edges may still have no strength to withstand shearing forces in the early phases, tissue engagement and forces should only be applied from healthy tissue towards the scar:
  o Use gentle circles or 'J' strokes at a touch grading of not more than 3
  o Use gentle stretching techniques along the direction of the scar (longitudinal)
  o Use only enough force to engage the elastic tissue barrier.

As healing progresses through the remodeling phase towards full maturity, the wound develops strength to withstand tissue loading and progressively more shearing forces perpendicular to the scar. Aims now move towards:

- Restoring normal tissue barriers:
  - o Stretch vertically above and below the scar. Start stretching tissue along and perpendicular to the scar.
  - o Use wringing 'S' bends, 'J' strokes, firm circles, and scar lifting techniques. Engage the tissue barrier and move through the elastic barrier towards the anatomical barrier. Grading of touch can progressively be increased safely towards a grading of 6.
  - o Take the scar between your fingers and gently lift, stretch, and vibrate.
- Restoring tissue gliding between deeper fascial and muscle layers progressively working from superficial to deep. **Do not skip layers.**
  - o Using massage, myofascial or combined massage or manual techniques, progressively increase loading, shearing, amplitude and time until full anatomical barriers in all layers have been restored to as close to pre-surgery levels as possible.

Finish treatment with light effleurage of the area, routing fluids towards lymphatic drainage pathways.

Peritoneal and visceral adhesions

Adhesions develop rapidly after damage to the peritoneum during surgery, infection, trauma or irradiation. They are difficult to detect and evaluate objectively, as they may form in areas not directly linked to the original surgical incision or may develop between structures not accessible to the palpating hand.

The manual evaluation of visceral adhesions depends heavily on the palpation skills of the therapist and a sound knowledge of the visceral anatomy and its variations. Only superficial adhesions between the abdominal wall, parietal peritoneum and immediate underlying viscera may be palpable. The only investigation to date which has shown promise in identifying deep adhesions is the use of cine-MRI (Van Goor 2007).

The following further complicates the interpretation of palpation findings:
- Pain associated with the adhesion may manifest itself in another location up to 35% of the time
- Dense, thick adhesions (possibly palpable) are associated with the least intense pain

- Movable filmy adhesions (mostly non-palpable) are associated with the most intense pain (Van Goor 2007).

Evaluation and treatment principles follow the same guidelines when testing and engaging the internal tissue barrier. These barriers are, however, very subtle as the visceral environment is highly mobile without bony or muscular support. The effectiveness of treatment does not necessarily lie in the selection of a technique, but in the mobilization of the abdominal cavity as a unit.

- For dense and thick adhesions, engaging and moving the tissue barrier would be the treatment approach. These adhesions are tough and do not respond well to manual techniques alone.
- Movable and filmy adhesions do not have a palpable tissue barrier, and a generalized mobilization of the abdominal environment may be enough to disconnect mobile organs from the peritoneum.

Cautions

Therapists must use their training and best judgment when deciding whether or not to proceed with scar massage. While treatment is most effective when a scar is still in its immature phase, it is also a wise time to seek physician permission. It is always good practice to monitor the response of scar tissue to determine the appropriateness and effectiveness of massage intervention. Warning signs of potential scar problems include limited range of motion, new onset of joint restrictions, banding of scar tissue with movement, or blanching with stretching of the scar tissue

A few additional cautions for immature scars include:
- Take extreme care with radiated tissues, as the skin is delicate and can break easily
- Aside from friction massage, do not continue if your actions cause pain or increase tissue redness
- Never perform massage on any open lesions.

In many cases the problem may be irreversible with scars becoming so fixed and strong that only surgery will release the adhesion. In established fixed scars, where no tissue gliding is possible by manual means, treatment is aimed at creating more soft tissue space and flexibility in the surrounding tissue. In many cases adhesive scarring may affect quality of life adversely; however, open, positive discussion with adequate explanation and intervention may vastly diminish the patient's anxiety, suffering and disability, making scar work a rewarding field in manual therapy.

References

Andrade C-K, Clifford P 2008 Outcome-based massage, from evidence to practice, 2nd edn. Wolters Kluwer, Philadelphia

ASRM Committee 2013 Pathogenesis, consequences, and control of peritoneal adhesions in gynecologic surgery: a committee opinion. Fertil Steril 99:1550–1555, doi:10.1016/j.fertnstert.2013.02.031

Atiyeh B S 2007 Nonsurgical management of hypertrophic scars: evidence-based therapies, standard practices, and emerging methods. Aesth Plast Surg 31:468–492

Bouffard N A et al 2008 Tissue stretch decreases soluble TGF-β and type-1 procollagen in mouse subcutaneous connective tissue: evidence from ex vivo and in vivo models. J Cell Physiol 214:389–395

Chaitow L, DeLany J 2008 Clinical application of neuromuscular techniques, vol 1. The upper body, 2nd edn. Churchill Livingstone Elsevier, Edinburgh

Curties D 1999 Breast massage. Curties-Overzet Publications, Toronto

Ellis H 2007 Postoperative intra-abdominal adhesions: a personal view. Colorectal Dis 9 (Suppl 2):3–8

Ergul E, Korukluoglu B 2008 Peritoneal adhesions: facing the enemy. Int J Surg 6:253–260 doi:10.1016/j.ijsu.2007.05.010

Fourie WJ, Robb K 2009 Physiotherapy management of axillary web syndrome following breast cancer treatment: discussing the use of soft tissue techniques. Physiotherapy 95:314–320 doi:10.1016/j.physio.2009.05.001

Hedley G 2010 Notes on visceral adhesions as fascial pathology. J Bodyw Mov Ther 14:255–261 doi: 10.1016/j.jbmt.2009.10.005

Kania A, Boersen-Gladman K 2013 The physiological perspective of burn scar tissue and the integration of Massage Therapy into a multi-disciplinary burn rehabilitation program. Available online at http://www.massagetherapycanada.com/content/view/1411/38/. Accessed 5 August 2013

Lederman E 1997 Fundamentals of manual therapy. Churchill Livingstone, Edinburgh

Lee T S et al 2009 Prognosis of the upper limb following surgery and radiation for breast cancer. Breast Cancer Res Treat 110:19–37

Lewit K, Olsanska S 2004 Clinical importance of active scars: abnormal scars as a cause of myofascial pain. J Manipulative Physiol Ther 27:399–402

Myers BA 2012 Wound management: principles and practice, 3rd edn. Pearson Education, New Jersey

Ogilvie-Harris DJ, Choi CH 2000 Arthroscopic management of degenerative joint disease. In: Grifka J, Ogilvie-Harris DJ (ed) Osteoarthritis: fundamentals and strategies for joint-preserving strategies. Springer-Verlag, Berlin

Piedade SR, Pinaroli A, Servien E, Neyret P 2009 Is previous knee arthroscopy related to worse results in primary total knee arthroplasty? Knee Surg Sports Traumatol Arthrosc 17:328–333 doi 10.1007/s00167-008-0669-9

Roques C 2002 Massage applied to scars. Wound Repair Regen 10(2):126–128

Shin T M, Bordeaux JS 2011 The role of massage in scar management: a literature review. Dermatol Surg 38:414–423 doi: 10.1111/j.1524–4725.2011.02201.x

Stedman's Medical Dictionary, 22nd edn 1972 Williams & Wilkins, Baltimore

Van Goor H 2007 Consequences and complications of peritoneal adhesions. Colorectal Dis 9 (Suppl. 2):25–34

Villeco JP 2012 Edema: a silent but important factor. J Hand Ther 25:153–62 doi: 10.1016/j.jht.2011.09.008

Chapter 19

MASSAGE THERAPY AND FASCIA

Sandy Fritz

Introduction - Overview: Massage Therapy

Massage therapy falls under the umbrella of manual therapy (Jonas 2005, *Mosby's Medical Dictionary* 2009). According to the *Massage Therapy Body of Knowledge* document (MTBOK 2010) *'Massage therapy is a healthcare and wellness profession involving manipulation of soft tissue.'*

Since fascia is an anatomical structure with physiological function, massage can be adapted to address fascia function and dysfunction. In general, manual therapies, of which massage is a type, can be described as soft tissue based and joint-based. Massage therapy targets soft tissue and logically affects fascia through the same proposed biologically plausible mechanisms associated with other soft tissue targeted manual therapy techniques that use manual mechanical force application in numerous strain directions to treat injuries and somatic dysfunctions (Eagan et al. 2007, Simmonds 2012). This chapter introduces and expands on the variations in applied mechanical load that together make up massage methodology.

Application of mechanical force

The methods of massage described in this chapter introduce one or a combination of the five types of mechanical force into the body to achieve a therapeutic benefit (Fig. 19.1). The five kinds of force that can affect body tissues are compression, tension, bending, shear, and torsion:

- **Compressive forces** occur when two structures are pressed together. As massage load moves into the tissue layers, compressive force is created.
- **Tension forces** (also called tensile forces) occur when two ends of a structure are pulled in opposite directions. Tension force is used during massage with applications that drag, glide, lengthen, and stretch tissue.
- **Bending forces** are a combination of compression and tension. One side of a structure is exposed to compressive forces as the other side is exposed to tension forces. Bending occurs during many massage applications. Force is applied across the fiber or across the direction of the muscles, tendons or ligaments, and fascial sheaths.
- **Shear forces** is a sliding force, and significant friction is often created between the structures that slide against each other.
- **Torsion forces** are best understood as twisting forces. Massage introduces torsion forces through application of methods that knead and twist soft tissues.

For example compression, shear and tension forces are combined as an approach to treat myofascial trigger points as follows: apply pressure on the trigger point while moving tissues containing the trigger point back and forth and at the same time elongating the tissue.

There are seven alterations in application that can modify the intensity of the massage application. Modifiers of the intensity of the mechanical force on the soft tissue include:

- **Depth of pressure** (compressive force) can be light, moderate, deep, or variable. Pressure

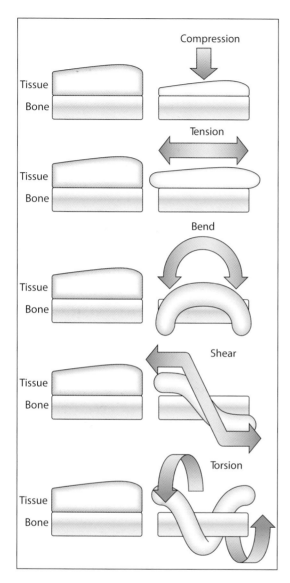

FIGURE 19.1 Five types of mechanical forces.

• **Drag** is the amount of pull (stretch) on the tissue (tensile force). Dry skin has a high resistance to slip; therefore, mechanical forces, primarily tension, can drag tissue in various directions without slipping. Lubricant is used during massage to increase slip and thus reduce drag. As tissue is dragged it will eventually encounter bind. The sensation of bind comes from tissue being restrained from motion, i.e. it can no longer easily be moved by force application. One of the most noticeable differences in massage when compared with other manual therapy approaches is the use of a lubricant to reduce drag on the skin during application. Because drag is necessary to load

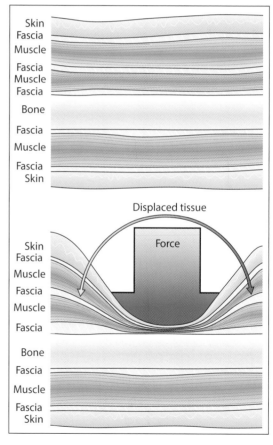

FIGURE 19.2 Massage applications systematically generate force through each tissue layer. This provides a graphic representation of the application of force. It begins with light, superficial application and progresses with increased pressure to the deepest layer.

must be delivered through each successive tissue layer, displacing the tissue to reach the deeper layers without damage to the tissues or discomfort for the client (Fig. 19.1). The deeper the pressure, the broader the base of contact with the surface of the body. More pressure is required to address thick, dense tissue than delicate thin tissue. Tissue layers begin at the skin surface and include superficial fascia, and multiple muscle and associated deep fascia layer until the bone is reached.

Box 19.1

Sensing bind

'Bind' is shorthand for what is noted when tissues reach or pass their end-of-range. A barrier is reached or is surpassed, and tissues modify from an 'ease' state to 'bind'. Soft tissue, including fascia, display increased density, or tension, as the point of 'bind' is reached.

Activity 1

1. The end of a cloth, tissue, piece of paper, rubber band, etc. should be held with one hand, with the other hand holding the other end, with the material in between
2. Keep one hand still and begin to slowly pull the material with the other
3. When you feel a tiny tug on the hand that is still, you have reached (or have just gone beyond) bind – you have passed the barrier of resistance.

Activity 2

1. Using one of your hands, grasp the lower edge of your shirt or blouse at one of the side seams
2. Pull the shirt down a little and then hold it still
3. Side bend away from the side being held down
4. When you feel the tug in the hand holding the shirt down you have reached (or have just gone beyond) the point of bind.

The following is a suggested scale for determining drag:

0: no drag
1: moves tissue but not to bind
2: moves tissue to bind
3: maximum drag– moves tissue past bind (stretch).

---

tissue with tension forces, modifying massage by reducing lubricant and increasing drag is one of the main changes made in massage therapy to specifically address fascia. To experience the sensation of bind, follow the activities in Box 19.1 (Fig. 19.2).

- Direction means that the massage may proceed from the center of the body outward (centrifugal) or from the extremities inward to the center of the body (centripetal). It can proceed from proximal to distal attachments of the muscle (or vice versa) following the muscle fibers, transverse to the tissue fibers, or in circular motions. The direction of massage that specifically targets fascia would follow the directional pattern in Figure 19.3.
- **Rhythm** refers to the regularity of application of the technique. A method that is applied at regular intervals is considered even, or rhythmic. A method that is disjointed, or irregular, is considered uneven, or non-rhythmic.
- **Frequency** is the rate at which the method repeats itself within a given time frame. In general, each method is repeated about three times

before the practitioner moves or switches to a different approach. Frequency is adapted to target fascia by increasing the number of times the method repeats.

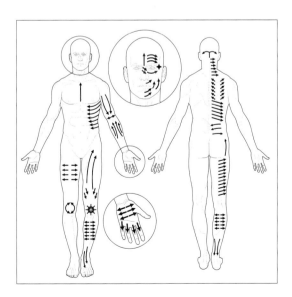

FIGURE 19.3 Direction of massage application to target fascia.

- **Duration** is the length of time the method is applied or that the technique remains in one location. A logical scale for application in a specific location is:
  - Short duration: 10 seconds
  - Moderate duration: 30 seconds
  - Long duration: 60 seconds.

  For a whole massage session:
  - Short duration: 5–15 min
  - Moderate duration: 15–30 min
  - Long duration: 45–60 min.
- **Speed** is how slow or fast a method is applied. Speed of application can be fast, slow, or variable. A logical scale for speed is:
  - Slow: 10–30 seconds from beginning to end of stroke
  - Moderate: 5–10 seconds from beginning to end of stroke
  - Fast: 2–5 seconds from beginning to end of stroke.

Massage methods

Massage methods involve the nine general approaches used to create the five mechanical forces that act on the soft tissue. The methods are adapted to achieve a variety of outcomes by the seven modifiers of depth of pressure, drag, direction, rhythm, frequency, duration and speed.

- **Holding** involves holding tissue without movement. Holding can be applied by simply laying hands on the surface of the skin or becoming the method used to hold soft tissue at the resistance barrier during what is often called myofascial release (Fig. 19.4).
- **Compression** involves use of compressive force without slip, commonly applied at a 90° angle to the tissue. Compression is an aspect of all massage application to determine pressure depth, from very light to deep, followed by a lift or release of force, or the compressive force can be sustained through the excursion (length) of the massage stroke.
- **Gliding/stroking** (effleurage) involves gliding movements that create tension forces. The pressure produce by adding compression may range through the tissue layers from

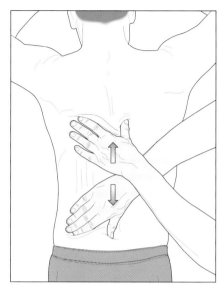

FIGURE 19.4 Gliding with drag.

superficial to deep. Depending on the amount of lubricant used during application of gliding, the drag component can be minimal or maximal. Drag is an important quality when addressing fascia, therefore use of lubricant is minimal (Fig. 19.4).

- **Kneading** (petrissage) involves lifting, rolling, squeezing, and releasing tissue, most commonly using rhythmic alternating pressures and introduce bending and torsion forces. This method is helpful in supporting sliding of fascia layers (Fig. 19.5).
- **Lifting** involves pulling tissue up and away from its current position and can introduce bending and tension forces. Lifting is an effective method for separating fascial layers (Fig.19.6).
- **Percussion** (tapotement) involves alternating or simultaneous rhythmic striking movement of the hands against the body, allowing the hand to spring back after contact, controlling the impact. While these methods are commonly included in massage it is one of the least effective for force application into fascia.
- **Vibration/oscillation** involves shaking, quivering, trembling, swinging, or rocking movements most commonly applied with the fingers, the full hand, or an appliance. Shaking is quite

include warming, rolling, wringing, linear, stripping, cross-fiber, chucking, and circular friction. Most friction strokes are administered with little or no lubricant. However, excess friction (shearing force) may produce an inflammatory irritation that causes many soft tissue problems. Friction can be used to address locally adhered tissues (Fig. 19.7).

- **Movement and mobilization** application (joint movement, stretching, and traction) entails shortening and/or lengthening of soft tissues with movement at one or more joints. Variations include active movements (the client moves structures without the practitioner's help), passive movements (the therapist moves the structures without the client's help), resistive movement (the client moves structures against resistance provided by the therapist), and active assisted movement (the client moves structures with support and assistance from the therapist). Stretching introduces forces of bend, torsion, and tension that mechanically affect connective tissue. Longitudinal stretching pulls connective tissue in the direction of the fiber configuration. Cross-directional stretching pulls the connective tissue against the fiber direction. Cross-directional stretching focuses on the tissue itself and does not depend on joint movement. Variations include pin and stretch, where the massage therapist identifies dysfunctional tissue and then drags and holds that tissue at bind (pin) while

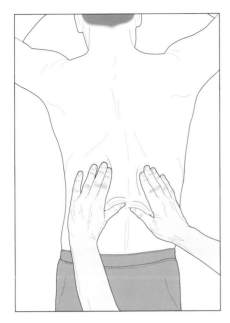

FIGURE 19.5 Kneading stroke.

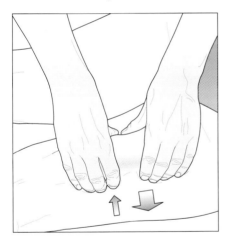

FIGURE 19.6 Lifting with the addition of movement/shaking to increase fascia layer separation.

effective in moving tissue layers over each other and should be used more often when addressing fascia during massage.

- **Friction** involves rubbing one surface over another, with little or no surface glide creating both compressive and shearing forces. Pressure may range from superficial (light) to deep, providing friction effects between various tissue levels. Examples of friction

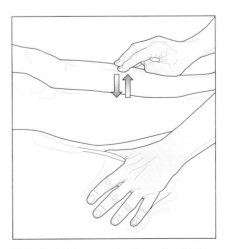

FIGURE 19.7 An example of cross fiber friction.

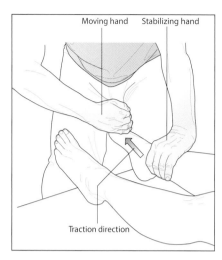

Moving hand   Stabilizing hand

Traction direction

FIGURE 19.8 Example of movement/
mobilization with stretching.

moving the adjacent joint or tissue into a stretch position with the result of loading the area beyond bind to create the therapeutic effect. Active release is similar to pin and stretch where the massage therapist identifies dysfunctional tissue and then drags and holds that tissue at bind (pin). The difference is that the client actively moves the adjacent joint into a stretch position (Fig. 19.8)

Adaptation of massage for specific fascia application

The main modification a massage therapist uses to assess and address fascia more specifically is a choice of methods relying on compression, gliding, holding, kneading, lifting, shaking, friction and stretching, modified by drag, speed, and duration so that mechanical force application affects the fascia. There is a general agreement that the approaches which target fascia should be applied either away from bind or into bind, both of which require sufficient drag on tissues (Chaudhry et al. 2008, Eagan et al. 2007, Findley 2011, Meltzer & Standley 2010). Creating drag on tissue during massage requires that little or no lubricant is used in the targeted areas. Speed is slow and duration is long. Direction is also a factor and often across the tissue fibers.

Massage outcomes

Everything moves in the body, and parts must slide over and around other parts. Lubricating fluid secreted by the body allows structures to slide. The layers of loose connective tissue within deep fasciae have been found to have layered distribution of hyaluronan (HA). Abundant in the extracellular matrix, HA also contributes to tissue hydrodynamics, movement and proliferation of cells, and participates in a number of cell surface receptor interactions. Advances in scientific equipment have made it possible to study a layer of hyaluronan fluid, which allows sliding between deep fascia and muscle. The deep fascia has a layer of HA between fascia and the muscle and within the loose connective tissue that divided different fibrous sublayers of the deep fascia. The HA within the deep fascia facilitates the free sliding of two adjacent fibrous fascial layers, thus promoting the normal function associated with the deep fascia. Researchers believe that the basis of the common phenomenon known as 'myofascial pain' is related to changes when HA assumes a more packed configuration with increased density altering tissue sliding (Findley 2011, Stecco et al. 2011).

In muscle or myofascia, part of the fascia is anchored to bone (or another structure) and part is free to slide. If tissues cannot slide as they are supposed to, inflammation and reduced range of motion (ROM) and strength can result. As part of the cycle of dysfunction, the lack of sliding motion may be the result of inflammation, with the latter being the causal factor.

Fascia is formed by crimped/wavy collagen fibers and elastic fibers arranged in distinct layers; the fibers are aligned in a different direction in each layer. These fibers are embedded in the gelatin-like ground substance. Superficial fascia can be stretched because of the wavy nature of the fiber structure and the elastic fibers, which allow the fascia to return to its original resting state. Subcutaneous fascia (tissue containing body fat that is located under the skin but on top of muscle) forms a very elastic sliding membrane that is essential for thermal regulation, metabolic exchanges, and protection of vessels and nerves.

Deep fascia is stiffer and thinner (resembling duct tape) than subcutaneous fascia. Deep fascia surrounds and compartmentalizes the muscles and forms the structures that attach soft tissues to bone. This type of fascia also forms a complex latticework of connective tissue, resembling struts, crossbeams, and guy wires, that helps maintain the structural integrity and function of the body. The richly innervated fascia is maintained in a taut resting state, known as fascial tone, as a result of the different muscular fibers that pull on it (somewhat like a trampoline). This resting state enables the free nerve endings and receptors in the fascial tissue to sense any variation in the shape of the fascia (and therefore any movement of the body) (Schleip et al. 2005). Changes in the gliding /sliding of the fascia (e.g. too loose, too tight, or twisted) cause altered movement and thus tissue adaptation. Various techniques in massage and other bodywork methods that target the fascia involve the same components. Any form of application such as massage that deforms (changes the shape of) the tissue has the potential to affect the fascia.

Fascia has contractile cells, which respond to the application of mechanical force, and smooth muscle cells, which are controlled by the autonomic nervous system. The fascial tonus (tone) may therefore be influenced and regulated by the state of the autonomic nervous system. Any intervention targeting the fascia also is an intervention influencing the autonomic system and vice versa (Henley et al. 2008). The smooth muscle cell contraction is most likely controlled by the sympathetic aspect of the autonomic nervous system, but confirming research is sparse. If the sympathetic nervous system is the regulator, then its activation would increase the overall fascial tension (Klingler et al. 2004). Sympathetic activation is a stress response. Might a massage that reduces the fight-or-flight response (sympathetic dominance) and supports relaxation (parasympathetic dominance) influence fascia?

Assessment

The general application of massage is the assessment process. The underlying principles are as-

sessment of ease and bind, and massage therapy is an excellent platform for soft tissue and movement assessment. This aspect of massage is **not** treatment but looks and feels like a massage that is pleasurable and achieves the outcome of general relaxation. In a general full body massage soft-tissue and joint mobility is assessed for motion restriction by palpation and/or joint movement. During joint movement assessment it is important to identify the physiological barrier where the client experiences appropriate stiffness, and the pulling sensation into the area being stretched acts as a protective mechanism, preventing movement to the anatomical limits and potential injury. Assessment indicates if there is a pathological barrier that may be one of two types:

- Where pain and stiffness occurs when joint movement assessment identifies reduced ROM or hypomobility
- Where a lack of resistance is experienced when normal ROM is reached during assessment indicating hypermobility.

When moving a joint during assessment it is important to stay within the normal physiological barriers, and if limits of ROM are identified, to gently and slowly encourage the joint to increase its ROM. It may take multiple sessions supported by client self-stretching to see sustained results. Expect flexibility to increase gradually.

During general massage the therapist identifies areas of tightness/bind where the normal sliding of fascia does not occur. The quality of the fascia can generally be assessed by noting the pliability of the skin and subcutaneous layers. Thickened, adhered fascia is less mobile, and the skin will glide only a short distance before feeling tight (bind). If the client has requested that alterations in fascia are addressed, and has sufficient adaptive capacity to respond positively to the interventions, and there are no contraindications for treatment, then massage application is modified to create change in the dysfunctional fascia.

Treatment during massage

Focused tension (stretching) of the tissues appears to be an effective mechanical force for influencing the fascia. The force applied during massage must move the tissue until it binds, at which point addition force is applied to move the tissue sufficiently to engage the resistance barrier. The tissue is held at this point until a softening is felt. The tissue is again moved to the bind/resistance barrier and the process is repeated one or two more times. In this author's experience, the resistance barrier is typically engaged for 15–60 seconds before the tissue softens, and three to four repetitions are usually sufficient to affect, but not over-stress, the tissue or the client. The goal of the mechanical force applied to that area allows the tissues to normalize by becoming more pliable: through a change in the water content; by sending signals to adjacent and distant areas of the body; and, likely, through many more mechanisms waiting to be identified through research into mechanotransduction.

Treatment interventions

Direct and indirect connective tissue methods

Both direct and indirect connective tissue methods have been shown to reverse the inflammatory effects in cells that have been strained repetitively. A direct technique moves the restricted tissue into the barrier caused by binding. An indirect technique moves the tissue away from the restrictive barrier to a point of ease. Changing the strain pattern in cells (indirect, away from the bind or direct, toward the bind) may result in improvement in symptoms. It may take only 60 seconds for changes to occur (Meltzer & Standley 2010).

Methods

Indirect functional techniques are very gentle and safe. Rather than being treated as a specific modality, functional indirect methods need to be incorporated into the massage application, regardless of whether the focus is soft tissue or joint restriction. These methods, rather than engaging and attempting (by whatever means) to overcome resistance (bind), do the exact opposite. The soft tissue or joint is taken to the point of maximum ease. The massage practitioner simply maintains the joint or tissue in this ease position (see chapters 11 and 16 in particular). No further treatment is provided at this point, and after 30–60 seconds the position is gently released and reassessed for an increase in mobility. Breathing can enhance the ease position and is incorporated by having the client inhale and exhale, typically holding the breath for a few seconds in the direction that further contributes to the ease of tissue tension. Because indirect functional techniques are noninvasive methods, they should be the first approach attempted to normalize tissue and joint movement.

Direct functional techniques are the opposite of indirect methods. These methods begin at the restriction barrier (bind) and move into the resistance. Direct methods are more invasive then indirect methods. Because these methods produce changes by increasing the intensity of the mechanical force application to move tissue beyond the point of bind, the potential for adverse effects is increased. Stretching is considered a direct technique because it engages bind and moves through it.

A modification that incorporates indirect methods and more aggressive direct stretching, involves moving back and forth between the ease position and the bind position. This can be described as indirect/direct. First, the ease position is identified and held, as previously described. Then the restrictive barrier of a joint or tissue is engaged in each plane of motion and is held taut at the barrier until softening occurs. The corrective activating force allows movement slightly through the restrictive barrier, and this position is held for 15–60 seconds, until the tissue softens. It is effective to alternate two or three times between direct and indirect application.

Tissue movement methods

The process is as follows:
1.   Make firm but gentle contact with the skin. This is best accomplished with the tissues relaxed

2. Increase downward, or vertical, pressure slowly until resistance is felt; this barrier is soft and subtle

3. Maintain downward pressure at this point; now add horizontal drag until the resistance barrier is felt again

4. Sustain horizontal pressure and wait

5. The tissue will seem to creep, unravel, melt, slide, quiver, twist, or dip, or some other movement sensation will be apparent

6. Follow the movement while gently maintaining tension on the tissues and encouraging the pattern as it undulates though various levels of release

7. Slowly and gently release first the horizontal force, and then the vertical force

8. Kneading and lifting applied in the direction of the restriction can be used to reassess and further treat areas where dysfunction remains.

Stretching

During stretching method, the client should experience a pulling sensation in the shortened soft tissue and but never a pain or strain in the joint or other part of the body that is not being stretched. Do not stretch any jointed area beyond anatomical barriers. Only stretch areas of hypomobility. If assessment identifies hypermobility do not stretch. Instead, some sort of strengthening approach is required.

Stretching procedures

- Only stretch tissues when they are warm and pliable.
- Begin the stretch sequence by using massage to prepare the tissues.
- Stabilize the body so only the target area moves during stretching.
- Move the area to the pathological barrier and back off a bit.
- Instruct the client to breathe in (inhale) right before the stretch and then breathe out (exhale) slowly as you move them into stretch.
- Stretching should always be done within the comfortable limits of the range of movement of the client.
- Stretching should be controlled and performed at a slow pace.

- A stretch does not need to be held longer than 20 seconds and performed in sets of 2-5 repetitions with a 15–30 second rest in between each stretch.
- Static stretches are done so that the joints are placed in the outer limits of the available painless ROM and held.
- Dynamic stretching occurs when opposing muscles are used to produce the force to stretch the short tissues. Considered active.

Muscle energy techniques (MET), explained in Chapter 13, involve a voluntary contraction of the client's muscles in a specific and controlled direction, at varying levels of intensity, against a specific counterforce applied by the therapist. Muscle energy procedures have a variety of applications and are considered active techniques in which the client contributes the corrective force. The amount of effort may vary from a small muscle twitch to a maximal muscle contraction. The duration may be a fraction of a second to several seconds. All contractions begin and end slowly, gradually building to the desired intensity. An increased tolerance to stretch that results from MET application is now considered to be the mechanism involved.

Ease/indirect and bind/direct methods can be combined with muscle energy methods. During muscle energy application, muscles (contractions) are actively used to support the desired tissue response. The muscle tissue is held in a specific position; the client then pushes slowly in a controlled manner against a counterforce supplied by the massage therapist.

Example of a massage sequence to target fascia (Fig. 19.9)

1. Place crossed hands over tissue and meld hands to the skin.

2. Separate hands moving tissue to and just into bind. Do not slip.

3. Forearms can be used. Place on the tissue and meld to it.

4. Separate arms moving tissue to and just into bind.

5. Small areas of tissue can be stretched by placing the short tissue between the fingers of both

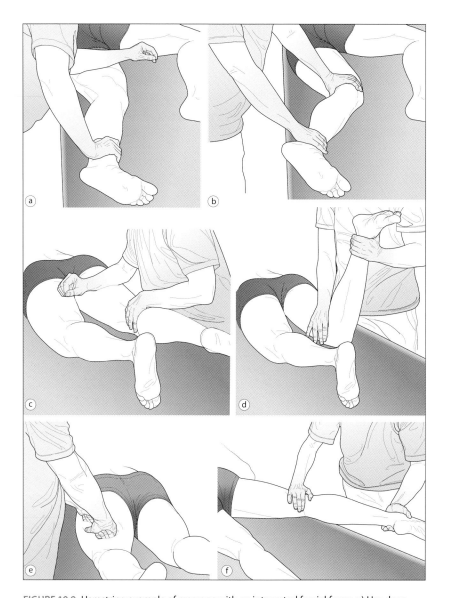

FIGURE 19.9 Hamstring example of massage with an integrated fascial focus. a) Use deep, broad-based gliding with compression force while moving the leg into knee flexion and extension. b) Apply inhibitory pressure at the distal attachments with movement. c) Apply compression at the proximal attachments to create inhibitory pressure. d) Apply inhibitory pressure at the distal attachments. e) Apply deep, slow compression to the belly of the muscle. f) Provide active assisted stretching; this also can be a position for muscle energy methods or active resisted movement.

hands, and then without slipping separate tissues into the bind.

6. Stabilize tissue at one end of the target area and hold fast. Then slowly glide, with drag maintaining tension on the tissues at all times.

7. Use shear forces to move tissue in and out of bind.

8. Use bending force to move tissue into bind (skin rolling).

9. Grasp, lift, and pull to create combined loading to move tissue into and out of bind.

10. Use torsion force to twist tissue into and out of bind.

11. Stretching methods take tissue into bind. Hold at the ends of the area to be stretched and move away to create tension force.

12. Traction applies tension force to the tissues surrounding a joint. Grasp firmly above and below the joint and move hands apart to create tension force into bind.

13. Pin and stretch variation. Move target tissue from ease position toward bind and hold in place.

14. As the target tissue is held fixed, move the joint area to create the tension force into the bind.

15. Active release variation. Compress target tissue while in ease and then move from ease to bind position.

16. Client moves the jointed area away while the tissue is fixed to create the tension force to move tissues into bind.

References

Chaudhry H et al 2008 Three-dimensional mathematical model for deformation of human fasciae in manual therapy. J Am Osteopath Assoc 108(8): 379–390

Eagan T et al 2007 Importance of strain direction in regulating human fibroblast proliferation and cytokine secretion: a useful in vitro model for soft tissue injury and manual medicine treatments. JMPT 30(8):584–592

Findley T 2011 Fascia research from a clinician/scientist's perspective. Int J Ther Massage Bodywork 4(4):1–6

Henley C et al 2008 Osteopathic manipulative treatment and its relationship to autonomic nervous system activity as demonstrated by heart rate variability: a repeated measures study. Osteopath Med Prim Care 2(1):7–8

Jonas WB 2005 Mosby's dictionary of complementary and alternative medicine. Elsevier Mosby, St Louis

Klingler W et al 2004 European Fascia Research Project Report 2005. Paper presented at Fifth World Congress on Low Back and Pelvic Pain, Melbourne Australia, November 10–16

Meltzer K, Standley 2010 In vitro modeling of repetitive motion injury and myofascial release. J Bodyw Mov Ther 14(2):162–171

Mosby's Medical Dictionary, 8th edn 2009 Elsevier, St Louis

MTBOK 2010 Version 1 of the Massage Therapy Body of Knowledge. Massage Therapy Body of Knowledge. Available online at: http://mtbok.org. Accessed 25 May 2013

Schleip R et al 2005 Active fascial contractility: fascia may be able to actively contract in a smooth muscle-like manner and thereby influence musculoskeletal dynamics. Med Hypotheses 65(2):273–7

Simmonds N 2012 A theoretical framework for the role of fascia in manual therapy. J Bodyw Mov Ther 16(1):83–93

Stecco C et al 2011 Hyaluronan within fascia in the etiology of myofascial pain. Surg Radiol Anat 33(10):891–6

Chapter 20

TRIGGER POINT RELEASE METHODS INCLUDING DRY NEEDLING

César Fernández-de-las-Peñas

Introduction

In clinical practice, trigger point (TrP) release methods cover several manual therapies aimed at eliminating or inactivating TrPs. The latter are mainly described as hypersensitive spots in a taut band of a skeletal muscle painful on stimulation that elicit referred pain (Simons et al. 1999). TrP release methods include direct techniques such as massage, ischemic compression, TrP pressure release, or strain–counterstrain (Dommerholt & McEvoy 2010), and also indirect interventions, e.g. spray and stretch, passive stretching, muscle energy techniques (MET), neuromuscular approaches and/or myofascial induction. Direct techniques are those targeted at connective tissues related to the TrP by applying pressure directly over the TrP, whereas indirect techniques are those targeted at connective tissues related to the taut band and surrounding tissues, including fascia (Dommerholt & McEvoy 2010). An alternative release method is TrP dry needling (TrP-DN; Dommerholt & Fernández-de-las-Peñas 2013). This technique inserts acupuncture filiform and fine needles into the TrP area with the aim of inactivating the TrP. All TrP release methods are complementary because they usually act on different connective tissue levels, including the taut band, TrP area, muscle tissue, and surrounding fascia.

Overview

Throughout history TrPs have been referred to by different names (myogelosis, fibrositis, etc.). Although various definitions of TrPs are used among different disciplines, the most commonly accepted definition maintains that *'TrPs are hy-persensitive spots in a taut band of a skeletal muscle that are painful on compression, stretch, overload or contraction of the tissue which respond with a referred pain'* (Simons et al. 1999). Based on their clinical experience, different authors have modified TrP release methods (Simons et al. 1999, Chaitow 2007, Fernández-de-las-Peñas et al. 2011). Different TrP release methods, depending on the amount of pressure applied, presence-absence of pain, duration of the application, position of the tissue (shortened or lengthened), or presence-absence of active contraction are clinically proposed for TrP treatment (Fernández-de-las-Peñas & Pilat 2011).

Several mechanical and neurophysiological mechanisms have been proposed to explain the effects of the different TrP release methods and it is likely that all of them act at the same time.

From a mechanical viewpoint, it has been suggested that mechanical stimulation exerted by TrP release methods can equalize the length of the muscle sarcomeres, can induce longitudinal or transverse mobilization of the taut band, or can induce changes in muscle properties (Dommerholt & McEvoy 2010, Fernández-de-las-Peñas et al. 2011).

- Potential neurophysiological mechanisms include spinal reflex effects inducing muscle relaxation, muscle hyperemia, stimulation of the gate control theory, or activation of the descending inhibitory pain mechanisms (Dommerholt & McEvoy 2010).

- These mechanisms are also involved in TrP-DN; however, considering that TrP-DN is a painful intervention and it represents a nociceptive input to the central nervous system (CNS), it is more plausible that the neurophysiological mechanisms are highly relevant for TrP-DN (Dommerholt & Fernández-de- las-Peñas 2013).

- Finally, recent theories also include mechanisms to the surrounding fascial tissue as it is suggested that TrP release methods, including TrP-DN, can change viscoelastic properties or behavior of the fascial tissue (Langevin 2013). The interaction between TrPs and fascia is based on the premise that muscle perimysium has a high density of myofibroblasts, a common cell found in connective tissue (Schleip et al. 2005), and the role of hyaluronanic acid in myofascial pain (Stecco et al. 2011).

Some systematic reviews have found moderate evidence supporting the use of some TrP release methods for immediate pain relief of TrPs and limited evidence for long-term pain relief; however, it is difficult to draw any clinical conclusion since most studies have investigated single modalities, whereas multimodal approaches are usually used by clinicians (Vernon & Schneider 2009). More recent studies have reported that the integration of TrP release methods, including TrP-DN, within multimodal manual therapy programs is effective for some chronic pain conditions such as heel pain, ankle sprain, fibromyalgia syndrome, n eck pain, etc. Future studies are needed to determine the efficacy of TrP release methods included in a biopsychosocial treatment of chronic pain.

Objectives

Rather than explaining TrP as a local pathological/anatomical muscle problem, current theories focus on the nociceptive nature of TrPs and their role in perpetuating sensitization mechanisms. The clinical aims of any TrP release method are the inactivation of muscle-associated sensory and motor symptoms and the decrease of nociceptive barrage to the CNS (Fernández-de-las-Peñas et al. 2011). TrP release methods are applied by numerous healthcare professionals, including osteopaths, physicians, chiropractics, physical therapists, dentists, or massage therapists, among others, dependent upon the country and local jurisdictional regulations.

Since there are different TrP release methods, these approaches can be applied in any condition where the muscle or fascial tissues are involved in their etiology. For instance, several studies have included the application of ischemic compression, TrP pressure release, neuromuscular intervention, or myofascial induction in the management of shoulder pain, heel pain, ankle pain, chronic pelvic pain, or tension-type headache.

Assessment

All TrP release methods aim to inactivate active TrPs. The first step in the clinical reasoning process to determine which TrP release method should be used, is the accurate diagnosis of a TrP. In fact, correct TrP diagnosis requires manual ability, training, and clinical practice to develop a high degree of reliability in the clinical examination. Typical signs and symptoms include: 1) presence of a hyperirritable spot in a palpable taut band in a skeletal muscle (when accessible to palpation); 2) palpable local twitch response on snapping palpation or DN of the TrP area (when possible); and 3) presence of referred pain elicited by stimulation of the TrP. Additional helpful signs for the diagnosis include muscle weakness, pain on contraction, pain on stretching, a jump sign, autonomic phenomena, or motor disturbances (Simons et al. 1999). Although Gerwin et al. (1997) concluded that some muscles are more reliably examined than others, there is no general consensus on the reliability of TrP diagnosis.

TrPs are mainly identified through manual palpation. Clinicians can use either a flat palpation where the finger or thumb presses the muscle against underlying bone tissue, or a pincer palpation in which a particular muscle is palpated between the clinician's fingers. Taut band can be identified by palpating perpendicular to the fiber direction, which can elicit a local twitch response (strumming palpation). Once the taut band is located, the clinician moves along the taut band to find a discrete area of intense pain and, sometimes, hardness, which will elicit referred pain.

Once the clinician has localized the TrP, the intervention will depend on the irritability of the tissue, the accessibility of the muscle, and the symptoms. For instance, in patients with higher levels of pain and irritability, the clinician can choose indirect release methods targeting the taut band (e.g. longitudinal strokes or myofascial induction) or pain-free compression methods (e.g. TrP pressure release or strain–counterstrain). In such a patient, the application of TrP-DN may not be the first choice because of the DN-related pain. On the contrary, in patients with lower irritability of the CNS, TrP-DN can be the first therapeutic option, or compression interventions at the pain threshold level applied over the TrP. Nevertheless, clinicians should use a biopsychosocial clinical reasoning to determine which TrP release method is the most suitable for a particular patient

Mechanisms

Any therapeutic intervention should be evidence-informed and based on scientific evidence, clinicians' judgments, expertise, and clinical decision-making (Dommerholt 2012). It is difficult to determine the exact therapeutic mechanism involved in TrP release methods since mechanical and neurophysiological mechanisms are involved at the same time. In fact, TrP release methods are complementary since they can act at different tissue levels including taut band, TrP region, muscle tissue, and surrounding fascia. The therapeutic aim of TrP release methods is to stop the vicious cycle of the evidence-informed integrated TrP hypothesis (Simons et al. 1999). The updated version of this etiological hypothesis is the most comprehensive framework currently available to explain the TrP formation and to guide the therapeutic management (Gerwin et al. 2004). According to this hypothesis, any TrP release method should focus on decreasing TrP-related symptoms by reversing the observed hypoxia and low pH, and by decreasing the excitability of the muscle nociceptors.

- From a mechanical viewpoint, it has been proposed that TrP release methods that compress the muscle in a vertical or perpendicular manner equalize the length of the muscle sarcomeres. This effect would be increased if the muscle contracts at the same time (Fernández-de-las-Peñas et al. 2011). Either TrP release intervention can be applied along or across the TrP taut band. By applying these interventions, clinicians will exert transverse or longitudinal mobilization to the taut band and surrounding fascia.

- It is important to note that the mechanical effects of TrP release methods also involve changes in the viscoelastic properties and/or behavior of surrounding fascia (Langevin 2013). In fact, longitudinal strokes applied along the taut band seem to be very similar neuromuscular technique approaches (Chaitow & DeLany 2008).

- It has been suggested that the application of a continuous mechanical stimulus, particularly compression or stretching, to soft connective tissue induces a piezoelectric effect, which modifies the 'gel' state of the connective tissue to a more solute state. In fact, it has been demonstrated that to produce lasting changes in viscoelastic properties of fascia, mechanical stimulus should be applied for up to 60 seconds (Chaudhry et al. 2007).

- Hou et al. (2002) investigated the time required for application of TrP pressure release and reported that this intervention is generally applied for 90 seconds. Therefore, it is plausible that compression interventions aimed at the TrP also induce changes in the surrounding fascia. In such a scenario, some authors have proposed that TrP release methods participate in a similar manner to fascial approaches, involving mechanotransduction processes (Dommerholt 2012).

- It is also likely that Fascial Manipulation® should play a greater role in TrP release as suggested by Stecco (2004). Similarly, connective tissue relaxation appears to require a static stretching to the fascia that is sustained for at least 10 minutes (Langevin 2013).

From a neurophysiological point of view, several theories have been also proposed.

- Hou et al. (2002) suggested that pain relief may result from reactive hyperemia in the TrP area or a spinal reflex mechanism inducing muscle relaxation. The reactive hyperemia can be related to the reversal of the hypoxia present in the TrP area with the consequent increase in muscle circulation (Gerwin et al. 2004).

- In addition, muscle relaxation induced by the mechanical stimulus can activate spinal reflex mechanisms including the gate control (Dommerholt & McEvoy 2010).

- The activation of the gate control is elicited by stimulation of αδ-sensory afferent fibers by the nociceptive mechanical stimulation induced by the TrP release intervention. This activation provokes segmental nociceptive effects over the TrP (Fernández-de-las-Peñas et al. 2011).

- The segmental antinociceptive effect is based on the premise that active TrPs are a source of peripheral nociception since the concentrations of bradykinin, calcitonin gene-related peptide, substance P, tumor necrosis factor-α, interleukins 1β, IL-6, and IL-8, serotonin, and norepinephrine were significantly higher near active TrPs than near latent TrP or non-TrP points (Shah et al. 2008). It is not known whether the therapeutic effects of all the TrP release methods, particularly the reduction in referred pain, are related to a reduction of nociceptive afferences to the dorsal horn neurons.

- A second potential neurophysiological mechanism is the activation of brain areas, particularly descending inhibitory pain mechanisms (Niddam 2009). It seems that nociceptive stimulus applied to the TrP area activates the pain neuromatrix.

- These mechanisms are also mainly involved in TrP-DN; however, considering that TrP-DN is a painful intervention, and therefore represents a nociceptive input to the nervous system, neurophysiological mechanisms are more relevant (Dommerholt & Fernández-de-las-Peñas 2013).

- It is known that TrP-DN reduces segmental nociceptive input (Srbely et al. 2010). In fact, although no study has investigated the effect of TrP-DN in activation of cortical areas, there is evidence suggesting that the insertion of a needle into acupuncture and non-acupuncture points involves the activation of the limbic system and the descending inhibitory pathways (Dommerholt & Fernández-de- las-Peñas 2013)

- Nevertheless, the mechanical effect of the needling over the fascia should be not ignored, since every time a needle is inserted through the skin towards a TrP, the needle passes through multiple levels of fascia (Langevin 2013).

- Stretching connective tissue with a (rotating) needle has been shown to stretch and reduce the tissue tension, flatten fibroblasts and re-model the cytoskeleton. Therefore, mechanical stimulation by a needle may activate mechanotransduction (Langevin 2013).

- Because clinicians induce different movements to the needle during needling, i.e. rotation or in-and-out, it is possible that collagen bundles adhere to the needle, creating a small 'whorl' of collagen in the immediate vicinity of the needle (Langevin 2013). Therefore, acupuncture needles can be used to create sustained and localized stretching of subcutaneous and deeper connective tissue layers.

Protocol

Various TrP release methods can be used in clinical practice depending on the patient´s features and clinical experience. They differ in the amount of pressure used, presence/absence of pain, duration of the technique, position of the tissues, and employment, or not, of active contraction (Fernández-de-las-Peñas et al. 2011, Fernández-de-las-Peñas & Pilat 2011). Several systematic reviews investigating the effectiveness of TrP release methods (Vernon & Schneider 2009) and DN (Furlan et al. 2005, Tough et al. 2009) have been published. The conclusion in relation to manual release methods is that there is evidence supporting their use for short-term relief but not for medium- and long-term follow-ups. The effectiveness of TrP-DN is controversial since one Cochrane Review found evidence for its use in patients with low back pain (Furlan et al. 2005), but a more recent review concludes that there is limited evidence for TrP-DN when compared with standardized care (Tough et al. 2009). Nevertheless, it is difficult to draw clinical conclusions from current evidence since most studies investigated TrP release methods or DN as single modalities, whereas multimodal approaches are practiced by clinicians. In fact, current research supports that pain is produced by the brain when there is a perception of bodily danger requiring specific action. Therefore, consideration of the patient's overall situation is critical for a therapeutic approach. The effects of TrP release methods including TrP-DN cannot be considered independently of the biopsychosocial model and must be approached from a pain science perspective, as it is no longer sufficient to consider any TrP release method strictly as a tool to address local muscle pathology (Dommerholt & Fernández-de-las-Peñas 2013).

In the author's clinical practice, the pressure level, duration of application, and position of the tissue (shortened, stretched) will depend on the degree of sensitization of the CNS presented by the patient and the irritability of the TrP.

- Hou et al. (2002) suggest alternative compression approaches using low pressure, below pain threshold, for prolonged periods of time (i.e. 90 seconds) or high pressure over the pain threshold (pain tolerance) for shorter periods of time (i.e. 30 seconds).
- Clinicians should consider that TrP release methods also involve changes in the viscoelastic properties or behavior of surrounding fascia when they are applied for a duration of at least up to 60 seconds (Chaudhry et al. 2007).
- Table 20.1 summarizes clinical application of different forms of TrP compression: ischemic compression, pressure release, strain–counterstrain or positional release therapy and pulsed or intermittent compression.
- TrP release methods based on compression interventions can be applied in several chronic and acute pain conditions, including mechanical neck pain, shoulder pain, elbow pain, hip pain, knee pain, temporomandibular pain, headaches, fibromyalgia, and whiplash, with the aim to decrease the pain, improve restricted range of motion and/or improve function.
- The manual technique depends on the degree of CNS irritability of the patient: in patients with high levels of sensitivity, pain-free TrP release methods can be used, e.g. strain–counterstrain or positional release therapy, whereas in patients with low levels of sensitivity use of more intense interventions are possible, e.g. ischemic compression (Fig. 20.1a).
- Another TrP release method is massage, which can be performed along (longitudinal strokes) or across (transverse strokes) the taut band. The application of longitudinal strokes along the taut band is sometimes associated with neuromuscular approaches (Chaitow & Delany 2008). See Chapter 15.
- In this particular approach, longitudinal strokes (glides, slides) are performed over the taut band containing TrPs. The strokes are generally applied with the thumb (Fig. 20.1b), elbows, or knuckles. In muscles where taut bands can be grasped with pincer palpation, the strokes can be applied with a pincer grip (Fig. 20.1c). Again, the degree of pressure and the speed of gliding will depend on the irritability and tone of the tissue. In the author's clinical experience the best result comes from repetitive strokes (6–10 times) over the affected tissue.

Table 20.1 Different compressive trigger point (TrP) release

	Muscle position	Degree of compression	Time of pressure	Duration of the technique
Ischemic compression	Fully lengthened	Sufficient to induce moderate pain between 3 and 6–7 (where 10 is maximum)	Until pain decreases by around 50–75%	Up to 90 seconds
TrP pressure release	Partially lengthened or neutral	Usually pain-free (first perception of tissue barrier)	Until the therapist perceives TrP or taut band release	Up to 90 seconds
Strain–counterstrain	Neurologically silent (usually shortened)	Reduction of pain by around 70–80%	Constant throughout	90 seconds
Pulsed ischemic compression	Neutral or at the 'first sign of resistance' barrier, i.e. no lengthening	5 seconds compression to induce pain at level 5–6 followed by 3 seconds no pressure – repeated until local or referred pain change or reduction in tissue resistance	5 seconds pressure, 3 seconds no pressure, repeated	Up to 90 seconds - or until change in pain is reported, or taut band release perceived

NPRS: Numerical Pain Rate Scale (0–10).

- Since TrPs are located in active tissues, i.e. muscle or fascia, some patients will benefit from dynamic interventions. In these approaches the clinician will apply any TrP release method, e.g. TrP pressure release or longitudinal strokes, combined with contraction or stretching of the affected muscle (Fernández-de-las-Peñas et al. 2011).
- One possible combination is that during a manual compression, the patient is asked to move the segment through a range of motion. A dynamic technique involves a longitudinal stroke applied by the clinician along the taut band while the patient is asked to move the segment (Fig. 20.1d).
- The mechanisms of these techniques are still unknown, but may be related to activation of the intra-fascial Pacinian/Paciniform and the Ruffini mechanoreceptors, which are found in all types of dense proper connective tissues (Schleip et al. 2005).
- Stretching approaches are also included in TrP release methods: passive stretching (the therapist passively stretches the affected muscle without participation of the patient), active stretching (the patient actively stretches the muscle without participation of the therapist), spray/stretch, or post-isometric relaxation/contract–relax–release (MET).
- MET involve the accurate localization of forces to the muscle barrier (first sign of resistance of the TrP taut band), an isometric contraction of the muscle against an unyielding counterforce supplied by the therapist, followed by patient relaxation and engagement of a new tissue barrier, or stretching past the previous barrier. The force and duration of the isometric contraction will adapt to the irritability of the tissues ranging from 3 to 9 seconds (see Ch. 13).
- The therapeutic mechanism of the muscle energy interventions may be the combination of a temporary elongation of the connective tissue and plastic changes in the connective tissues. A final non-manual TrP release method involves TrP-DN. It is recommended that patients are lying down during any needling procedures, because of the risk of autonomic responses. For every muscle, anatomical landmarks should

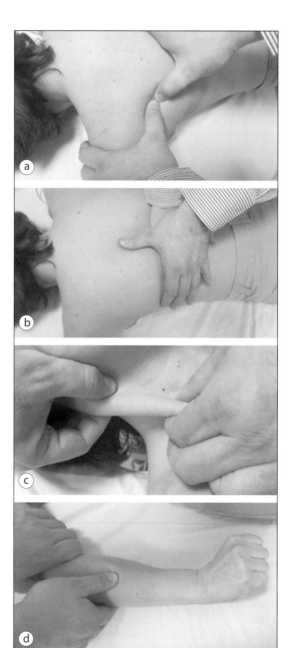

FIGURE 20.1 Different trigger point (TrP) release methods. (a) Ischemic compression intervention targeted at infraspinatus TrPs. (b) Longitudinal stroke along the taut band over paraspinal muscle TrPs. (c) Centrifugally longitudinal stroke with a pincer palpation along the taut band on the sternocleidomastoid muscle Trps. (d) Dynamic intervention: longitudinal stroke along the taut band of extensor wrist muscle TrPs as the patient simultaneously and actively extends the wrist.

be first identified, including the margins of the muscle and any relevant bony structures, i.e. the medial and lateral borders of the scapula and the scapular spine when DN infraspinatus muscle TrPs are treated.

- Although no consensus exists whether disinfection of the skin is necessary, cleaning the surrounding skin with alcohol before any TrP-DN intervention is common practice (Dommerholt & Fernández-de-las-Peñas 2013).

- For TrP-DN, acupuncture needles in tubes are recommended. The tube is placed on the skin overlying the TrP and the needle is quickly tapped into the skin. The tube is removed, and the needle is moved in and out into the region of the TrP by drawing the needle back to the sub-

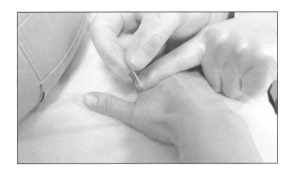

FIGURE 20.2 Trigger point dry needling (TrP-DN) over adductor pollicis muscle TrP.

cutaneous tissue (never outside of the skin) and redirecting it (Fig. 20.2).

Exercise

- The clinician, following a clinical reasoning based on the clinical history of the patient, suspects the presence of a TrP in the right sternocleidomastoid muscle. The patient suffers from unilateral headaches located over the temple and the orbit.

- The clinician palpates the right sternocleidomastoid muscle with a pincer palpation all along the muscle searching for the presence of active TrPs. During the examination, the muscle exhibits two painful points in the muscle belly.

- One of these points elicits referred pain to the head at 6 seconds on compression by the therapist. This referred pain reproduces the headache of the patient (i.e. it is an active TrP). The other point does not refer pain, there is only local pain and tenderness on palpation.

- The clinician decides to treat the active TrP with manual release methods. The first attempt would be the application of an ischemic compression technique. The muscle is grasped with a pincer palpation over the TrP and the clinician compresses the muscle until moderate pain appears. The compression is maintained at this level of pressure.

- After 15 seconds of compression the patient comments that the compression elicits re-

ferred pain to the head and is highly uncomfortable. The clinician decides to reduce the intensity of the intervention, and to maintain the compression level at the tissue resistance (i.e. TrP pressure release).

- Therefore, the compression is maintained at the tissue resistance level, which is mainly asymptomatic for the patient.

- After 20 seconds, the tissue resistance eases and the clinician again increases the level of compression until the next tissue barrier is reached. This procedure is repeated 3–4 times.

- After the compression intervention, manual palpation of the TrP does not elicit referred pain but the right sternocleidomastoid muscle is still tender and slightly painful because of the TrP taut band. The clinician then decides to apply a longitudinal stroke along the taut band away from the TrP.

- The clinician grasps the muscle with a pincer palpation at the TrP area with both hands. The pressure should be applied at the tissue resistance for 5–10 seconds.

- At this moment, a longitudinal stroke along the taut band is applied centrifugally away from the TrP. The speed of the stroke is gentle and smooth at the tissue barrier level. This procedure can be repeated 3–4 times.

- The objective of TrP-DN is to elicit local twitch responses, which are an indication that the TrP is indeed inactivated (Hong 1994). In some muscles or patients, if the local twitch responses are not clearly elicited, the presence of referred pain during TrP-DN can be also considered an indicator of a successful needling (Dommerholt & Fernández-de-las-Peñas 2013).
- Following TrP-DN, hemostasis must be accomplished to prevent and/or minimize local bleeding. It should be noted that TrP-DN (and all trigger point deactivation procedures) should be accompanied by other interventions to restore and maintain range of motion and to facilitate the return to normal function.

References

Chaitow L 2007 Positional release techniques. Churchill Livingstone, Edinburgh

Chaitow L, DeLany J 2008 Clinical application of neuromuscular techniques, 2nd edn. Vol 1: The upper body. Churchill Livingstone, Edinburgh

Chaudhry H et al 2007 Viscoelastic behaviour of human fasciae under extension in manual therapy J Bodywork Mov Ther 11:159–167

Dommerholt J 2012 Trigger point therapy. In: Schleip R, Finley T, Chaitow L, Huijing P (eds) Fascia in manual and movement therapies. Churchill Livingstone Elsevier, Edinburgh

Dommerholt J, McEvoy J 2010 Myofascial trigger point release approach. In: Wise CH (ed) Orthopaedic manual physical therapy: from art to evidence. FA Davis, Philadelphia

Dommerholt J, Fernández-de-las-Peñas C (eds) 2013 Trigger point dry needling: an evidenced and clinical-based approach. Churchill Livingstone Elsevier, London

Fernández-de-las-Peñas C et al 2011 Manual treatment of myofascial trigger points. In: Fernández-de-las-Peñas C, Cleland J, Huijbregts P (eds) Neck and arm pain syndromes: evidence–informed screening, diagnosis, and conservative management. Churchill Livingstone Elsevier, London, pp 451-61

Fernández-de-las-Peñas C, Pilat A 2011 Soft tissue manipulation approaches to chronic pelvic pain (external). In:

Chaitow L, Lovegrove R (eds) Chronic pelvic pain and dysfunction: practical physical medicine. Churchill Livingstone Elsevier, London

Furlan AD et al 2005 Acupuncture and dry-needling for low back pain. Cochrane Database Syst Rev 1:CD001351

Gerwin RD et al 1997 Inter-rater reliability in myofascial trigger point examination. Pain 69:65–73

Gerwin RD et al 2004 An expansion of Simons' integrated hypothesis of trigger point formation. Current Pain Head Reports 8:468–475

Hong CZ 1994 Lidocaine injection versus dry needling to myofascial trigger point. The importance of the local twitch response. Am J Phys Med Rehabil 73:256–63

Hou CR et al 2002 Immediate effects of various physical therapeutic modalities on cervical myofascial pain and trigger-point sensitivity. Arch Phys Med Rehabil 83:1406–14

Langevin HM 2013 Effects of acupuncture needling on connective tissue. In: Dommerholt J, Fernández-de-las-Peñas C (ed) Trigger point dry needling: an evidenced and clinical-based approach. Churchill Livingston Elsevier, pp 29–32

Niddam DM 2009 Brain manifestation and modulation of pain from myofascial trigger points. Current Pain Headache Report 13:370–5

Schleip R et al 2005 Active fascial contractility: fascia may be able to contract in a smooth muscle-like manner and thereby influence musculoskeletal dynamics. Med Hyp 65:273–7

Shah J P et al 2008 Biochemicals associated with pain and inflammation are elevated in sites near to and remote from active myofascial trigger points. Arch Phys Med Rehabil 89:16-23

Simons DG et al 1999 Travell & Simons' Myofascial pain and dysfunction: the trigger point manual: the upper half of body. Williams & Wilkins, Baltimore

Simons DG 2002 Understanding effective treatments of myofascial trigger points. J Bodywork Mov Ther 6:81–8

Srbely JZ et al 2010 Dry needle stimulation of myofascial trigger points evokes segmental anti-nociceptive effects. J Rehabil Med 42:463–468

Stecco L 2004 Fascial manipulation for musculoskeletal pain. Piccin, Padova

Stecco C et al 2011 Hyaluronan within fascia in the etiology of myofascial pain. Surgical Radiol Anat 33: 891–6

Tough EA et al 2009 Acupuncture and dry needling in the management of myofascial trigger point pain: a systematic review and meta-analysis of randomised controlled trials. Eur J Pain 13: 3–10

Vernon H, Schneider M 2009 Chiropractic management of myofascial trigger points and myofascial pain syndrome: a systematic review of the literature. J Man Physiol Ther 32: 14–24

Index

Note: Page numbers followed by b, t, and f indicate box, tables, and figures respectively.